Reflexive Polymers and Hydrogels

Understanding and Designing Fast Responsive Polymeric Systems

Reflexive Polymers and Hydrogels

Understanding and Designing Fast Responsive Polymeric Systems

Edited by
Nobuhiko Yui, Randall J. Mrsny, and Kinam Park

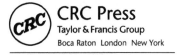

CRC Press
Taylor & Francis Group
Boca Raton London New York

CRC Press is an imprint of the
Taylor & Francis Group, an **informa** business

CRC Press
Taylor & Francis Group
6000 Broken Sound Parkway NW, Suite 300
Boca Raton, FL 33487-2742

First issued in paperback 2020

ISBN 13: 978-0-367-57839-8 (pbk)
ISBN 13: 978-0-8493-1487-2 (hbk)

This book contains information obtained from authentic and highly regarded sources. Reasonable efforts have been made to publish reliable data and information, but the author and publisher cannot assume responsibility for the validity of all materials or the consequences of their use. The authors and publishers have attempted to trace the copyright holders of all material reproduced in this publication and apologize to copyright holders if permission to publish in this form has not been obtained. If any copyright material has not been acknowledged please write and let us know so we may rectify in any future reprint.

**Visit the Taylor & Francis Web site at
http://www.taylorandfrancis.com**

**and the CRC Press Web site at
http://www.crcpress.com**

Cover image: *Canon #8* by Jennifer C. Hsieh. This work represents changes in a reflexive system over time as it cycles repetitively with an underlying chaotic nature.

Library of Congress Cataloging-in-Publication Data

Reflexive polymers and hydrogels : understanding and designing fast responsive polymeric
systems / edited by Nobuhiko Yui, Randall Mrsny, and Kinam Park.
p. cm.
Includes bibliographical references and index.
ISBN 0-8493-1487-9 (alk. paper)
1. Polymers. I. Yui, Nobuhiko. II. Mrsny, Randall J., 1955- III. Park, Kinam.

TA455.P58.R43 2004
620.1'92—dc22   2003065368

Library of Congress Card Number 2003065368

Preface

Smart materials designed to alter their properties in response to specific stimuli have been important parts of recent advances in the field of material sciences. These materials, typically polymers, can be based upon novel synthetic structures or may use materials obtained from natural sources. Various smart materials have been developed that can respond to even minute environmental changes. While the responsive properties of smart materials are thermodynamic in nature, their spectrum of applications expands dramatically once the component of kinetic control can be incorporated into their response profiles.

Despite significant advances in smart materials and the obvious importance of the kinetic aspects of their responses, only a limited number of studies have addressed the potentially powerful combination of thermodynamic and kinetic regulation of a smart material. This book brings together a collection of works and discussions that consider both thermodynamic and kinetic properties of smart materials. *Instant response* is written in Chinese characters as "瞬發" (pronounced "shun-patsu" in Japanese, "shun-fa" in Chinese, and "soon-bal" in Korean), but English has no equivalent term. For lack of a suitable term to describe materials whose properties can be modified in a rapid, repetitive, and responsive fashion, we have coined the term *reflexive systems*.

The chapters of this book have been organized to examine components of reflexive systems found in nature, to consider the theoretical limitations of reflexive systems, to characterize the current status of artificially prepared materials that may produce both thermodynamic and kinetic response events, and to explore potential future applications of such systems. Chapters in the first section of the book focus on systems found in nature (both in plants and animals) with an emphasis on molecular mechanisms. The second section investigates model systems in which selected interactions of specific reflexive system components are evaluated to determine theoretical limits of response rates and cycle times. The third section recapitulates and focuses on the functions observed in natural systems using synthetic polymers and conditions. Examples of available synthetic systems known to have fast responsive properties or that may benefit greatly by having fast responsive properties are discussed.

We, the editors, are most appreciative of the superb, insightful contributions made by the chapter authors of this book. We would also like to acknowledge the endless support of the staff members at CRC Press, in particular Alice Mulhern and Christine Andreasen for their careful editing of the chapters. It is our hope that this book will serve as a springboard for thought and experimentation toward the identification of novel reflexive systems that more closely emulate natural reflexive systems. We feel that it is only a matter of time for the development of truly biomimetic materials and that progress in the area of reflexive systems will facilitate that goal.

Nobuhiko Yui
Randall J. Mrsny
Kinam Park

Preface

Editors

Nobuhiko Yui, Ph.D., is a professor in the School of Materials Science, Japan Advanced Institute of Science and Technology, Ishikawa. Dr. Yui earned his Ph.D. in polymer chemistry from Sophia University, Japan, in 1985. He then joined the Institute of Biomedical Engineering of Tokyo Women's Medical College as an assistant research professor. While at Tokyo Women's Medical College, he spent a year as a doctoral research fellow at the University of Twente, the Netherlands. In 1993, Dr. Yui became an associate professor at the Japan Advanced Institute of Science and Technology; he became a full professor in 1998.

Dr. Yui is a member of the Controlled Release Society (CRS), the American Chemical Society, the New York Academy of Sciences, the Japanese Chemical Society, the Japan Society of Polymer Science, the Japan Society of DDS (Drug Delivery Systems), the Japanese Society for Biomaterials, the Japanese Society for Artificial Organs, and the Japanese Society for Tissue Engineering. He serves as a board member of the Japanese Society for Artificial Organs, the Japan Society of DDS, and the Japanese Society for Tissue Engineering. He is on the Board of Directors of the Japanese Society for Biomaterials, the Board of Scientific Advisors of the CRS, and the Editorial Board of the *Journal of Biomaterials Science, Polymer Edition*.

Dr. Yui served as the general secretary for the first, second, and third Asian International Symposia on Biomaterials and Drug Delivery Systems, which succeeded in strengthening Asian research interests in biomaterials and drug delivery systems (1996–2002). He helped organize the sixth World Biomaterials Congress Workshop entitled "Supramolecular Approach to Biological Functions" in 2000. He edited a book entitled *Supramolecular Design for Biological Applications* for CRC Press in 2002. He received the Award for Outstanding Research from the U.S. Society for Biomaterials in 1985, the 49th Worthy Invention Award from the Science and Technology Agency of Japan in 1990, the Young Investigator Award from the Japanese Society for Biomaterials in 1993, the CRS–Cygnus Recognition Award for Excellence in Guiding Student Research from the CRS in 1997, and the Best Paper Award from the Japanese Society of Artificial Organs in 1997.

Dr. Yui is the author of more than 210 scientific papers. His current major research interests include the molecular designs of biodegradable and/or smart polymers with unique supramolecular structures.

Randall J. Mrsny, Ph.D., is a professor of biology and drug delivery at the Welsh School of Pharmacy in Cardiff, Wales. He earned a B.S. in biochemistry and biophysics from the University of California at Davis (UCD) in 1977. In 1981, he obtained a Ph.D. in cell biology and human anatomy based on studies performed at the UCD School of Medicine. From 1982 through 1987 he was a National Institutes of Health postdoctoral fellow at the Institute of Molecular Biology at the University of Oregon. After postdoctoral training, Dr. Mrsny joined ALZA Corporation where he headed the Peptide Biology Group until 1990. From 1990 through 2001, he headed the drug delivery/biology group at Genentech, Inc. He assumed his current faculty position in 2002 and simultaneously founded a drug delivery company known as Trinity BioSystems, Inc. in California where he holds the position of Chief Scientific Officer.

Dr. Mrsny has held a variety of editorial positions and is currently on the editorial boards of several journals. He has published widely in a variety of areas related to drug delivery. His current research focuses primarily on cellular and molecular events associated with epithelial cell functions in health and disease.

Kinam Park, Ph.D., is a professor in the Department of Biomedical Engineering and Pharmaceutics of Purdue University. He earned a Ph.D. in pharmaceutics from the University of Wisconsin in 1983. After postdoctoral training in the Department of Chemical Engineering at the same university, he joined the faculty at Purdue University in 1986 and was promoted to full professor in 1994. Since 1998, he has held a joint appointment in the Department of Biomedical Engineering.

Dr. Park is currently an associate editor and the book review editor of *Pharmaceutical Research*, and he serves on the editorial boards of various journals. He is the founder of Akina, a company specializing in controlled drug delivery formulations. His current research includes development of novel fast melting tablet formulations, application of the solvent exchange method for microencapsulation, synthesis of hydrotropic polymeric micelles, application of layer-by-layer coating methods for making drug-eluting stents, and elastic superporous hydrogels.

Contributors

Namjin Baek, Ph.D.
Akina, Inc.
West Lafayette, Indiana

Yong Woo Cho, Ph.D.
Akina, Inc.
West Lafayette, Indiana

Mitsuhiro Ebara, Ph.D.
Department of Applied Chemistry
Waseda University
Tokyo, Japan

Hiroshi Frusawa, Ph.D.
Department of Environmental Systems
  Engineering
Kochi University of Technology
Kochi, Japan

Rupali Gangopadhyay, Ph.D.
Chemical Sciences Division
Saha Institute of Nuclear Physics
Kolkata, India

Stevin H. Gehrke, Ph.D.
Departments of Chemical and
  Petroleum Engineering and
  Pharmaceutical Chemistry
The University of Kansas
Lawrence, Kansas

Richard A. Gemeinhart, Ph.D.
Departments of Biopharmaceutical
  Sciences and Bioengineering
University of Illinois
Chicago, Illinois

Jian Ping Gong, Ph.D.
Graduate School of Science
Hokkaido University
Sapporo, Japan

Chunqiang Guo, M.S.
Department of Biopharmaceutical
  Sciences
University of Illinois
Chicago, Illinois

Wim E. Hennink, Ph.D.
Department of Pharmaceutics
Utrecht Institute for Pharmaceutical
  Sciences
Utrecht, the Netherlands

Michio Homma, Ph.D.
Graduate School of Science
Nagoya University
Nagoya, Japan

Kunihiro Ichimuta, Ph.D.
Research Institute for Polymers and
  Textiles
Science University of Tokyo
Tokyo, Japan

Shin'ichi Ishiwata, Ph.D.
Department of Physics
School of Science and Engineering
Waseda University
Tokyo, Japan

Kohzo Ito, Ph.D.
Graduate School of Frontier Sciences
University of Tokyo
Chiba, Japan

Eduardo Jule, Ph.D.
Graduate School of Engineering
University of Tokyo
Tokyo, Japan

Nobuyuki Kansawa, Ph.D.
Faculty of Science and Technology
Sophia University
Tokyo, Japan

Kazunori Kataoka, Ph.D.
Graduate School of Engineering
University of Tokyo
Tokyo, Japan

Norihiro Kato, Ph.D.
Faculty of Engineering
Utsunomiya University
Utsunomiya, Japan

Akihiko Kikuchi, Ph.D.
Institute of Advanced Biomedical
  Engineering and Science
Tokyo Women's Medical University
Tokyo, Japan

Jong-Duk Kim, Ph.D.
Department of Chemical and
  Biomolecular Engineering
Korean Advanced Institute of Science
  and Technology
Daejeon, South Korea

Seiji Kurihara, Ph.D.
Faculty of Engineering
Kumamoto University
Kumamoto, Japan

Randall J. Mrsny, Ph.D.
Welsh School of Pharmacy
Cardiff University
Cardiff, Wales

Teruo Okano, Ph.D.
Institute of Advanced Biomedical
  Engineering and Science
Tokyo Women's Medical University
Tokyo, Japan

Tooru Ooya, Ph.D.
School of Materials Science
Japan Advanced Institute of Science and
  Technology
Ishikawa, Japan

Yoshihito Osada, Ph.D.
Graduate School of Science
Hokkaido University
Sapporo, Japan

Kinam Park, Ph.D.
Departments of Pharmaceutics and
  Biomedical Engineering
Purdue University
West Lafayette, Indiana

Nicholas A. Peppas, Ph.D.
Departments of Chemical, Biomedical
  Engineering and Pharmaceutics
University of Texas
Austin, Texas

Kiyotaka Sakai, Ph.D.
Department of Applied Chemistry
Waseda University
Tokyo, Japan

Teruo Shimmen, Ph.D.
Graduate School of Science
Himeji Institute of Technology
Hyogo, Japan

Madoka Suzuki, M.Sc.
Department of Physics
School of Science and Engineering
Waseda University
Tokyo, Japan

Takahide Tsuchiya, Ph.D.
Faculty of Science and Technology
Sophia University
Tokyo, Japan

Cornelus F. van Nostrum, Ph.D.
Department of Pharmaceutics
Utrecht Institute for Pharmaceutical
  Sciences
Utrecht, the Netherlands

Jan Hein van Steenis, Ph.D.
Department of Pharmaceutics
Utrecht Institute for Pharmaceutical
  Sciences
Utrecht, the Netherlands

Toshiharu Yakushi, Ph.D.
Graduate School of Science
Nagoya University
Nagoya, Japan

Seung Rim Yang, Ph.D.
Department of Chemical and
  Biomolecular Engineering
Korean Advanced Institute of Science
  and Technology
Daejeon, South Korea

Etsuo Yokota, Ph.D.
Graduate School of Science
Himeji Institute of Technology
Hyogo, Japan

Ryo Yoshida, Ph.D.
Graduate School of Engineering
University of Tokyo
Tokyo, Japan

Nobuhiko Yui, Ph.D.
School of Materials Science
Japan Advanced Institute of Science and
  Technology
Ishikawa, Japan

Contents

Section I

Learning from Natural Systems

Section I

1 Learning from Nature: Examples of Rapid, Repetitive, Responsive Biological Events

Randall J. Mrsny

CONTENTS

INTRODUCTION

A wide range of potential biomedical applications of polymers have been described in the literature. One very exciting subset of these applications involves efforts to mimic some of the rapid, repetitive, responsive biological events (RRRBEs) observed in various tissues and organs of the body. Such events allow the body to perform critical tasks associated with homeostasis as well as adaptation. For example, the body must maintain a constant supply of critical nutritive factors to all of its areas yet must be able to increase or decrease the levels of these factors systematically or locally in accordance with changes in the demand for these factors.

Complex systems regulate hemodynamic parameters and allow the body to adapt to changing needs. Other RRRBEs can be observed in systems where the body must react to stimuli as well as filter responses to specific external signals. Olfactory events serve as examples of such systems.[1] A new odor is easily detected initially, but with time that odor stimulus is filtered (even muted) to provide for increased acuity to new odors even in the continued presence of the initial odor. Both systems, blood flow and odor sensation, are extremely complex. Fortunately, studies have been able to break down such complex systems into incremental biological functions of individual RRRBEs. Such simplified systems may be potentially mimicked by polymeric processes.

The success of current and future applications of polymeric systems that mimic RRRBEs will require overcoming a number of challenges. One challenge is that these systems sufficiently portray a desired biological event. It may not be necessary to match the RRRBE exactly; rather it may be sufficient to emulate its critical functions. Identifying the critical parameters of such events demands an appreciation of not only the biological principles of the event in question but also, and maybe more importantly, an understanding of the intent of the RRRBE function. It is the goal of this chapter to discuss both of these issues — the critical factors of such events in light of the action that the event is acting to achieve.

The examples presented were selected specifically to provide a perspective of several types of RRRBEs observed in the body. Some of these events have already been modeled in various ways using polymeric systems. Others have not yet been solved. However, from the discussion of these systems, it is hoped that the reader will obtain a better understanding of how nature has solved problems related to RRRBEs and possibly how to apply these principles in instances where polymeric systems may find applications.

GENERAL PRINCIPLES

The body performs such a wide range of tasks that it would be impossible to even begin to describe them here. These events occur inside cells, outside cells, and even between cells, and they occur at every possible level of sophistication. Many events appear simple and thus quite direct, i.e., rising glucose levels result in the increased release of insulin from the beta cells of the pancreatic islets. Thus, such events might be readily modeled using a polymeric system that can respond to a glucose signal with the release of insulin. However, this superficial assessment of the role of islet beta cells does not accurately describe the true complexity of the system in which the cells participate.[2]

Glucose recognition by islet beta cells initiates an extensive network of intra-cellular signaling events that leads to outcomes much more complex than simply secreting insulin.[3] From a pharmaceutical perspective, the connection of glucose to insulin secretion can be sufficient for a therapeutic application.[4] Thus, a polymeric system that primarily emulates such an outcome may not need to follow the entire pathway of the events required to achieve that outcome in the body. With this in mind, we wish to introduce a new descriptor of polymeric systems designed to emulate RRRBEs. In essence, such systems should be able to respond to a stimulus to provide a simple response rather than the complex and interactive network of events that typically occurs in the body. Therefore, the term *multi-reflexive* was introduced to describe polymeric systems that produce the rapid, repetitive, and responsive events similar to those observed in the body, yet work in the absence of more complex networks of events that commonly occur following such stimuli.

The term *multi-reflexive* was selected due to connotations of the root components that discriminate function and capabilities of these types of polymers. Reflex events involve direct outcomes that occur in the absence of a higher level of responding network or cognitive events. Since it is highly unlikely that current polymeric technologies would be able to respond more elaborately than in a purely reflexive fashion, *reflexive* seemed a more accurate term than *responsive*. The term *multi* refers to the desired action of such systems to potentially affect specific types of events at several levels of responses. In some instances, it may be desirable for the system to transition repeatedly between two physical states — rapidly producing multiple all-or-none events. In other cases, the system may provide the desired action through a graded response rather than an all-or-none outcome. Such a system could allow a stimulus to provide varied levels of responses through opening one to many portals of release for a substance to be delivered. Although these two types of responses are not mutually exclusive, and it is likely that combinations of such events would be attractive in certain cases, each represents the concept that polymers can provide multiples of release and/or modification events. These are only a few examples of how multi-reflexive polymeric systems might function. The types of polymer systems being developed are likely to provide a tremendous variety of polymer-based delivery systems that might be used to emulate RRRBEs.

In order to emulate RRRBEs through the use of multi-reflexive polymeric systems, it is important to understand the critical elements of the desired outcome. Further, it is important to establish a system that responds only to a desired stimulus and at a threshold where premature, undesirable events will not occur. These two issues represent difficult challenges for multi-reflexive polymeric systems because they do not typically have the sophistication of RRRBEs where networks of events can act to guard against subthreshold activation events and where a combination of low-level stimuli can provide an augmented, and thus sufficient, stimulus for system activation. For example, nerves can discriminate varied levels of stimuli that might be simultaneously delivered from several factors.[5] The release of a neurotransmitter from an adjacent cell may be insufficient to activate an action potential in a nerve unless it is of a certain magnitude or it is presented in the presence of another stimulus such as heat or another neurotransmitter, etc.[6] Additionally, a response to factors that normally induce an action potential may be completely muted in the presence of another type of neurotransmitter whose function is to evaluate the stimulus in another way and to determine signal validity. Nerves are constantly modulating their synaptic interactions to provide a very complex level of cell function modification.[7] These types of responses are frequently bidirectional to provide feedback information.[6] As one might imagine, a multi-reflexive polymeric system may never be able to achieve such levels of complexity. Therefore, the remainder of this chapter will be devoted to examples of RRRBEs that are deconstructed in an effort to find situations where multi-reflexive polymeric systems might be applicable and, more importantly, successful. The intent of this approach is to highlight mechanisms used to achieve the speed and sophistication of responses observed for many RRRBEs of the body.

LESSONS FROM NERVES

Nervous tissue is comprised of a number of cell types with very different phenotypes and functions.[6] At the heart of nervous tissue is one cell type — the neuron — although, here again, a wide range of subtypes of such cells exist that relate primarily to their anatomic locations and whether they perform specialized functions. The other cell types present in nervous tissue support the functions of neurons.[8]

In general, these mixtures of cells (neurons and supporting cells) are organized into circuits to provide pathways for the passage of information through a series of electrical disturbances induced by chemical stimuli.[9] Some nerve cells do more than passing on information; they also act as sensors.[10] Thus, in one cell the sensation of a stimulus can produce the response of releasing neurotransmitters to communicate sensed information to the next neuron. Looking at an individual nerve cell with such capabilities provides the opportunity to analyze a RRRBE that responds to chemical stimuli.

Nerve cells produce RRRBEs by establishing a large potential energy in the form of chemical gradients across their plasma membranes and by having mechanisms to release the gradients very rapidly.[11] Ions are what nerve cells use to establish these potential energies and these energies can, in turn, be thought of as measures of electrical work.[12] The resting membrane potential of a nerve cell is typically between 30 and 70 mV (let us assume the average is approximately 60) and the inside of the neuron is more negative than its extracellular environment (or roughly −60 mV for the average nerve). This potential is established by sequestering K^+ and excluding Na^+ and Cl^- ions relative to the extracellular environment. Increasing or decreasing the relative differences of these ion gradients results in a proportional change in the resting potential of the nerve. The classical Nernst equation that takes into account factors such as charge valency, concentration, and permeability for each ion at a given temperature can be used to provide a close approximation of this resting potential. Additional (but subtle) factors including charge density, distribution, and local water content that may be affected by polycharged matrices could act to shift this resting potential (and its ability to be altered during an action potential) slightly.

Two properties of the nerve cell allow for the rapid loss of these ion gradients and the generation of what is known as action potential: the ion gradients (mentioned above) and the selective permeability of those ions across the plasma membrane. Although several nearly simultaneous events occur, the transient increase in Na^+ permeability across the nerve cell plasma membrane depolarizes the plasma membrane and acts to conduct the action potential. Initially, a few Na^+ channels open and as Na^+ moves inward (down its concentration gradient), the membrane depolarizes further and more Na^+ channels open.[13] As Na^+ ions move inward, a series of K^+ channels opens to allow this ion to flow rapidly down its concentration gradient and out of the cell.[14] Thus, the established ion gradients of the nerve cell and selective ion permeability across the plasma membranes of the ions involved in those gradients work together to make the action potential a very fast event. The actual action potential can occur in less than a millisecond. Other physical and chemical properties of the nerves allow this action potential to be transmitted long distances, up to a meter, with almost the same speed. The focus for this discussion is that at the site of stimulation, nerves can respond rapidly due to the establishment of ion gradients.

The fact that nerves can quickly regenerate these ion gradients makes the system capable of repetition on a rapid time scale. A hypothetical polymeric system emulating some aspects of the rapid and repetitive actions of a nerve is shown in Figure 1.1.

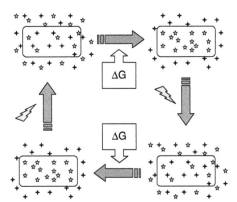

FIGURE 1.1 Cartoon of a cyclic system capable of selectively sequestering components and excluding others (horizontal arrows) to establish potential energies through concentration gradients. This event requires the input of energy into the system (ΔG). Rapid release of these gradients (vertical arrows) through the action of stimuli (lightning bolts) results in their loss until the system is recharged. One can envision that each cycle could result in the release of some factor or agent. This type of system is analogous to situations where the stimulus of a nerve impulse induces an action potential in an adjacent nerve for information propagation or in a muscle cell to induce a contraction. Similarly, a soluble factor like a hormone could act as a stimulus to affect a cell's membrane potential to initiate a cellular event such as granule secretion (described on p. 9 of this chapter).

Before re-establishing these gradients, a nerve cell is refractory to another stimulus. With extended repetitions of stimulating action potentials, the intensity of response can lessen and the refractory period of a nerve can lengthen. These changes occur because of the mechanism used to re-establish the resting state of the nerve cell. A series of ion pumps functions to move Na^+, K^+, and Cl^- to establish the gradients described above. These pumps use energy in the form of adenosine triphosphate (ATP) to move these ions against their respective gradients.[15] Extended use of a neuron does two things. Initially, if the repeated stimulus comes faster than the time required for the ion pumps to re-establish gradients, the uptake of ions tends to become less and less complete and the intensity of response is lessened. Further, if the systems involved in the generation of ATP are not given sufficient time or nutrients to maintain critical levels, the refractory period will lengthen to whatever time is required to allow for the re-establishment of these ion gradients under the conditions of limited ATP supply.

The responsive aspect of the nerve action potential highlights a critical aspect of all RRRBEs: the establishment of a threshold required to activate this all-or-none event. For nerves, the value of the threshold required to initiate an action potential appears to depend upon the relative numbers of Na^+ and K^+ ion channels at rest (resting ion channels) and those that gate these ions (gating ion channels) across the plasma membrane. Any stimulus will open ion channels in the plasma membrane. If that stimulus is sufficient to counteract the mechanisms that actively maintain ion gradients across the plasma membrane, then an action potential will ensue, but this outcome reflects a complex arrangement of competing forces.[16] If, however, the stimulus cannot sufficiently depolarize the membrane no action potential is observed.

While the actions (and functions) of nerves require them to use this all-or-none method of activation, many biological systems have a need to provide graded responses to different levels of stimulus. In the nervous system, this is achieved by a complex series of regulating neurons that act through sensory or motor nerve pathways to fine-tune the magnitude of a response. In most cases, the magnitude of response is correlated with the number of nerves that have undergone an action potential that feeds back to the same response element. Such an approach leads us to the next RRRBE example: muscle.

LESSONS FROM MUSCLES

Muscle in the human body is found in three basic forms: striated, cardiac and smooth. Although all three have similar functions of contractions through organized structures of actin and myosin filaments, for simplicity, only the striated form will be discussed here. To understand how muscle functions as a RRRBE, it is important to first appreciate its organizational elements. Under the ionic conditions inside cells, that is low Na^+ and high K^+ ion content, and in the presence of ATP,[17] individual globular actin (G-actin) proteins can form filaments (F-actin).

An important role is also played by Mg^{2+} ions in this process of G-actin $\rightarrow$ F-actin. Because the association region of G-actin interacts with itself, the noninteracting region protrudes in a helical manner from the forming filament. Myosin, a much larger protein than actin, ends up interacting to establish, in many ways, a type of structure similar to F-actin.[18] Initially, two myosin molecules dimerize through extensive interactions along their long heavy chain tails. As these tail regions form larger (300 to 400) oligomers, the two globular heads of each myosin dimer are positioned in a helical arrangement about its surface with spacing of ~14 nm.[19] Driven by ATP hydrolysis, these arranged myosin heads can move along actin filaments through specific interactions with the protruding actin domains that are also arranged in a helical fashion. During this movement, each myosin molecule hydrolyzes 5 to 10 ATP molecules per second. The sliding movements of actin and myosin against each other provide the basis for muscular contraction. Many factors can regulate these events of ATP hydrolysis and thus muscle contraction.[20]

For the actin–myosin system to perform useful work when it hydrolyzes ATP (i.e., to induce a muscle contraction), it must be organized into a structure that is anchored in some way. This is achieved through the function of a large range of structural proteins and leads to the organization of what are known as myofibrils. These myofibrils are organized further into myofibers that are bundled together to form muscles that are typically attached to bony structures through terminal tendons.

Let us stay focused in the actin-myosin system of the myofibril since this is the basic unit of contraction and therefore provides the lessons of interest as an RRRBE. The "walking" of myosin heads along the anchored actin filaments occurs through a cycle of actions associated with ATP hydrolysis.[19] ATP is thought to weaken the binding of myosin to actin and relax their interactions. As ATP is hydrolyzed, the myosin head is thought to pivot and allow for a reassociation in a more contracted state prior to the release of the produced adenosine diphosphate (ADP) and binding of ATP that acts to reposition the myosin fiber along the actin fiber. Thus, repeated ATP hydrolysis events act to continuously reposition myosin heads (and myosin fibers) along the actin fibers in accordance to their projecting structures that are arranged in specific helical patterns.

The issue that a muscle must overcome to function efficiently is coordination. Each muscle contains millions of myofibrils that must work in unison to provide useful muscular activity. Since muscle contraction is controlled by nerve activation, one way to achieve this would be to have nerves going to every myofibril of a muscle and fire all the nerves simultaneously. It should be immediately apparent that this solution is not viable because the space occupied by nerves would immediately increase to the point where the body would have no room for anything but nerves. Instead, the body sends signals to a muscle through a much smaller number of neurons, and this requires the muscle to dissipate the information in a rapid and efficient manner.[21] That signal, however, must be assisted in some way because simple diffusion events would otherwise require much longer times of muscle contraction (and relaxation) than required for survival. To solve this task, the muscle uses several unique systems, employs Ca^{2+} ions as activating signals, and takes advantage of critical aspects associated with the parameters that control actin–myosin contraction.

Recall that each muscle cell contains a large number of myofibrils surrounded by a plasma membrane. The transverse tubule (T-tubule) is a specialized organization of the plasma membrane that protrudes deep into the cell body and associates with one of the anchoring regions of the organized actin–myosin complex. An extensive, continuous membrane system, the sarcoplasmic reticulum (SR), is found at the surface of each myofibril within a muscle cell. The SR, which acts as a reservoir of Ca^{2+} ions sequestered from the muscle cell cytoplasm and myofibrils, establishes a close association with T-tubules through an organization of voltage-sensing Ca^{2+} channels at terminal cisternae of the SR.[22] Depolarization of the plasma membrane of each myofiber through the actions of neurons leads to an opening of these voltage-gated Ca^{2+} channels and a rapid release of Ca^{2+} into the cytoplasm. A rise in cytosolic Ca^{2+} concentration triggers the binding of actin to the myosin–ADP complex to stimulate the subsequent events of muscle contraction.

Because each membrane depolarization is conducted along the T-tubule to the SR membrane within milliseconds, every myofibril in a cell can contract simultaneously. Figure 1.2 depicts an analogous polymer system and shows the localized sequestering and release of an agent, similar to the activity of Ca^{2+} in muscle cells. This contraction will continue until the Ca^{2+} levels are decreased through the actions of a Ca^{2+} ATPase present in the SR membrane that acts to extract this ion from the cytoplasm, placing it back into the SR against a concentration gradient.

Re-establishment of the Ca^{2+} gradient into the SR provides for the repetitive nature of muscle contraction. Like nerve function, muscle contraction ultimately requires energy in the form of ATP for the actual contraction event and also for recharging the SR Ca^{2+} gradient.[22] Also similar to the action potential of a nerve, the capacity for a muscle to contract repetitively is dictated by the rate of ion gradient re-establishment and maintenance ATP levels.

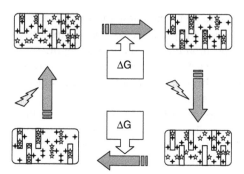

FIGURE 1.2 Cartoon of a cyclic system having an internal structure (or organization) capable of selectively sequestering components while excluding others (horizontal arrows) to establish potential energies through concentration gradients. This event requires the input of energy into the system (ΔG). Rapid release of these gradients (vertical arrows) through the action of a stimulus (lightning bolt) results in their loss until the system is recharged. One can envision that with each cycle, the system either releases some agent or alters one of its physical properties. This type of system describes what occurs in the transverse tubules of the sarcoplasmic reticulum system of muscle. An important feature of this system is how the entire matrix of the muscle can be accessed quickly and efficiently through the dissemination of a signal into invaginations into the matrix of the responding material. The invaginations in this figure are represented by the small rectangles where stars are sequestered prior to a stimulus.

With respect to the responsive aspect of this system, the Ca^{2+} ion appears to act as the regulating signal. Sufficient nerve stimulus leading to sufficient plasma membrane and T-tubule depolarization is required to achieve a threshold level of released Ca^{2+} from the SR of the cell.

LESSONS FROM ENDOCRINE TISSUES

The body utilizes a variety of factors that are secreted from a cell in one location of the body to act upon themselves (autocrine factors), adjacent cells (paracrine factors), or cells at distant sites (endocrine factors). Although a wide range of protein and peptide molecules that fit into these categories have been identified, those that have achieved the most clinical success are endocrine factors administered as replacement and augmentation therapies.

Two of the best-known examples are insulin and human growth hormone (hGH). Most insulin administered today is now a human form of the protein, but this was not always the case. Porcine- and bovine-derived proteins dominated the treatment field for several decades. Nonhuman forms of growth hormone were never found to be helpful due to the induction of a potent immune response to these nonself proteins. When considering the administration of insulin or hGH for applications involving multi-responsive polymeric systems, it is important to appreciate some of the complexities associated with the biologies of these two proteins.

Insulin is the predominant anabolic hormone that promotes glucose utilization and thus prevents or regulates episodes of hyperglycemia. It is released from the pancreas continuously at baseline levels and sporadically in postprandial spikes.

Since its actions to reduce blood concentrations of glucose can lead to life-threatening situations, it is not surprising that a variety of endocrine systems exist to oppose, or rather modulate, insulin action. Some of these counter-regulatory hormones include epinephrine, glucagon, growth hormone, and cortosol. Somatostatin, through its actions involving inhibition of glucagon secretion, acts to increase the severity and duration of insulin-induced hypoglycemia, pointing to the important role glucagon plays in reversing the hypoglycemic actions of insulin. Both insulin and glucagon are secreted from islet cells of the endocrine pancreas.[23] Their primary function in regulating blood glucose occurs at the liver where a large amount of sugar substrate is stored in the form of glycogen. Insulin acts to remove sugar from the blood and to add it to these stores while glucagon acts to break down established stores to release sugar into the blood. Although systemic administration of these two hormones is the most common form of delivery and provides for the peripheral actions at muscle and fat cells, a primary target for their actions is the liver.

Growth hormone also appears to use the liver as a primary site of action. Following release from the anterior pituitary gland into the systemic circulation, growth hormone activates receptors in the liver to stimulate the secretion of insulin-like growth factor I (IGF-I) which goes on to accelerate body growth.[24] Absence of growth hormone during childhood results in dwarfism; over-secretion leads to childhood gigantism and adult acromegaly.

The release of growth hormone is induced by the actions of growth hormone-releasing hormone (GHRH) secreted by the hypothalamus. An opposite action is produced by somatostatin, another hypothalamic factor. A complex series of environmental and biological factors that include sleep, stress, other hormones, and events such as hypoglycemia regulate the releases of GHRH and somatostatin. Thus, growth hormone release proceeds under a complex set of controls. The typical release pattern for growth hormone in growing children, as observed by serum levels, is a series of small pulses throughout the day with a consistent surge about 2 h long that occurs 1 to 2 h after sleep begins. This surge, however, can be variable and debate continues about the use of growth hormone therapy in children of small stature who are not necessarily growth hormone-deficient.[24]

Growth hormone and insulin are stored in secretion granules adjacent to the plasma membranes within acidophilic somatotrophs of the anterior pituitary and the beta cells of the islets of Langerhans in the pancreas, respectively. Mechanisms of regulated secretion of these granules, i.e., a graded amount of granule release based upon a certain level of stimulus, again identify Ca^{2+} ions having an important function. The bigger issue, however, is the practical aspect of how this quantized release of material is achieved by these cells. An idealized polymeric system using this principle is shown in Figure 1.3. The first aspect to consider is that these cells release packets (not one or two molecules) of hormone with each stimulation event. Considering parameters of body distribution and desired pharmacokinetic profiles, release of packets of material makes more sense when considering the quantities of hormone needed to achieve desired systemic levels.

Packaging proteins at high concentrations at 37°C, however, tends to produce tremendous storage problems for formulation scientists.[25] How does the body resolve this issue? One way is freshness. These proteins are continuously synthesized and

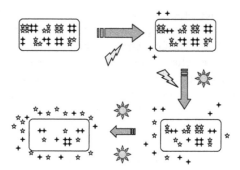

FIGURE 1.3 Cartoon of a system capable of repeatedly responding to an external stimulus (lightning bolt or sun) with the release (arrows) of a sequestered agent or factor. Without the ability to synthesize or sequester that agent or factor following each stimulus, the system is not cyclic in nature (noted by the decreased sizes of the arrows). Although not depicted here, such a loss could result in a shrinkage or even collapse of the system's physical structure. One can also envision a system that selectively releases more than one agent or factor, shown here by the two different agents and two different forms of stimulus. Such a system might be able to release a quantity of factor or agent relative to the amount of stimulus (where two suns rather than only one are used for activation). Endocrine cells show all these capabilities in the secretion mechanisms of protein hormones. Thus, this system models the selected release of discrete packets of two different drugs from one system where the release of each is under the selective control of specific stimuli and the quantity released responds to the amount of stimulus applied.

released and the lifetime of an intracellular package of growth hormone or insulin can be measured in hours, not months. Thus, these biological systems are repetitive — limited only by the rate of resynthesis of hormone (a rate much slower than recovery of Ca^{2+} or ATP levels). Another trick used by a cell is to dehydrate these storage packages or granules, potentially reducing the frequencies of degrading events facilitated by water and increasing the protein concentrations within the granules.[26] When significant amounts of water have been removed from the granules, the protein can precipitate in a manner that will render it biologically inactive. In the case of insulin, Zn^{2+} ions appear to coordinate with the protein and stabilize it in a form that can regain biological activity after rehydration, such as following release.[27] Similar observations have been made for growth hormone and this approach of producing a precipitated complex between the protein and Zn^{2+} has been used in several polymeric delivery systems.[28,29] Thus, formulation scientists can partially recreate conditions associated with protein storage at high concentrations within granules and the release of the protein following exocytosis.

Responses in these systems are typically driven by the actions of an external stimulator. The rapid nature of these secretion events, however, is not facilitated by the actions of nerves or SR structures, but rather by the ready access of stimulating factors to the surfaces of these granule-laden endocrine cells. In both cases, in the anterior pituitary and in the Langerhans islets in the pancreas, blood is in direct contact with the surfaces of these cells by the establishment of sinusoidal vascular systems.

This direct surface interaction eliminates the requirement to transport stimulants and hormones across endothelial barriers. Because of this, release of these hormones is more similar to an intravenous (i.v.) injection than a subcutaneous (s.c.) injection. Recreation of such a system is very difficult using multi-reflexive polymeric systems since it is very difficult to place such a system within a blood stream. Instead, such systems are usually positioned in s.c. or intramuscular (i.m.) spaces, thus reducing the abilities of stimulators to reach the material and impeding the speed of dissemination through the body of factors released from these systems.

CONCLUSIONS

The examples used here to describe RRRBEs have been greatly simplified to allow for a focused discussion of selected aspects of these processes. Many more components and feedback systems involved in these processes were not discussed. Instead, the discussion concentrated on how nature has established systems capable of rapidly responding to repetitive stimuli to produce biological outcomes. Only the essential parameters of these systems were described in order to better portray the potential applications of these concepts to multi-reflexive polymeric systems that are being evaluated for biomedical use. The body also uses a range of organizational relationships to augment its RRRBE capabilities that were not discussed at length in this review. For example, a method of stimulus distribution is frequently used to recruit multiple sites to act in unison. One example of this is the way a single nerve spreads over a number of muscle fibers to coordinate their contractions. Alternately, molecules can be released locally from endocrine tissues to modulate and coordinate a response following a stimulus from a systemically circulating hormone.

Several basic themes seem to hold about the RRRBEs described. Their rapid nature is commonly established by a chemical gradient, frequently by an ion that can be released without the expenditure of additional energy. Alternately, materials are packaged into structures that are poised to be released and stimulated to do so in a system in which minimal time is lost to the movement of the factors across biological barriers. The repetitive nature of these systems lies primarily with the fact that the cells involved act to re-establish these gradients of components through the expenditure of energy (in the form of ATP). These systems are set up to keep pace with their normal rates of repetition, but replacement can become a problem if the rate of use becomes too great. Finally, the examples provided demonstrate some of the possible means by which the body establishes responsive systems that can provide graded outcomes through the controlled summation of individual all-or-none events.

REFERENCES

1. Rawson, N.E. and G. Gomez, Cell and molecular biology of human olfaction, *Microsc. Res. Tech.*, 2002, 58(3), 142–151.
2. Routh, V.H., Glucose-sensing neurons: are they physiologically relevant? *Physiol. Behav.*, 2002, 76(3), 403–413.

3. Alrefai, H. et al., The endocrine system in diabetes mellitus, *Endocrine*, 2002, 18(2), 105–119.
4. Bouldin, M.J. et al., Quality of care in diabetes: understanding the guidelines, *Am. J. Med. Sci.*, 2002, 324(4), 196–206.
5. Cometto-Muniz, J.E. et al., Chemosensory detectability of 1-butanol and 2-heptanone singly and in binary mixtures, *Physiol. Behav.*, 1999, 67(2), 269–276.
6. Fields, R.G. and B. Stevens-Graham, New insights into neural glia communications, *Science*, 2002, 298(5593), 556–561.
7. Cohen-Cory, S., The developing synapse: construction and modulation of synaptic structures and circuits, *Science*, 2002, 298(5594), 770–776.
8. Nedergaard, M., T. Takano, and A.J. Hansen, Beyond the role of glutamate as a neurotransmitter, *Nat. Rev. Neurosci.*, 2002, 3(9), 748–755.
9. Martin, K.A., Microcircuits in visual cortex, *Curr. Opin. Neurobiol.*, 2002, 12(4), 418–425.
10. Sheng, M. and M.-J. Kim, Postsynaptic signaling and plasticity mechanisms, *Science*, 2002, 298(5594), 776–780.
11. Hartwell, L.H. et al., From molecular to modular cell biology, *Nature*, 1999, 402 (Suppl. 6761), C47–C52.
12. Veech, R.L., Y. Kashiwaya, and M.T. King, The resting membrane potentials of cells are measures of electrical work, not of ionic currents, *Integr. Physiol. Behav. Sci.*, 1995, 30(4), 283–307.
13. Strichartz, G.R. et al., Therapeutic concentrations of local anaesthetics unveil the potential role of sodium channels in neuropathic pain, *Novartis Found. Symp.*, 2002, 241, 189–201 (see discussion, 202–205 and 226–232).
14. Chiu, S.Y. et al., Analysis of potassium channel functions in mammalian axons by gene knockouts, *J. Neurocytol.*, 1999, 28(4–5), 349–364.
15. Scheiner-Bobis, G., The sodium pump: its molecular properties and mechanics of ion transport, *Eur. J. Biochem.*, 2002, 269(10), 2424–2433.
16. Burke, D., M.C. Kiernan, and H. Bostock, Excitability of human axons, *Clin. Neurophysiol.*, 2001, 112(9), 1575–1585.
17. Carlier, M.F., Actin polymerization and ATP hydrolysis, *Adv. Biophys.*, 1990, 26, 51–73.
18. Miroshnichenko, N.S., I.V. Balanuk, and D.N. Nozdrenko, Packing of myosin molecules in muscle thick filaments, *Cell Biol. Int.*, 2000, 24(6), 327–333.
19. Huxley, H.E., Past, present and future experiments on muscle, *Philos. Trans. R. Soc. Lond. B Biol. Sci.*, 2000, 355(1396), 539–543.
20. Reid, M.B., Invited review: redox modulation of skeletal muscle contraction: what we know and what we don't, *J. Appl. Physiol.*, 2001, 90(2), 724–731.
21. Personius, K.E. and R.J. Balice-Gordon, Activity-dependent synaptic plasticity: insights from neuromuscular junctions, *Neuroscientist*, 2002, 8(5), 414–422.
22. Lamb, G.D., Voltage-sensor control of Ca^{2+} release in skeletal muscle: insights from skinned fibers, *Front. Biosci.*, 2002, 7, 834–842.
23. Means, A.L. and S.D. Leach, Lineage commitment and cellular differentiation in exocrine pancreas, *Pancreatology*, 2001, 1(6), 587–596.
24. Macklin, R., Ethical dilemmas in pediatric endocrinology: growth hormone for short normal children, *J. Pediatr. Endocrinol. Metab.*, 2000, 13 (Suppl. 6), 1349–1352.
25. Perez, C. et al., Recent trends in stabilizing protein structure upon encapsulation and release from bioerodible polymers, *J. Pharm. Pharmacol.*, 2002, 54(3), 301–313.
26. Verdugo, P., Mucin exocytosis, *Am. Rev. Respir. Dis.*, 1991, 144(3, Pt. 2), S33–S37.

27. Grodsky, G.M. and F. Schmid-Formby, Kinetic and quantitative relationships between insulin release and 65ZN efflux from perfused islets, *Endocrinology*, 1985, 117(2), 704–710.
28. Johnson, O.L. et al., The stabilization and encapsulation of human growth hormone into biodegradable microspheres, *Pharm. Res.*, 1997, 14(6), 730–735.
29. Okumu, F.W. et al., Sustained delivery of human growth hormone from a novel gel delivery system: SABER, *Biomaterials*, 2002, 23(22), 4353–4358.

2 Seismonastic Movements in Plants

Nobuyuki Kanzawa and Takahide Tsuchiya

CONTENTS

PLANT MOVEMENTS

The sessile nature of plants has provided for unique adaptations to their surrounding environments. Over their evolutionary course, plants have survived by changing their functional or structural properties. Animals, being mobile, can change their circumstances to an extent, but plants do not have brains, nervous systems, or muscles. Plants are not, however, static; they are able to respond to a variety of environmental stimuli. They perform various macroscopic and microscopic movements in response to intrinsic and extrinsic stimuli.

Plant movements are generally of two types: tropistic and nastic (Figure 2.1). Tropism is an irreversible growth response toward (positive tropism), or away from (negative tropism), an external stimulus. Tropism has a clear connection between the direction of movement and the movement of the controlling external stimulus. The most familiar type is phototropism, a response to light. Phototropism is thought to be caused by an increase in growth rate on the shaded side and a concomitant decrease in growth rate on the lighted side of a plant shoot (Cholodny–Went theory), (Cholodny, 1927; Went, 1928). Lateral transport of a growth factor from the lighted side to the shaded side is thought to contribute to this differential growth rate. Blue light appears to be involved in the early steps of the signal transduction pathway for phototropism (Briggs, 1992; Kiss et al., 2002; Lin, 2002; Palmer et al., 1993a). Molecular biological analysis has revealed that phototropin, a photoreceptor, undergoes

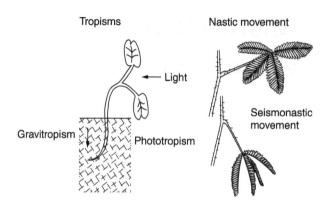

FIGURE 2.1 Plant movements: tropism and nastic movement.

autophosphorylation in blue light, and this results in activation of a phosphorylation cascade. It is believed that the phototropin-activated phosphorylation cascade is necessary for phototropic movement (Christie and Briggs, 2001; Palmer et al., 1993b; Reymond et al., 1992).

Gravitropism, another example of tropism, was first described 200 years ago (Knight, 1806). This response to gravity contributes to the upward growth of shoots by ensuring proper positioning of the leaves for efficient light gathering, and to the downward growth of roots for absorption of water and mineral ions from soil (Chen et al., 1999). The mechanism accepted at present for gravitropism involves the redistribution of gravity susceptors. In higher plants, settling of amyloplasts to the bottom of specialized cells (statocytes), is believed to create susceptors for gravity (Sack, 1991). Cells that detect the direction of gravity start to elongate in that direction.

An auxin gradient is believed to be a mediator for the gravity-stimulated elongation. Differential growth patterns induced by gravity stimulation are explained by the redistribution of auxin from the upper to the lower side (Young et al., 1990). Auxin stimulates rapid cell elongation in shoots and inhibits it in roots, resulting in upward curving of shoots and downward bending of roots. Cell elongation stimulated by auxin is thought to be regulated by expression of auxin-responsive genes (Hagen and Guilfoyle, 2002); however, it is not clear how auxin modulates expression of genes contributing to gravitropic curvature.

Opening and closing movements of many flowers and the responses of leaves to changes in temperature and light are nastic movements. Nastic and tropic movements are similar in that they are responses to external stimuli. However, unlike tropisms, nastic movements are reversible and are independent of the direction of the external signal. Nastic movements occur in a genetically determined manner and direction; they are not accompanied by cell growth. Therefore, a plant can respond repeatedly to the same stimulus repeatedly applied in a short period.

The most familiar example of nastic movement is nyctinastic movement, which is observed in *Samanea saman,* a tree in the *Mimosa* family. The plant opens its leaves and leaflets during the day and closes them at night. This movement is controlled by a biological clock, with a cycle of approximately 24 h, and is regulated by turgor changes in the motor organs of the plant. The motor organ for leaf movement is a pulvinus located at the base of the leaf or leaflet. Another well-studied example of nyctinastic movement is the opening and closing of leaf stomata. A variety of signals including hormones such as abscisic acid, light, humidity, and water status influence stomatal movement. This movement controls the uptake of CO_2 for photosynthesis and the loss of water vapor during transpiration.

Another example of nastic movement is the seismonasty (thigmonasty), of *Mimosa pudica*. Leaflets and sometimes entire leaves close or bend suddenly in response to touch or shaking or to electrical, thermal, or chemical stimuli. As with nyctinastic movement (also exhibited by *M. pudica*), seismonastic movement is generally explained by a sudden change in turgor pressure in motor cells of the pulvinus at the base of each leaf or leaflet.

SEISMONASTIC MOVEMENT IN *M. PUDICA*

Mimosa pudica L. responds to mechanical, thermal, electrical, and chemical stimuli with rapid bending of leaves and petioles. Like those of other *Mimosa* family members, leaves of *M. pudica* close at night or in darkness and open during the day or in light. Thus, the sensitive *M. pudica* has the ability to perform both seismonastic and nyctinastic movements.

Plant movement has fascinated scientists for centuries. Robert Hooke discussed muscular action in his famous book, *Micrografia* (Hooke, 1665); Charles Darwin was interested in *M. pudica* (Darwin, 1880). In the 18th century, de Mairan reported that leaves of *M. pudica* continued periodic movement even in constant darkness (de Mairan, 1927). Circadian rhythms have been found in most organisms and they are known to be regulated by internal molecules known as a clock genes or proteins (Dunlap, 1999; Staiger, 2002).

Movement of *Mimosa* leaves and leaflets is driven by changes in the curvature of the pulvinus. Folding of leaves and bending of petioles are caused by rapid shrinkage of the lower sides of motor cells of the pulvinus. Stimulation of a leaf causes an electrical signal to spread up the petioles. Subsequently, the electrical signal turns into a chemical signal that makes certain cell membranes become more permeable to K^+ and Cl^- ions. The increased permeability of the cell membranes causes ions to move from the symplasts into the apoplasts. Water accompanies the ions into the apoplasts by osmosis. This phenomenon is known as plasmolysis. As a result of plasmolysis, the protoplasts will shrink and this makes the leaflets or petioles droop.

STRUCTURE OF PULVINUS

In the early 20th century, the primary pulvinus was found to consist of motor cells surrounding the xylem and phloem. The fine structure of the *Mimosa* motor cell was characterized well in a series of studies by Toriyama (Toriyama and Sato, 1969) and Fleurat-Lessard (Fleurat-Lessard, 1990). As shown in Figure 2.2, a pulvinus contains a central vascular core consisting of xylem and phloem surrounded by 20 to 30 layers of parenchyma (motor), cells and a layer of epidermal cells.

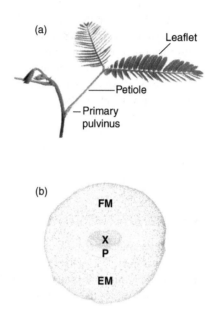

FIGURE 2.2 *Mimosa pudica* (a) and a transverse section of a primary pulvinus (b). The pulvinus contains a central vascular core consisting of xylem (X), and phloem (P). The core is surrounded by flexor motor (FM) and extensor motor (EM) cells.

Motor cells are roughly round in transverse section (15 to 20 μm), and are slightly elongated in longitudinal section (25 to 30 μm). Walls of flexor cells are three to four times thicker than those of extensor cells. This thickness is the only significant difference between motor cells and is easily recognized by light microscopy. Motor cells have vacuoles of two types. The large central vacuole can occupy more than 80% of the total cell volume, and the tannin vacuole is located near the nucleus (Figure 2.3). The central vacuole contains mainly inorganic salts and water and plays a role in the storage of metabolites and nutrients for maintenance of cytosolic homeostasis. The tannin vacuole is believed to function as a Ca^{2+} store (Toriyama and Jaffe, 1972; Turnquist et al., 1993). Calcium ion may be the secondary signal for initiating ion fluxes and associated water fluxes from vacuoles and cytoplasm into the apoplast. According to Fleurat-Lessard (Fleurat-Lessard, 1988), spherical central vacuoles shrink in response to the external stimuli, and tannin vacuoles separate into smaller vacuoles after curvature changes.

SIGNAL TRANSDUCTION

Living plant cells have negative resting membrane potentials. A nonequilibrium distribution of ions across the plasma membrane causes the potential difference. It is thought that when a cell receives a chemical or a physical stimulus, conformation of ion channels in the plasma membrane is altered. This conformational change

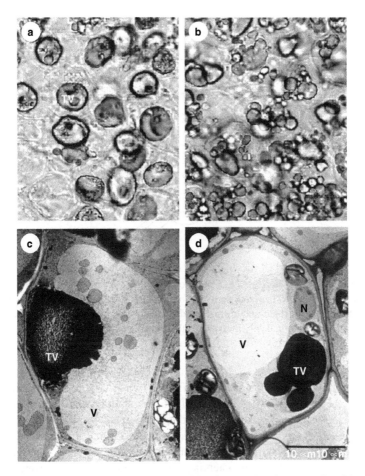

FIGURE 2.3 Light (a and b) and electron (c and d) micrographs of motor cells of the primary pulvinus of *M. pudica* in transverse section. The large central vacuole (V) and tannin vacuole (TV) are shown before bending (a and c). The vacuoles changed shape after bending (b and d). N = nucleus.

results in changes in the rates of ion migration through the membrane and thereby affects the electrical potential difference. The potential difference can change from a negative to a more positive value (depolarization). This change produces an action potential that can be propagated from cell to cell. Subsequent to depolarization, the original resting potential is re-established (repolarization).

Plant physiologists have investigated the propagation of action potentials in plants since the early 20th century. Ricca and Snow showed that an extract from *M. pudica* was able to induce closing of leaves in a dose-dependent manner (Ricca, 1916; Snow, 1924). They hypothesized that signal transduction substances are involved in the propagation of action potentials in plants. However, in 1926, Bose used isolated vascular bundles of a fern to show that excitation in both phloem and xylem is conducted similarly to excitation in frog nerve (Bose, 1926).

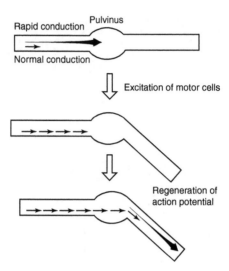

FIGURE 2.4 Rapid and normal signal conduction. Rapid conduction of an action potential occurs everywhere in the leaf and stem. Action potentials are initiated by many stimuli. A wound stimulus causes rapid and normal conduction of action potentials. Rapid conduction stops at the pulvinus; normal condition passes through slowly and regenerates action potential on the other side of the pulvinus.

In *M. pudica*, Houwink and Shibaoka found two types of electric signals (Houwink, 1935; Shibaoka, 1962; Shibaoka, 1966). Wounding, cutting, or burning can generate a slow signal. The speed of conduction is related to the velocity at which water moves in the xylem (normal conduction), suggesting the presence of signal transduction substances. In contrast, stimulation by cooling or by electrical means produces only a rapid action potential (rapid conduction). Moreover, the rapid conduction signal is interrupted at the pulvinus, whereas the normal conduction signal passes through. When a normal conduction signal passes through a pulvinus, a rapid conduction signal is generated on the other side of the pulvinus after a delay (Shibaoka, 1991) (Figure 2.4). The current path of signal conduction is still uncertain; it may pass through either companion and phloem parenchyma cells (Samejima and Shibaoka, 1983) or mature sieve elements (Fromm and Eschrich, 1988a; Fromm and Eschrich, 1990). Thus, the normal conduction signal stimulates the release of leaf movement factor into the vascular tissue, and the factor appears to alter the plasma membrane and subsequently induce the excitation of an action potential.

In 1983, Schildknecht isolated and determined the structure of the leaf movement factor (turgorin), of *M. pudica* (Schildknecht, 1983). He assumed that this leaf-movement substance is common to all nyctinastic plants and that leaf movement is controlled by changes in the internal concentration of turgorin. Recent investigation reveals that, in addition to turgorin, *M. pudica* contains opening and closing substances (Ueda and Yamamura, 1999; Ueda and Yamamura, 2000). Interestingly, Ueda and Yamamura reported the leaves of *M. pudica* can be kept open at night by treating with the opening factor; however, no significant effect of the factor was observed on the rapid seismonastic movement (Ueda and Yamamura, 1999). This observation shows that the nyctinastic movement of *Mimosa* is regulated by a mechanism different from that of the seismonastic movement.

IONS IMPLICATED IN TURGOR CHANGE

Motor organs in the pulvini move by turgor changes in the motor cells resulting from the excitation-induced movement of ions into and out of the cells (Satter and Galston, 1981). Potassium ions are accumulated in pulvinar motor cells and are involved in osmoregulation (Kiyosawa, 1979; Satter et al., 1974; Satter et al., 1970; Toriyama, 1955). The movement of K^+ out of motor cells during curvature change has been demonstrated by means of isotopically labeled K^+ (Allen, 1969) and by the micro-ashing technique (Toriyama, 1955). It was shown by cryo-ultramicrotome technique that K^+ is lost from extensor cells into the apoplasts and into the flexor cells of *S. saman* (Campbell et al., 1981).

The K^+ effluxes are accompanied by Cl^- effluxes during nyctinastic movement (Satter et al., 1977), whereas in *M. pudica*, Cl^- appears not to be the K^+ counterion (Fromm and Eschrich, 1988b).

Changes in cytosolic Ca^{2+} concentration during seismonastic movement were monitored by staining with alizarin-red sulfate. A loss of Ca^{2+} from the tannin vacuole during the curvature change and reabsorption of Ca^{2+} by the tannin vacuole during recovery were observed. It was hypothesized that release of Ca^{2+} from the tannin vacuole is associated with shrinkage of the central vacuole which is caused by Ca^{2+}-induced contraction of fibrous protein within the vacuole (Toriyama and Jaffe, 1972). However, using a Ca^{2+} channel blocker and chelating agents, Campbell and Thomson showed that influx of Ca^{2+} from the apoplast is accompanied by efflux of K^+ from the symplast. The effect of Ca^{2+} displacement on K^+ migration is still unsettled. It was shown with whole-cell patch clamp techniques that the elevation of cytoplasmic Ca^{2+} promotes the rundown of outward-rectifying K^+ channels in the plasma membranes of *Mimosa* protoplasts (Stoeckel and Takeda, 1995).

When ions accumulate in motor cells, the water potential decreases and consequent water uptake induces cell swelling, whereas reverse ion fluxes lead to turgor loss and cell shrinkage (Figure 2.5). We used nuclear magnetic resonance (NMR), imaging to study the displacement of water in a pulvinus of *M. pudica*. Water in the extensor half of the pulvinus was transferred to the flexor half (Tamiya et al., 1988). Recently, vacuolar membrane aquaporin, a water-pump, was found in the central vacuolar membranes of *Mimosa* motor cells. Expression of the protein seems to increase with functional maturation of the motor organ (Fleurat-Lessard et al., 1997). Fast water efflux through the water pump seems to be essential for rapid shrinkage of motor cells (Morillon et al., 2001). Plasma membrane aquaporins were identified in *S. saman*, and their role in nyctinastic movement of the plant was reported (Moshelion et al., 2002).

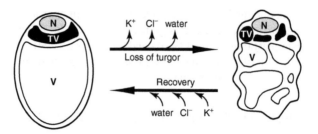

FIGURE 2.5 Change in motor cell shape. Motor cells contain two types of vacuoles: a central vacuole (V) and a tannin vacuole (TV). Efflux of K^+ and Cl^- ions accompanied by water occurs in response to stimuli. During shrinkage, both vacuoles change their shapes. N = nucleus.

ACTIN AND ACTIN-BINDING PROTEINS

Actin is one of the most abundant proteins that can form a dynamic filament network in eukaryotic cells. Actin filaments (F-actins), are polymers composed of monomeric globular actins (G-actins), and are important elements of the cytoskeletons of both muscle and nonmuscle cells. F-actin networks play crucial roles in cell morphology, motility, and cytokinesis (Pollard and Cooper, 1986). Not only in animals but also in plants, actin cytoskeletons are important for physiological phenomena (Baluska et al., 2001; Gibbon et al., 1999; Vidali et al., 2001).

A role for actin filaments in growth control of higher plant cells is well defined in pollen tubes and root hairs (Baluska et al., 2000; Staiger, 2000; Vidali et al., 2001). Growth in pollen tubes and root hairs requires the delivery of wall precursor-containing vesicles to the tip-growth zone. It has been proposed that these vesicles move along the actin filament. Thus, actin filaments in plants provide the driving force for cytoplasmic streaming and also control the direction of cytoplasmic movement (Kamiya, 1986). See Shimmen and Yokota, Chapter 5, this volume.

Recent investigations revealed dynamic reorganization of the actin cytoskeleton during opening and closing movements of guard cells of leaf stomata (Eun and Lee, 1997; Hwang and Lee, 2001; Kim et al., 1995). Stomatal movement is a microscopic example of nyctinastic movement, and its role in gas exchange and conservation of water is controlled by diurnally regulated changes in cell turgor. Immunofluorescence techniques revealed that actin filaments in guard cells radiate outward from the stomatal pore in daylight and disappear at night. Actin filaments in guard cells appear to be involved in signal transduction for stomatal movement. This was verified by treatment with cytochalasin D and phalloidin. These actin-affecting drugs inhibited stomatal movement by disrupting or inhibiting the reorganization of actin filaments in guard cells (Eun and Lee, 1997; Hwang and Lee, 2001).

Actin is also known to serve as a cytoskeleton in *M. pudica* motor cells. Actin inhibitors (cytochalasin B and phalloidin), prevent the bending movement of *Mimosa* leaves, suggesting that actin filaments are involved in the seismonastic movement of the plant (Fleurat-Lessard, 1988; Fleurat-Lessard et al., 1988). Studies with transmission electron microscopy have shown that the network of actin filaments becomes highly disordered in motor cells exposed to these drugs (Fleurat-Lessard et al., 1993).

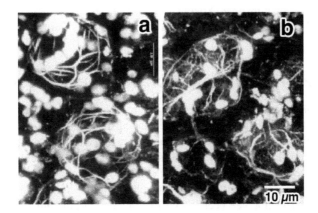

FIGURE 2.6 Immunofluorescence images of the actin cytoskeleton in motor cells in the extensor half of a primary pulvinus. (a) Long and thick actin filaments before bending; (b) change into short and thin filaments after bending.

As shown in Figure 2.6, distribution of the actin cytoskeleton changes drastically in the motor cells in the extensor half of the pulvinus during the bending of the petiole. Before movement, long and thick fiber-like fluorescences (bundles of actin filaments), are observed throughout the cytoplasm; after movement, only thin and short filaments are observed. In contrast, in the upper motor cells (flexor half of the pulvinus), redistribution of the actin network is minimal, in correspondence to the slight shape changes during the movement.

Recent investigations have focused on molecular mechanisms regulating the actin cytoskeletons in the motor cells. In animals, formation and stability of actin filaments are controlled by actin-binding proteins that affect actin nucleation, actin monomer sequestration, and actin filament (F-actin), severing, capping, and bundling (Korn, 1982; Pollard and Cooper, 1986; Stossel et al., 1985). Several actin-binding proteins have also been identified biochemically and via molecular biological techniques. They are thought to be responsible for modulating changes in actin organization and the dynamics of plant cell morphogenesis and development (McCurdy et al., 2001; Staiger, 2000; Staiger et al., 2000).

In a recent study of *M. pudica*, we showed the presence of a protein similar to the gelsolin family proteins. The protein severs actin filaments in a Ca^{2+}-dependent manner (Yamashiro et al., 2001), as do other gelsolin family proteins (Kwiatkowski et al., 1986). Since Ca^{2+} concentration in the cytoplasms of motor cells increases during bending movement (Toriyama and Jaffe, 1972), the gelsolin family proteins may play a role in the reorganization of the actin cytoskeletons of the motor cells. Interestingly, a villin (member of the gelsolin family)-like protein (P-135-ABP), (Nakayasu et al., 1998; Yokota and Shimmen Ki, 1998) has been reported to promote formation of actin filament bundles in pollen tubes and root hairs (Tominaga et al., 2000; Yokota and Shimmen, 1999). However, the actin filament-modulating activity of P-135-ABP is insensitive to Ca^{2+} concentration; it is regulated in a Ca^{2+}- and calmodulin-dependent manner (Yokota et al., 2000). These findings strongly suggest that gelsolin family proteins are regulators of the reorganization of actin filaments in plant cells.

PHOSPHORYLATION OF TYROSINE RESIDUES

Protein phosphorylation is the most common mechanism for cellular regulation in eukaryotic systems (Hunter, 1987). It is well established that protein serine/threonine and tyrosine phosphorylation and dephosphorylation cycles play pivotal roles in cell signaling in animals (Hunter, 1995). In higher plants, serine/threonine phosphorylation plays a key role in the regulation of plant growth and development; however, little is known about the role of tyrosine phosphorylation. This is because a tyrosine-specific kinase has not yet been identified in plants, although tyrosine-specific phosphatases exist in plants (Luan, 2002; Stone and Walker, 1995).

Some evidence indicates protein tyrosine kinase activity in peas (Torruella et al., 1986), tobacco (Suzuki and Shinshi, 1995), maize (Trojanek et al., 1996), and coconuts (Islas-Flores et al., 1998). Dual-specific kinases that phosphorylate tyrosine are present in plants (Ali et al., 1994; Cho et al., 2001; Hirayama and Oka, 1992; Mu et al., 1994; Rudrabhatla and Rajasekharan, 2002; Sessa et al., 1996; Ulm et al., 2001). Dual-specific protein kinases are able to phosphorylate both tyrosine and serine/threonine residues (Lindberg et al., 1992). There are few reports of a putative physiological role for tyrosine phosphorylation in plants. For example, tyrosine phosphorylation of plant profilin in the common bean (*Phaseolus vulgaris*), is thought to regulate actin cytoskeletal dynamics by changing in its affinity to actin (Guillen et al., 1999).

We reported that actin in motor cells of *M. pudica* is phosphorylated before curvature movement and dephosphorylated afterward. Treatment with phenylarsine oxide, an inhibitor of protein tyrosine phosphatase, inhibits bending movement of the plant (Kameyama et al., 2000) (Figure 2.7). This finding was surprising and novel. Moreover, we proved that the phosphorylation of actin–tyrosine residues was related to the reorganization of the actin cytoskeleton, although the importance of the tyrosine phosphorylation of actin-binding proteins was known (Guillen et al., 1999).

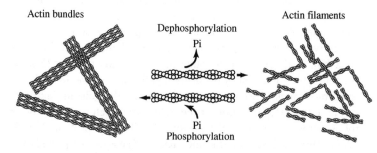

FIGURE 2.7 Actin cytoskeleton in a motor cell. A phosphorylation and dephosphorylation cycle of the tyrosine residues of actin regulates the actin cytoskeleton.

Phosphorylation of actin was observed in mammalian cells and in lower eukaryotes. Stimulation of fibroblasts with epidermal growth factor, for example, induces rapid phosphorylation of serine residues in cortical actin (van Delft et al., 1995). Actin–fragmin kinase isolated from *Physarum polycephalum* phosphorylates actin threonine residues *in vivo* during the transformation from plasmodia into a dormant mass called the *sclerotium* (De Corte et al., 1996; Furuhashi and Hatano, 1992; Furuhashi et al., 1998; Gettemans et al., 1992; Gettemans et al., 1993). In *Dictyostelium* amoebae, phosphorylation of tyrosine-53 of actin is associated with a cell shape change into a dormant spore form in response to environmental stress (Howard et al., 1992; Howard et al., 1993; Jungbluth et al., 1995; Kishi et al., 1998).

We assume that a phosphorylation and dephosphorylation cycle of tyrosine residues of *Mimosa* actin regulates reorganization of the actin cytoskeletons of motor cells. However, the effects of tyrosine phosphorylation on the affinity of actin for binding proteins or on the physiological properties of actin have not been determined. Recent evidence indicates that tyrosine dephosphorylation is a part of cell signaling for the opening and closing movements of guard cells in *Commelina communis* (MacRobbie, 2002). The stomatal movement is believed to have the same mechanism as the curvature movement of the *Mimosa* petiole. These findings indicate that a phosphorylation and dephosphorylation cycle of actin tyrosine residues plays a crucial role in both seismonastic and nyctinastic movements.

CONCLUSION

The work of many plant physiologists has provided a clear macroscopic outline of the seismonastic movement of *M. pudica*. However, molecular mechanisms underlying the movement are not known yet. For example, we do not understand how the electric signal is converted into the physical motion. Many people including scientists are interested in the seismonastic movement of *M. pudica* because the rapid bending in response to stimuli is so remarkable. However, the rapid bending makes analysis of the seismonastic movement difficult. Diethylether and cold anesthesia are applied to observe the cell structure of pulvini at rest. New techniques such as high pressure quick-freezing and molecular biological analysis will soon resolve the problem of observing processes during rapid movement.

REFERENCES

Ali, N., Halfter, U., and Chua, N.H. (1994), Cloning and biochemical characterization of a plant protein kinase that phosphorylates serine, threonine, and tyrosine, *J. Biol. Chem.*, 269, 31626–31629.

Allen, R.D. (1969), Mechanism of the seismonastic reaction in *Mimosa pudica*, *Plant Physiol.*, 44, 1101–1107.

Baluska, F., Jasik, J., Edelmann, H.G., Salajova, T., and Volkmann, D. (2001), Latrunculin B-induced plant dwarfism: plant cell elongation is F-actin-dependent, *Dev. Biol.*, 231, 113–124.

Baluska, F., Salaj, J., Mathur, J., Braun, M., Jasper, F., Samaj, J., Chua, N.H., Barlow, P.W., and Volkmann, D. (2000), Root hair formation: F-actin-dependent tip growth is initiated by local assembly of profilin-supported F-actin meshworks accumulated within expansin-enriched bulges, *Dev. Biol.*, 227, 618–632.

Bose, J.C. (1926), *The Nervous Mechanism of Plants*, Longmans, Green & Co., London.

Briggs, W.R. (1992), What remains of the Cholodny–Went theory? It's alive and well in maize, *Plant Cell Environ.*, 15, 763.

Campbell, N.A., Satter, R.L., and Garber, R.C. (1981), Apoplastic transport of ions in the motor organ of *Samanea*, *Proc. Natl. Acad. Sci. USA*, 78, 2981–2984.

Chen, R., Rosen, E., and Masson, P.H. (1999), Gravitropism in higher plants, *Plant Physiol.*, 120, 343–350.

Cho, H.S., Yoon, G.M., Lee, S.S., Kim, Y.A., Hwang, I., Choi, D., and Pai, H.S. (2001), A novel dual-specificity protein kinase targeted to the chloroplast in tobacco, *FEBS Lett.*, 497, 124–130.

Cholodny, N. (1927), Wuchshormone und Tropismen bei den Pflanzen, *Biol. Zentralbl.*, 47, 604–626.

Christie, J.M. and Briggs, W.R. (2001), Blue light sensing in higher plants, *J. Biol. Chem.*, 276, 11457–11460.

Darwin, C. (1880), *The Power of Movement in Plants*, John Murray, London.

De Corte, V., Gettemans, J., Waelkens, E., and Vandekerckhove, J. (1996), *In vivo* phosphorylation of actin in *Physarum polycephalum*: study of the substrate specificity of the actin–fragmin kinase, *Eur. J. Biochem.*, 241, 901–908.

de Mairan, M. (1927), *Observation Botanique*, Histoire de l'Académie Royale de Sciences, Paris, pp. 35–36.

Dunlap, J.C. (1999), Molecular bases for circadian clocks, *Cell*, 96, 271–290.

Eun, S.O. and Lee, Y. (1997), Actin filaments of guard cells are reorganized in response to light and abscisic acid, *Plant Physiol.*, 115, 1491–1498.

Fleurat-Lessard, P. (1988), Structural and ultrastructural features of cortical cells in motor organs of sensitive plants, *Biol. Rev.*, 63, 1–22.

Fleurat-Lessard, P. (1990), Structure and ultrastructure of the pulvinus in nyctinastic legumes, in Satter, R.L., Gorton, H., and Vogelmann, T., Eds., *The Pulvinus: Motor Organ for Leaf Movement*, American Society of Plant Physiologists, Rockville, MD, pp. 101–129.

Fleurat-Lessard, P., Frangne, N., Maeshima, M., Ratajczak, R., Bonnemain, J.L., and Martinoia, E. (1997), Increased expression of vacuolar aquaporin and H+-ATPase related to motor cell function in *Mimosa pudica* L., *Plant Physiol.*, 114, 827–834.

Fleurat-Lessard, P., Roblin, R., Bonmort, J., and Besse, C. (1988), Effect of colchicine, vinblastine, cytochalasin B and phalloidin on the seismonastic movement of *Mimosa pudica* leaf and on motor cell ultrastructure, *J. Exp. Bot.*, 39, 209–221.

Fleurat-Lessard, P., Schmit, A.C., Vantard, M., Stoeckel, H., and Roblin, G. (1993), Characterization and immunocytochemical distribution of microtubules and F-actin filaments in protoplasts of *Mimosa pudica* motor cells, *Plant Physiol. Biochem.*, 31, 757–764.

Fromm, J. and Eschrich, W. (1988a), Transport processes in stimulated and non-stimulated leaves of *Mimosa pudica* II. Energesis and transmission of seismic stimulations, *Trees*, 2, 18–24.

Fromm, J. and Eschrich, W. (1988b), Transport processes in stimulated and non-stimulated leaves of *Mimosa pudica*. III. Displacement of ions during seismonastic stimulations, *Trees*, 2, 65–72.

Fromm, J. and Eschrich, W. (1990), Seismonastic movements in *Mimosa*, in Satter, R.L., Gorton, H., and Vogelmann, T., Eds., *The Pulvinus: Motor Organ for Leaf Movement*, American Society of Plant Physiologists, Rockville, MD, pp. 25–43.

Furuhashi, K. and Hatano, S. (1992), Actin kinase: a protein kinase that phosphorylates actin of fragmin–actin complex, *J. Biochem. (Tokyo)*, 111, 366–370.

Furuhashi, K., Ishigami, M., Suzuki, M., and Titani, K. (1998), Dry stress-induced phosphorylation of *Physarum* actin, *Biochem. Biophys. Res. Commun.*, 242, 653–658.

Gettemans, J., De Ville, Y., Vandekerckhove, J., and Waelkens, E. (1992), *Physarum* actin is phosphorylated as the actin–fragmin complex at residues Thr203 and Thr202 by a specific 80 kDa kinase, *EMBO J.*, 11, 3185–3191.

Gettemans, J., De Ville, Y., Vandekerckhove, J., and Waelkens, E. (1993), Purification and partial amino acid sequence of the actin-fragmin kinase from *Physarum polycephalum*, *Eur. J. Biochem.*, 214, 111–119.

Gibbon, B.C., Kovar, D.R., and Staiger, C.J. (1999), Latrunculin B has different effects on pollen germination and tube growth, *Plant Cell*, 11, 2349–2363.

Guillen, G., Valdes-Lopez, V., Noguez, R., Olivares, J., Rodriguez-Zapata, L.C., Perez, H., Vidali, L., Villanueva, M.A., and Sanchez, F. (1999), Profilin in *Phaseolus vulgaris* is encoded by two genes (only one expressed in root nodules), but multiple isoforms are generated *in vivo* by phosphorylation on tyrosine residues, *Plant J.*, 19, 497–508.

Hagen, G. and Guilfoyle, T. (2002), Auxin-responsive gene expression: genes, promoters and regulatory factors, *Plant Mol. Biol.*, 49, 373–385.

Hirayama, T. and Oka, A. (1992), Novel protein kinase of *Arabidopsis thaliana* (APK1), that phosphorylates tyrosine, serine and threonine, *Plant Mol. Biol.*, 20, 653–662.

Hooke, R. (1665), *Micrographia*, Dover Publications, New York (reprint).

Houwink, A.L. (1935), The conduction of excitation in *Mimosa pudica*, *Recl. Trav. Bot. Neerl.*, 32, 51–91.

Howard, P.K., Sefton, B.M., and Firtel, R.A. (1992), Analysis of a spatially regulated phosphotyrosine phosphatase identifies tyrosine phosphorylation as a key regulatory pathway in *Dictyostelium*, *Cell*, 71, 637–647.

Howard, P.K., Sefton, B.M., and Firtel, R.A. (1993), Tyrosine phosphorylation of actin in *Dictyostelium* associated with cell-shape changes, *Science*, 259, 241–244.

Hunter, T. (1987), A thousand and one protein kinases, *Cell*, 50, 823–829.

Hunter, T. (1995), Protein kinases and phosphatases: the yin and yang of protein phosphorylation and signaling, *Cell*, 80, 225–236.

Hwang, J.U. and Lee, Y. (2001), Abscisic acid-induced actin reorganization in guard cells of dayflower is mediated by cytosolic calcium levels and by protein kinase and protein phosphatase activities, *Plant Physiol.*, 125, 2120–2128.

Islas-Flores, I.I., Oropeza, C., and Hernandez-Sotomayor, S.M. (1998), Protein phosphorylation during coconut zygotic embryo development, *Plant Physiol.*, 118, 257–263.

Jungbluth, A., Eckerskorn, C., Gerisch, G., Lottspeich, F., Stocker, S., and Schweiger, A. (1995), Stress-induced tyrosine phosphorylation of actin in *Dictyostelium* cells and localization of the phosphorylation site to tyrosine-53 adjacent to the DNase I binding loop, *FEBS Lett.*, 375, 87–90.

Kameyama, K., Kishi, Y., Yoshimura, M., Kanzawa, N., Sameshima, M., and Tsuchiya, T. (2000), Tyrosine phosphorylation in plant bending, *Nature*, 407, 37.

Kamiya, N. (1986), Cytoplasmic streaming in giant algal cells: a historical survey of experimental approaches, *Bot. Mag. Tokyo*, 99, 444–467.

Kim, M., Hepler, P.K., Eun, S.O., Ha, K.S., and Lee, Y. (1995), Actin filaments in mature guard cells are radially distributed and involved in stomatal movement, *Plant Physiol.*, 109, 1077–1084.

Kishi, Y., Clements, C., Mahadeo, D.C., Cotter, D.A., and Sameshima, M. (1998), High levels of actin tyrosine phosphorylation: correlation with the dormant state of *Dictyostelium* spores, *J. Cell Sci.*, 111, 2923–2932.

Kiss, J.Z., Miller, K.M., Ogden, L.A. and Roth, K.K. (2002), Phototropism and gravitropism in lateral roots of *Arabidopsis*, *Plant Cell Physiol.*, 43, 35–43.

Kiyosawa, K. (1979), Unequal distribution of potassium and anions within the *Phaseolus* pulvinus during circadian leaf movement, *Plant Cell Physiol.*, 20, 1621–1634.

Knight, T.A. (1806), On the direction of the radical and germen during the vegetation of seeds, *Philos. Trans. R. Soc. Lond. Biol. Sci.*, 99, 108–120.

Korn, E.D. (1982), Actin polymerization and its regulation by proteins from nonmuscle cells, *Physiol. Rev.*, 62, 672–737.

Kwiatkowski, D.J., Stossel, T.P., Orkin, S.H., Mole, J.E., Colten, H.R., and Yin, H.L. (1986), Plasma and cytoplasmic gelsolins are encoded by a single gene and contain a duplicated actin-binding domain, *Nature*, 323, 455–458.

Lin, C. (2002), Blue light receptors and signal transduction, *Plant Cell*, 14, S207-S225.

Lindberg, R.A., Quinn, A.M., and Hunter, T. (1992), Dual-specificity protein kinases: will any hydroxyl do? *Trends Biochem. Sci.*, 17, 114–119.

Luan, S. (2002), Tyrosine phosphorylation in plant cell signaling, *Proc. Natl. Acad. Sci. USA*, 99, 11567–11569.

MacRobbie, E.A. (2002), Evidence for a role for protein tyrosine phosphatase in the control of ion release from the guard cell vacuole in stomatal closure, *Proc. Natl. Acad. Sci. USA*, 99, 11963–11968.

McCurdy, D.W., Kovar, D.R., and Staiger, C.J. (2001), Actin and actin-binding proteins in higher plants, *Protoplasma*, 215, 89–104.

Morillon, R., Lienard, D., Chrispeels, M.J., and Lassalles, J.P. (2001), Rapid movements of plants organs require solute-water cotransporters or contractile proteins, *Plant Physiol.*, 127, 720–723.

Moshelion, M., Becker, D., Biela, A., Uehlein, N., Hedrich, R., Otto, B., Levi, H., Moran, N., and Kaldenhoff, R. (2002), Plasma membrane aquaporins in the motor cells of *Samanea saman*: diurnal and circadian regulation, *Plant Cell*, 14, 727–739.

Mu, J.H., Lee, H.S., and Kao, T.H. (1994), Characterization of a pollen-expressed receptor-like kinase gene of *Petunia inflata* and the activity of its encoded kinase, *Plant Cell*, 6, 709–721.

Nakayasu, T., Yokota, E., and Shimmen, T. (1998), Purification of an actin-binding protein composed of 115-kDa polypeptide from pollen tubes of lily, *Biochem. Biophys. Res. Commun.*, 249, 61–65.

Palmer, J.M., Short, T.W., and Briggs, W.R. (1993a), Correlation of blue light-induced phosphorylation to phototropism in *Zea mays* L., *Plant Physiol.*, 102, 1219–1225.

Palmer, J.M., Short, T.W., Gallagher, S., and Briggs, W.R. (1993b), Blue light-induced phosphorylation of a plasma membrane-associated protein in *Zea mays* L., *Plant Physiol.*, 102, 1211–1218.

Pollard, T.D. and Cooper, J.A. (1986), Actin and actin-binding proteins: a critical evaluation of mechanisms and functions, *Annu. Rev. Biochem.*, 55, 987–1035.

Reymond, P., Short, T.W., Briggs, W.R., and Poff, K.L. (1992), Light-induced phosphorylation of a membrane protein plays an early role in signal transduction for phototropism in *Arabidopsis thaliana*, *Proc. Natl. Acad. Sci. USA*, 89, 4718–4721.

Ricca, U. (1916), Solution d-un probleme de physiologie: la propagation de stimulus dans la sensitive, *Arch. Ital. de Biol.*, 65, 219–232.

Rudrabhatla, P. and Rajasekharan, R. (2002), Developmentally regulated dual-specificity kinase from peanut that is induced by abiotic stresses, *Plant Physiol.*, 130, 380–390.

Sack, F.D. (1991), Plant gravity sensing, *Int. Rev. Cytol.*, 127, 193–252.

Samejima, M. and Shibaoka, T. (1983), Identification of the excitable cells in the petiole of *Mimosa pudica* by intracellular injection of procion yellow, *Plant Cell Physiol.*, 24, 33–39.

Satter, R.L. and Galston, A.W. (1981), Mechanisms of control of leaf movements, *Annu. Rev. Plant Physiol.*, 32, 83–110.

Satter, R.L., Geballe, G.T., Applewhite, P.B., and Galston, A.W. (1974), Potassium flux and leaf movement in *Samanea saman*. I. Rhythmic movement, *J. Gen. Physiol.*, 64, 413–430.

Satter, R.L., Marinoff, P., and Galston, A.W. (1970), Phytochrome controlled nyctinasty in *Albizzia julibrissin*. II. Potassium flux as a basis for leaflet movement, *Am. J. Bot.*, 57, 916–926.

Satter, R.L., Schrempf, M., Chaudri, J., and Galston, A.W. (1977), Phytochrome and circadian clocks in *Samanea*: rhythmic redistribution of potassium and chloride within the pulvinus during long dark periods, *Plant Physiol.*, 59, 231–235.

Schildknecht, H. (1983), Turgorine, hormones of the endogenous daily rhythms of higher organized plants: detection, isolation, structure, synthesis, and activity, *Angew. Chem. Int. Ed. Engl.*, 22, 695–710.

Sessa, G., Raz, V., Savaldi, S., and Fluhr, R. (1996), PK12, a plant dual-specificity protein kinase of the LAMMER family, is regulated by the hormone ethylene, *Plant Cell*, 8, 2223–2234.

Shibaoka, T. (1962), Excitable cells in *Mimosa*, *Science*, 137, 226.

Shibaoka, T. (1966), Action potentials in plant organs, *Symp. Soc. Exp. Biol.*, 20, 49–74.

Shibaoka, T. (1991), Rapid plant movements triggered by action potentials. *Bot. Mag. Tokyo*, 104, 73–95.

Snow, R. (1924), Conduction of excitation in stem and leaf of *Mimosa pudica*, *Proc. R. Soc. B*, 96.

Staiger, C.J. (2000), Signaling to the actin cytoskeleton in plants, *Annu. Rev. Plant Physiol. Plant Mol. Biol.*, 51, 257–288.

Staiger, C.J., Baluska, F., Volkmann, D., and Barlow, P.W. (2000), *Actin: A Dynamic Framework for Multiple Plant Cell Function*, Kluwer, London.

Staiger, D. (2002), Circadian rhythms in *Arabidopsis*: time for nuclear proteins, *Planta*, 214, 334–344.

Stoeckel, H. and Takeda, K. (1995), Calcium-sensitivity of the plasmalemmal delayed rectifier potassium current suggests that calcium influx in pulvinar protoplasts from *Mimosa pudica* L. can be revealed by hyperpolarization, *J. Membr. Biol.*, 146, 201–209.

Stone, J.M. and Walker, J.C. (1995), Plant protein kinase families and signal transduction, *Plant Physiol.*, 108, 451–457.

Stossel, T.P., Chaponnier, C., Ezzell, R.M., Hartwig, J.H., Janmey, P.A., Kwiatkowski, D.J., Lind, S.E., Smith, D.B., Southwick, F.S., and Yin, H.L. (1985), Nonmuscle actin-binding proteins, *Annu. Rev. Cell Biol.*, 1, 353–402.

Suzuki, K. and Shinshi, H. (1995), Transient activation and tyrosine phosphorylation of a protein kinase in tobacco cells treated with a fungal elicitor, *Plant Cell*, 7, 639–647.

Tamiya, T., Miyazaki, T., Ishikawa, H., Iriguchi, N., Maki, T., Matsumoto, J.J., and Tsuchiya, T. (1988), Movement of water in conjunction with plant movement visualized by NMR imaging, *J. Biochem. (Tokyo)*, 104, 5–8.

Tominaga, M., Yokota, E., Vidali, L., Sonobe, S., Hepler, P.K., and Shimmen, T. (2000), The role of plant villin in the organization of the actin cytoskeleton, cytoplasmic streaming and the architecture of the transvacuolar strand in root hair cells of *Hydrocharis*, *Planta*, 210, 836–843.

Toriyama, H. (1955), Observational and experimental studies of sensitive plants. VI. The migration of potassium in the primary pulvinus, *Cytologia*, 20, 72–81.

Toriyama, H. and Jaffe, M.J. (1972), Migration of calcium and its role in the regulation of seismonasty in the motor cell of *Mimosa pudica* L., *Plant Physiol.*, 49, 72–81.

Toriyama, H. and Sato, S. (1969), Electron microscope observations of *Mimosa pudica* L. III. The fine structure of the central vacuole in the motor cell, *Proc. Jpn. Acad.*, 45, 175–179.

Torruella, M., Casano, L.M., and Vallejos, R.H. (1986), Evidence of the activity of tyrosine kinase(s), and of the presence of phosphotyrosine proteins in pea plantlets, *J. Biol. Chem.*, 261, 6651–6653.

Trojanek, J., Ek, P., Scoble, J., Muszynska, G., and Engstrom, L. (1996), Phosphorylation of plant proteins and the identification of protein-tyrosine kinase activity in maize seedlings, *Eur. J. Biochem.*, 235, 338–344.

Turnquist, H.M., Allen, N.S., and Jaffe, M.J. (1993), A pharmacological study of calcium flux mechanisms in the tannin vacuoles of *Mimosa pudica* L. motor cells, *Protoplasma*, 176, 91–99.

Ueda, M. and Yamamura, S. (1999), Leaf-opening substance of *Mimosa pudica* L.: chemical studies on the other leaf movement of *Mimosa*, *Tetrahedron Lett.*, 40, 353–356.

Ueda, M. and Yamamura, S. (2000), Chemistry and biology of plant leaf movements, *Angew. Chem. Int. Ed. Engl.*, 39, 1400–1414.

Ulm, R., Revenkova, E., di Sansebastiano, G.P., Bechtold, N., and Paszkowski, J. (2001), Mitogen-activated protein kinase phosphatase is required for genotoxic stress relief in *Arabidopsis*, *Genes Dev.*, 15, 699–709.

van Delft, S., Verkleij, A.J., Boonstra, J., and van Bergen en Henegouwen, P.M. (1995), Epidermal growth factor induces serine phosphorylation of actin, *FEBS Lett.*, 357, 251–254.

Vidali, L., McKenna, S.T., and Hepler, P.K. (2001), Actin polymerization is essential for pollen tube growth, *Mol. Biol. Cell*, 12, 2534–2545.

Went, F. (1928), Wuchsstoff und Wachstum, *Recl. Trav. Bot. Neerl.*, 25, 1–116.

Yamashiro, S., Kameyama, K., Kanzawa, N., Tamiya, T., Mabuchi, I., and Tsuchiya, T. (2001), The gelsolin/fragmin family protein identified in the higher plant *Mimosa pudica*, *J. Biochem. (Tokyo)*, 130, 243–249.

Yokota, E., Muto, S., and Shimmen, T. (2000), Calcium–calmodulin suppresses the filamentous actin-binding activity of a 135-kilodalton actin-bundling protein isolated from lily pollen tubes, *Plant Physiol.*, 123, 645–654.

Yokota, E. and Shimmen, T.T. (1998), Actin-bundling protein isolated from pollen tubes of lily: biochemical and immunocytochemical characterization, *Plant Physiol.*, 116, 1421–1429.

Yokota, E. and Shimmen, T. (1999), The 135-kDa actin-bundling protein from lily pollen tubes arranges F-actin into bundles with uniform polarity, *Planta*, 209, 264–266.

Young, L.M., Evans, M.L., and Hertel, R. (1990), Correlations between gravitropic curvature and auxin movement across gravistimulated roots of *Zea mays*, *Plant Physiol.*, 92, 792–796.

3 Contractile Systems of Muscles

Madoka Suzuki and Shin'ichi Ishiwata

CONTENTS

INTRODUCTION

The voluntary movements of the human body required for walking, running, eating, and talking are made possible by the organized movement of the muscle–skeleton (or muscle–connective tissue) system. The active component of this system is the *skeletal muscle,* both ends of which adhere to bone or elastic tissue through tendons. The states of contraction or relaxation of voluntary muscles are regulated in an all-or-nothing fashion by electric signals transmitted from neurons.

The contractile system of skeletal muscle constitutes a hierarchy from a single-molecule (protein) to a tissue (Figure 3.1). The contractile system is a highly ordered structure that supports physiological functions. The structures in the system range in size from 10 nm to about 1 cm. The former requires an electron microscope or scanning probe microscope such as an atomic force microscope (AFM) for us to observe, and the latter can be observed with our eyes and touched with our hands. Macroscopic muscle contraction results from the accumulated efforts of microscopic or nanoscopic assemblies of several kinds of muscle proteins such as a complex of

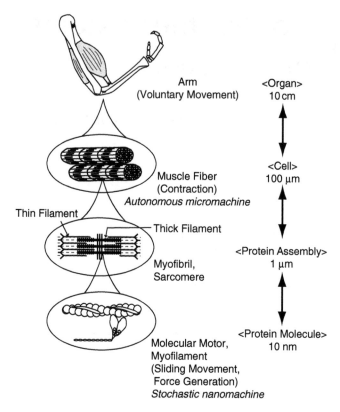

FIGURE 3.1 Hierarchy of muscle contractile system. The system ranging from a single molecular level on a nanometer scale to a tissue level on a centimeter scale constitutes a hierarchical structure. The hierarchy illustrated is common to all kinds of striated muscles, i.e., both skeletal and heart muscles.

actin and myosin (a mechano-enzyme), tropomyosin and troponin (regulatory proteins), and connectin/titin (an elastic protein). We stress here the one-to-one correspondence between the motile organs created by nature and the motile machines made by human beings. As shown in Figure 3.2, although necessary and sufficient conditions for constructing a motile system are common to both natural and artificial systems, the principles required to produce a motile system (software) and the materials to construct the framework (hardware) are very different. It is now possible to produce an artificial machine as small as a micrometer or even a few hundred nanometers so that the sizes are within the same order. However, the principle that generates force and movement in muscle is chemomechanical transduction. Force and movement in man-made micro- and nano-sized machines usually proceed via electromechanical transduction.

The working principles of artificial machines are fully clarified; for example, an automobile moves based on physical principles such as thermodynamics and mechanics. However, we do not yet fully understand the physical principles of mechanochemical energy transduction that operate in the molecular motors of muscles.

Automobile (Artificial Machine)	MECHANISM	Muscle (Natural Machine)
Computer and electric system	-Control System-	Nerve signal to the membrane
Spark ignition	-Trigger-	Ca^{2+} release from inner membrane system
Cylinder, Piston	-Engine-	Actin, Myosin (Mechano enzyme)
<Thermodynamics>		*<Mechanochemical coupling>*
Strokes of a piston	-Work Production-	Conformational change
Combustion of the mixture of gasoline and air	-Energy Conversion-	Hydrolysis of ATP
Power transmission	-Amplifying System-	Sarcomere repeat, Elastic component
Wheel rotation	-Movement as a Whole-	Contraction (Shortening)
<Rigid connection>		*<Flexible connection, Feedback>*

FIGURE 3.2 Necessary and sufficient conditions for constructing a motile system. Comparison of motile systems created by nature (muscle) and human beings (automobile). Necessary and sufficient conditions for constructing a motile system are common to natural and artificial systems, so that the systems have one-to-one correspondence. However, at least two significant differences exist: the principle of motility (force generation) and the materials.

Muscles require proteins; artificial machines require metals or chemical compounds. Every protein is a complex system composed of heterogeneous elements and possesses a flexibility (self-regulatory feedback mechanism) that can respond quickly to changes of environment. However, the methods of response and regulation of a man-made machine must be artificially designed and programmed beforehand.

In this chapter, we describe the structure and function of the muscle contractile system as a typical example of a biological fast responsive movement system that has a hierarchical structure. We also focus on the stochastic properties of molecular motors, i.e., nanoscopic systems composed of myosin and actin (also called stochastic bionanomachines). We would like to stress that flexibility is the essence of the structures and functions of constituent proteins — something very distinct from the characteristics of artificial machines.

MUSCLE CONTRACTILE SYSTEM

The structural and functional unit of the skeletal muscle is the *muscle fiber* (Figure 3.3). A muscle fiber is a long (e.g., 1 m in a giraffe) and thin (10 to 100 μm in diameter), cylindrical, multinucleus cell created by fusion. The fiber is surrounded by a cell membrane to which a nerve end is attached. The muscle fibers are assembled parallel to each other and form a bundle that is organized into muscle tissue.[1]

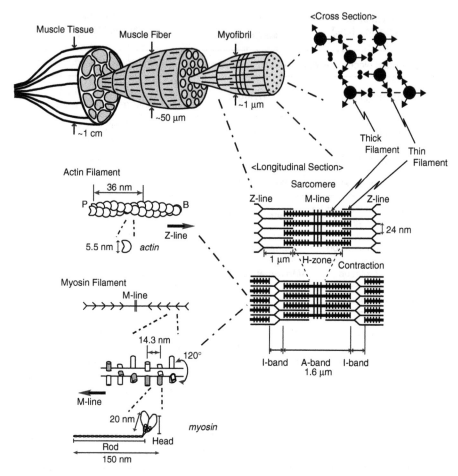

FIGURE 3.3 Muscle contractile system. The minimum structural and functional unit of the system is a sarcomere constructed from a lattice structure composed of thin and thick filaments that are, respectively, polar and bipolar helical polymers. Myosin is a long molecule having two head domains that bind to an actin filament to form a cross-bridge and hydrolyze ATP. Another domain called a rod is composed of a coiled–coil structure. The neck domain connects the head and rod domains. Actin is a horse hoof-shaped small molecule that polymerizes into a helical polymer; the end that attaches to the Z-line is called the B-end, and the other is the free P-end.

A muscle fiber is a parallel assembly of many *myofibrils* that constitute a contractile apparatus about 1 μm in diameter. Because myofibril has a striation pattern and neighboring myofibrils are assembled in phase, muscle fibers also have striation patterns. Striation patterns are common to skeletal and cardiac muscles, in contrast to smooth muscles that do not have such ordered periodical structures. Striation of myofibrils is attributable to the periodic alignment of the A-band, a structure about 1.6 μm long, and the I-band, a structure of variable width. The thick line crossing the center of each I-band is called the Z-line or Z-disk. A structural unit of the striation pattern is divided by the Z-lines and is called a sarcomere; it is usually 2 to 3 µm long.

The A-band consists of thick filaments, the centers of which are bundled at the M-line. The I-band is composed of a parallel array of thin filaments about 8 nm thick and 1 µm long. The thin filaments extend from the Z-line toward the center of the A-band and partially overlap the thick filaments in the A-band. The central region of the A-band in which the thin filaments are absent is called the H-zone. The two kinds of myofilaments construct a lattice structure. For example, in mammalian skeletal muscle, these filaments are hexagonally packed in a way that a single thin filament is surrounded by three thick filaments located at the corner of the triangular lattice (see Figure 3.3, top right).

Myosin and actin molecules are the main components of the thick and thin filaments, respectively. The thick filament is a bipolar polymer composed of about 300 myosin molecules; and their structures are symmetrical against the centers at which M-proteins are attached to form M-line structures. The thin filament is a polar helical polymer composed of actin molecules. The free ends of the thin filaments are called the P-ends to which capping proteins named tropomodulins attach.[2] The other (B) end attaches to the Z-line so that the thin filament lattice is fixed at the Z-line to form the I-Z-I brush, the structure of which is symmetrical against the Z-line. Myosin and actin molecules account for about 70% of the muscle proteins constituting the contractile apparatus.

MOLECULAR MECHANISMS OF MUSCLE CONTRACTIONS

SLIDING FILAMENT MECHANISM

The contraction of a myofibril can be explained by the *sliding-filament* mechanism.[3–5] The head part of a myosin molecule protruding from the surface of the thick filament forms a *cross-bridge* by interacting with the thin filament. The essence of the sliding-filament mechanism is that the cross-bridge changes its conformation accompanied by the hydrolysis of adenosine triphosphate (ATP) to generate force. The thick and thin filaments slide past each other while maintaining the total length of each filament (that is, the elasticity of the myofilaments is not taken into account in the sliding-filament mechanism).

The fact that the lengths of the thick and thin filaments remain constant during sliding and while generating force was first demonstrated by optical[3] and electron[4] microscopy. The length of the A-band was unchanged, whereas the widths of both the I-band and the H-zone changed in parallel. This demonstration was done under static conditions, that is, after relaxing a myofibril for optical microscopy and chemical fixation of the muscle preparation for electron microscopy under various sarcomere lengths. Thus, the length of the myofilament during shortening or generating force was not examined. The possibility that the repetition of local extension and shortening of myofilaments plays an important part in force generation has not been eliminated.

In practice, myofilaments are elastic, not rigid, bodies. For example, the flexural rigidity of actin filaments was estimated to be one to two orders of magnitude smaller than that of steel of the same size. This estimation was first demonstrated more than 30 years ago by S. Fujime, who measured and analyzed the frequency shifts of laser light scattered from filaments that fluctuated thermally in solution.[6] This technique (called quasielastic scattering of laser light or dynamic light scattering) revealed that the flexibility of actin filaments increased upon the binding of myosin in the absence of ATP (rigor condition)[7] and also in the presence of ATP (contraction condition).[8,9] The flexibility of the thin filaments reconstituted from purified actin and the regulatory proteins (tropomyosin and troponin) changed, depending on the concentration of free Ca^{2+} around micromolar levels (corresponding to a pCa value of 6). The filament became flexible when the pCa value was below about 6, which led to the binding of Ca^{2+} to troponin and accordingly the activation of the contractile system.[10] When the reconstituted thin filaments interacted with myosin molecules, the effect of Ca^{2+} on flexibility was remarkable.[8,9] The flexibility of reconstituted thin filaments interacting with myosin was largest (most flexible) in the presence of Ca^{2+} (pCa < ca. 6 corresponding to the contraction condition), but smallest (most rigid) in the absence of Ca^{2+} (pCa > ca. 6 corresponding to the relaxation condition) as if myosin molecules were absent. These effects of Ca^{2+} were reversible, suggesting that the flexibility of thin filaments may be involved in the regulatory mechanism and also in the contraction mechanism.

Since the imaging of single actin filaments became possible under fluorescence microscopy by labeling the filaments with a fluorescent dye,[11] the elastic modulus (inverse of the flexibility) of actin filaments could be measured by analyzing the bending Brownian motion (the longer the relaxation time of bending Brownian motion, the more flexible the filament). The flexural rigidity of actin filaments and reconstituted thin filaments thus obtained was consistent with that estimated using dynamic laser light scattering, about 10^{-17} dyn cm^2.[7,10–13]

The sliding-filament mechanism has been established,[5,14] but the detailed mechanism of contraction, the dynamic feature of myosin motors and actin, has yet to be clarified. There is a consensus that the elastic modulus of muscle fiber during contraction is attributable to both the cross-bridges and the thin filaments.[15] Low angle x-ray diffraction of muscle fibers has shown that the thin filaments extend by an order of 0.1% during force generation.[16,17] However, whether the flexibility of the thin filaments is directly involved in the mechanism of contraction (force generation) is still an open question.

The contractile system does not work solely by the actin–myosin motor system; contractile properties depend on several factors such as the elastic components organizing the contractile system and the geometry of the lattice structure of myofilaments. An elastic framework is needed to stabilize the lattice structures of myofilaments during force generation and transmit the generated force effectively to the ends of myofibrils (compare Figure 3.3). For example, both ends of the thick filaments are connected to the Z-line through an elastic protein called connectin/titin in each sarcomere. Connectin/titin is the largest protein in nature, with a molecular weight of about 3×10^6. When the sarcomere is stretched by about 30% of its resting length (or longer than about 3 µm), an extension of the connectin/titin molecules develops tension. This implies that the elastic force developed by this extension plays a role in maintaining the thick filament at the center of each sarcomere. The passive tension developed under relaxing conditions is called resting tension, and is attributable to the connectin/titin extension. Moreover, experimental evidence shows that cross-bridges are activated in response to muscle stretch, implying that connectin/titin-based passive tension modulates cross-bridge activity.[18,19] This property is considered significant in the Frank–Starling law (development of active tension in response to muscle stretch), which is known to be an essential element of the systolic function of the heart.

CROSS-BRIDGE MECHANISM

During the sliding of myofilaments and the generation of force, or even during force generation without sliding (isometric contraction: the total length of the fiber is adjusted to be constant during tension development), the repeated attachment and detachment of cross-bridges is accompanied by the hydrolysis of ATP. Huxley and Simmons studied the cross-bridge dynamics of single muscle fibers in relation to the molecular mechanism of force generation. The transient response of muscle fibers was analyzed by applying small stepwise changes of length during contraction. When muscle fiber under isometric contraction was suddenly shortened or stretched within 1 ms, tension was instantaneously dropped or elevated, and then recovered to the initial tension level. The degree of tension drop was proportional to the extent of shortening. The isometric tension diminished transiently when the extent of shortening per half a sarcomere became only about 4 nm; one possible interpretation is that the compliant parts of cross-bridges and/or the thin filaments were stretched by about 4 nm. The extension of the compliant part is the origin of the generated force.

Huxley and Simmons constructed a theoretical model of cross-bridge rotation (the lever-arm model)[20] that explains their results.[5] Their lever-arm model was recently supported by the measurement of the polarization of a fluorophore fixed to the neck region of myosin in muscle fibers that may monitor the orientation of cross-bridges.[21] Although the lever-arm mechanism seems established, it is possible that molecular motors may have other properties. To elucidate the essence of the molecular motor, we need to fully understand the cooperative behaviors of cross-bridges (described below) and the role of the dynamic properties of thin filaments (discussed above in relation to the flexibility changes of thin filaments).

SYNCHRONIZATION OF CROSS-BRIDGES

Under normal physiological solvent conditions, the state of the contractile system of muscle is regulated by concentrations of free Ca^{2+}. Contraction or relaxation will occur, depending on whether the pCa value is below or above about 6, respectively. When the conditions are set to be intermediate between those of contraction and relaxation, a third state known as spontaneous oscillatory contraction (SPOC) appears. Intermediate conditions are realized at a pCa value slightly above 6 (Ca-SPOC) for cardiac muscle or in coexistence with ATP, adenosine diphosphate (ADP), and inorganic phosphate (Pi) without Ca^{2+} (ADP-SPOC) for cardiac and skeletal muscle.

An example of ADP-SPOC observed in a single skeletal myofibril with both ends fixed at a pair of glass microneedles is shown in Figure 3.4. One of the two

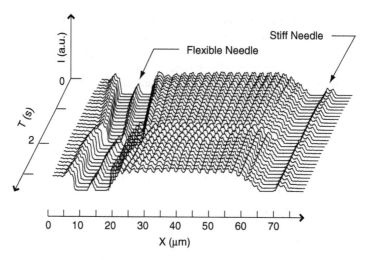

FIGURE 3.4 Time course of the image profile of a myofibril showing spontaneous oscillatory contraction (SPOC). The T, X, and I axes, respectively, represent the time course of the SPOC (every 0.1 s), the position along the myofibril, and the brightness of the phase-contrast image. Each end of the myofibril was fixed to a pair of glass microneedles. The glass microneedle on the left side is flexible so that the developed tension is represented by its deflection. The needle on the right side is rigid so that the myofibril can be quickly stretched or released by a stepwise move of this needle. Solvent conditions are 120 mM KCl, 4 mM MgCl$_2$, 0.2 mM ATP, 4 mM ADP, 4 mM Pi, 20 mM MOPS (pH 7.0), and 4 mM EGTA. Temperature = 25°C. (From Shimamoto, Y., M.S. thesis, Waseda University, Tokyo, 2003. With permission.)

microneedles is flexible so that its deflection can monitor tension generation. Under SPOC conditions, tension spontaneously oscillates and the length of each sarcomere oscillates in a sawtooth waveform consisting of rapid lengthening and slow shortening phases within 1 to 6 s, depending on solvent conditions. Further, the lengthening phase is propagated to adjacent sarcomeres one by one, creating a traveling wave along a myofibril (SPOC wave).

The necessary conditions for the sliding mechanism described do not hold during SPOC. That is, sarcomeres of longer lengths (smaller numbers of interacting cross-bridges) and those of shorter lengths (larger numbers of interacting cross-bridges) coexist in the same myofibril under the same external load, implying that the forces generated by different numbers of cross-bridges in every sarcomere must be balanced against each other. The SPOC phenomena strongly suggest that cross-bridges gain the ability to self-regulate their states through intermolecular interaction, that is, they gain intermolecular synchronization by assembling in an organized structure.

A-BAND MOTILITY ASSAY SYSTEM

We have recently developed a new motility system that locates in the hierarchical structure between the muscle contractile system and the *in vitro* motility assay system as shown in Figure 3.1. This system we designated the *A-band motility assay system* (or *bionanomuscle*) is prepared by selective removal of the thin filaments from a myofibril using gelsolin (an actin-binding protein that severs an actin filament and caps its B-end) as a molecular tool.[22] This system consists of exposed A-bands in which the thick filaments are supposed to maintain the filament lattice as in the intact myofibrils. By applying a single actin filament with the B-end attached to a polystyrene bead through gelsolin adhered to the surface of the bead and by trapping the bead with optical tweezers, the displacement of the bead from the trap center and the force generated on the actin filament can be measured.

It should be stressed again that one characteristic of the A-band motility assay system is that the ordered structure of thick filament lattice is kept native and other components that are expected to contribute to the contractile properties in the fibers such as connectin/titin have been removed. Thus, the physiological functions of these missing components can be investigated.

The time course showing the sliding movement of an actin filament in the A-band motility assay system revealed a considerable force fluctuation both in the rising phase of force generation and even in the steady phase in which the force generated by cross-bridges and the load applied by the optical tweezers are balanced (Figure 3.5). It was estimated that 20 to 30 cross-bridges (myosin molecules) interacted with the actin filament in this example. The result implies that the tension generated on each thin filament fluctuates at random even when working in the ordered structure of a myofilament lattice. This is attributable to the fact that the period of the force-generating state for each cross-bridge is very short (on the order of 1 ms) and the

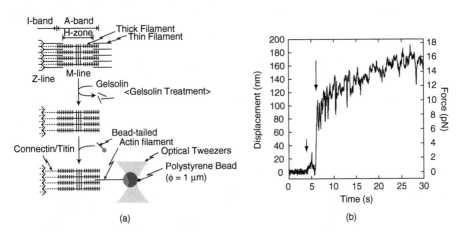

FIGURE 3.5 (a) A-band motility assay system. An exposed A-band is obtained by selective removal of thin filaments from a myofibril using gelsolin, an actin-binding protein that severs the actin filament. A single actin filament attached to a polystyrene bead 1 μm in diameter is brought into contact with the edge of the A-band by optical tweezers. (b) Time course of the displacement of the trapped bead interacting with the A-band. When the actin filament began to interact with the A-band, the filament was pulled into the A-band and the bead was pulled away from the trap center (ordinate = 0) at the distance indicated by a short arrow. The bead, once pulled back to the trap center, was pulled away again (long arrow) accompanied by a large force fluctuation of a few pN. The force fluctuation continued even at the steady phase where the force generated on the actin filament and the load applied by the optical tweezers were balanced (about 22 s).

proportion of the period of the force-generating state occupying one cycle of ATP hydrolysis (i.e., duty ratio) is small (less than 0.1). The chemical reaction occurs stochastically for each cross-bridge. The stochastic properties of force generation of molecular motors are shown in an *in vitro* motility assay as described below. However, in living muscle, where more than 10^5 cross-bridges work at the same time in parallel within a single myofibril, the fluctuation of tension is smoothed so that a steady force is developed.

We confirmed that the average tension level is proportional to the average length of overlap between the thin and thick filaments. These results suggest that, at least under normal contracting conditions, tension develops in proportion to the number of interacting cross-bridges, so myosin II molecular motors in skeletal muscles function as independent force generators.[14] Under certain conditions intermediate between contraction and relaxation, SPOC phenomena appear; cooperative force generation is expected to exist where cross-bridges are not independent of each other.

NANOSCOPIC SYSTEM OF MOTILITY

Single Molecular Mechanics of Molecular Motors

Progress in microscopic techniques has meant that it is now possible to manipulate single protein molecules and detect movements and the force generation of single molecular motors on the order of nanometers and piconewtons, respectively. Structural changes in the myosin of muscle (myosin II) occurring during interaction with actin can be examined via microscopic technique: Finer et al.[23] and Miyata et al.[24] showed that stepwise movements of about 10 nm were occasionally observable at low ATP concentrations, probably accompanying ATP hydrolysis. At physiological ATP concentrations, myosin II is easily detached from actin, so that it is difficult to examine the elementary processes of single myosin II motors under physiological conditions.[23,25]

Veigel et al. measured the mechanical transitions made by a single myosin head (nonmuscle compound called myosin I that may correspond to each head or subfragment-1 (S1) of myosin II) while it was attached to actin.[26] They found that the working stroke of myosin I was divided into two distinct steps: 6 nm followed by 5.5 nm. The initial movement after the attachment of the myosin head to the actin took fewer than 10 ms. They could not detect two separate steps for skeletal muscle myosin S1, because the second step that might have occurred was too small or too fast to be observed. However, they found that the tension rose in 5 ms and fell within 1 ms; and concluded that the S1 working stroke occurs within 5 ms of the binding of myosin to actin.

In a different type of experiment, Kitamura et al. showed that myosin S1 moved along an actin filament with approximately 5.3-nm steps.[27] They suggested that this result supports the idea that the movement of molecular motors occurs without large conformational changes within the motors, but is attributable to the change of the interaction potential or rather to the structural changes of actin. While the former mechanism has much data supporting it, more data will be needed to provide a similar level of support for the latter mechanism.

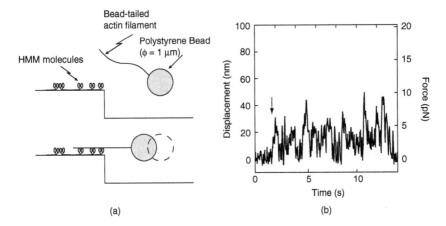

FIGURE 3.6 Tension measurements in an *in vitro* motility assay. (a) Schematic illustration of the *in vitro* motility assay system on a chemically-etched coverslip. HMM molecules adhere to the glass surface. A single actin filament attached to a polystyrene bead 1 μm in diameter is brought into contact with HMMs on the pedestal by optical tweezers. (b) Time course of the displacement of the trapped bead interacting with the HMMs. When the actin filament began to interact with the HMMs, the filament was pulled so that the bead was pulled away from the trap center (ordinate = 0) (indicated by arrow).

COMPARISON OF TENSION MEASUREMENT IN *IN VITRO* MOTILITY ASSAY AND A-BAND MOTILITY ASSAY

The microscopic measurement of tension development in an *in vitro* motility assay was first achieved by Kishino and Yanagida.[28] Using the same technique shown in Figure 3.6a, we measured the tension developed on a single actin filament by chymotryptic fragments of myosin (HMM) molecules adhered to a glass surface. As shown in Figure 3.6b, the developed tension fluctuated similarly to that obtained in the A-band motility assay (Figure 3.5b). The observation of such a large fluctuation in both systems is due to the small number of motors working on a single actin filament. These results demonstrate that the function of the molecular motor is stochastic at a single molecular level.

A substantial difference between the two systems is that the *in vitro* assay system is two-dimensional, whereas the A-band assay system is three-dimensional, so that actin filaments easily dissociate from the motor molecules under physiological ionic strength. The average tension per cross-bridge obtained at the lower ionic strength in the *in vitro* assay was less than half of that obtained at physiological ionic strength in the A-band motility assay. The smaller tension development in the *in vitro* assay was attributable to the two-dimensional arrangement of HMM molecules and also to the random orientation of the molecules. Further, in the A-band motility system, we found that stepwise movement (tension development) of an actin filament corresponded to the periodic arrangement of the cross-bridges within the thick filaments. Thus, we expect that the A-band motility assay system can bridge the gap between the regularly arranged organized structures of myofibrils and a randomly oriented single molecular system.

TEMPERATURE-PULSE MICROSCOPY (TPM) IN *IN VITRO* MOTILITY ASSAY: RESPONSE TO THERMAL ACTIVATION

A motor protein is a mechano-enzyme in that it responds to both mechanical perturbation and thermal activation. The way temperature affects the properties of muscle contraction has been studied. The rate of ATP hydrolysis is very sensitive to the temperature and increases about five times with a temperature increase from 22 to 30°C. The sliding velocity of actin filaments examined in an *in vitro* motility assay showed exactly the same temperature dependency, implying that the sliding movement is tightly coupled with the rate of ATP hydrolysis. On the other hand, the force in muscle fiber rose by a factor of two to three between 5 and 20°C, but only by a factor of about one or 1.5 between 20 and 40°C.

A protein is a biological machine that is too sensitive to bear a higher temperature than that for which it was originally designed, so it is highly desirable to restore the initial temperature as soon as measurements are finished in temperature-jump experiments to prevent thermal deterioration of biological samples and confirm the absence of deterioration. In a temperature-pulse microscopy (TPM) technique we devised, temperature (higher than 60°C at the peak) was elevated spatially (in a region of approximately 10 µm in diameter) and temporally (within about 10 ms) by illuminating a lump of metal particles using an infrared laser. A concentric temperature gradient was created around the lump of metal particles.[29] The speed of temperature elevation may be sufficiently high in TPM to make a square-wave temperature pulse with rise and fall times of less than 10 ms as the heat rapidly diffused into the surrounding medium (a coverslip and water) when the laser beam was cut. As temperature was monitored through the fluorescence intensity of the temperature-sensitive rhodamine phalloidin labeled to actin filaments in the sample chamber, temperature on a single actin filament could be imaged even when it was sliding. This TPM technique was applied to the thermal activation of the sliding movement and tension development of actomyosin motors in an *in vitro* motility assay.

At first we observed a reversible acceleration of the sliding movement by repetitive application of relatively long temperature pulses (0.5 to several seconds) and found that the sliding velocities reversibly reached two steady-state values within 1/30 s between 2 and 20 µm/s when the temperature jumped up and down between 18 and 40°C. Next, we examined how sliding movements responded to very short temperature pulses with durations of 1/16 to 1/128 s. When a laser pulse of 1/16 s was applied, an abrupt displacement of the actin filament occurred, which corresponded to a sliding velocity of about 26 µm/s. The average temperature during this illumination was estimated to be 45°C and the maximum temperature exceeded 60°C. When the duration of the temperature pulse was shortened, the degree of abrupt displacement correspondingly decreased, suggesting that steady-state sliding at the high temperature had been achieved at the shortest duration of 1/128 s.

As demonstrated by TPM, motor activity reversibly and quickly responded to thermal stimulus without being denatured, even when the temperature was raised above physiological level (up to double) if the duration was sufficiently short.

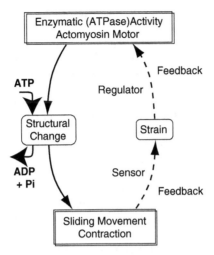

FIGURE 3.7 Spatiotemporal synchronization characteristic of a mechano-enzyme. A feedback loop is present between the enzymatic activity and the mechanical output in an assembly of nonprocessive motors.

CONCLUDING REMARKS

Molecular motors are mechano-enzymes that perform mechanical work using chemical energy produced by hydrolysis of ATP. Molecular motors in muscles work only in assemblies in which feedback loops are present.[30] As shown in Figure 3.7, structural changes of molecular motors occur accompanied by ATP hydrolysis and tension is generated, which results in force generation and sliding movement of the myofilament (shown by solid arrows).

Contraction in one part of a muscle produces strains on other motors located nearby (shown by dashed arrows), resulting in modulation of the enzymatic activity of the assembly of motors. Thus, this spatiotemporal synchronization within a protein assembly is characteristic of the mechano-enzymes, i.e., molecular motors of muscles. In essence, molecular motors of muscles might have been designed in nature as motors that respond quickly only to electric signals and mechanical stimuli from outside when working in assemblies. The next challenge in muscle research is to clarify the physical and chemical principles (corresponding to the physical principles or thermodynamics of a man-made machine) that govern force generation and synchronization of molecules.

REFERENCES

1. Engel, A.G. and Franzini-Armstrong, C., *Myology*, 2nd ed., McGraw Hill, New York, 1994.
2. Littlefield, R., Almenar-Queralt, A., and Fowler, V.M., Actin dynamics at pointed ends regulates thin filament length in striated muscle, *Nature Cell Biol.*, 3, 544–551, 2001.

3. Huxley, A.F. and Niedergerke, R., Interference microscopy of living muscle fibres, *Nature*, 173, 971–973, 1954.
4. Huxley, H.E. and Hanson, J., Changes in the cross-striations of muscle during contraction and stretch and their structural interpretation, *Nature*, 173, 973–976, 1954.
5. Huxley, A.F. and Simmons, R.M., Proposed mechanism of force generation in striated muscle, *Nature*, 233, 533–538, 1971.
6. Fujime, S., Quasi-elastic light scattering from solutions of macromolecules. II. Doppler broadening of light scattered from solutions of semi-flexible polymers, F-actin, *J. Phys. Soc. Jpn.*, 29, 751–759, 1970.
7. Fujime, S. and Ishiwata, S., Dynamic study of F-actin by quasielastic scattering of laser light, *J. Mol. Biol.*, 62, 251–265, 1971.
8. Oosawa, F., Fujime, S., Ishiwata, S., and Mihashi, K., Dynamic property of F-actin and thin filament, *Cold Spring Harb. Symp. Quant. Biol.*, 37, 277–286, 1973.
9. Ishiwata, S., Study on Muscle and Muscle Proteins: Principal Dynamic Properties of Actin Filament Studied by Quasielastic Scattering of Laser Light, Ph.D. thesis, Nagoya University, Japan, 1975.
10. Ishiwata, S. and Fujime, S., Effect of calcium ions on the flexibility of reconstituted thin filaments of muscle studied by quasielastic scattering of laser light, *J. Mol. Biol.*, 68, 511–522, 1972.
11. Yanagida, T., Nakase, M., Nishiyama, K., and Oosawa, F., Direct observation of motion of single F-actin filaments in the presence of myosin, *Nature*, 307, 58–60, 1984.
12. Fujime, S., Quasi-elastic scattering of laser light: a new tool for the dynamic study of biological macromolecules, *Adv. Biophys.*, 3, 1–43, 1972.
13. Isambert, H., Venier, P., Maggs, A.C., Fattoum, A., Kassab, R., Pantaloni, D., and Carlier, M.F., Flexibility of actin filaments derived from thermal fluctuations, *J. Biol. Chem.*, 19, 11437–11444, 1995.
14. Huxley, A.F., Muscle structure and theories of contraction, *Progr. Biophys. Biophys. Chem.*, 7, 255–318, 1957.
15. Higuchi, H., Yanagida, T., and Goldman, Y.E., Compliance of thin filaments in skinned fibers of rabbit skeletal muscle, *Biophys. J.*, 69, 1000–1010, 1995.
16. Huxley, H.E., Stewart, A., Sosa, H., and Irving, T.C., X-ray diffraction measurements of the extensibility of actin and myosin filaments in contracting muscle, *Biophys. J.*, 67, 2411–2421, 1994.
17. Wakabayashi, K., Sugimoto, Y., Tanak, Y., Ueno, Y., Takezawa, Y., and Amemiya, Y., X-ray diffraction evidence for the extensibility of actin and myosin filaments during muscle contraction, *Biophys. J.*, 67, 2422–2435, 1994.
18. Fukuda, N., Sasaki, D., Ishiwata, S., and Kurihara, S., Length dependence of tension generation in rat skinned cardiac muscle: role of titin in the Frank–Starling mechanism of the heart, *Circulation*, 104, 1639–1645, 2001.
19. Granzier, H. and Irving, T.C., Passive tension in cardiac muscle: contribution of collagen, titin, microtubules, and intermediate filaments, *Biophys. J.*, 68, 1027–1044, 1995.
20. Huxley, H.E., The mechanism of muscular contraction, *Science*, 164, 1356–1365, 1969.
21. Corrie, J.E.T., Brandmeier, B.D., Ferguson, R.E., Trentham, D.R., Kendrick-Jones, J., Hopkins, S.C., Van der Heide, U.A., Goldman, Y.E., Sabido-David, C., Dale, R.E., Criddle, S., and Irving, M., Dynamic measurement of myosin light-chain-domain tilt and twist in muscle contraction, *Nature*, 400, 425–430, 1999.

22. Suzuki, M., Fujita, H., and Ishiwata, S., New aspects of muscle contraction from the A-band motility assay system, *Biophys. J.*, 82, 362a, 2002 (Abstr.).

23. Finer, J.T., Simmons, R.M., and Spudich, J.A., Single myosin molecule mechanics: piconewton forces and nanometre steps, *Nature*, 368, 113–119, 1994.

24. Miyata, H., Hakozaki, H., Yoshikawa, H., Suzuki, N., Kinosita, K., Jr., Nishizaka, T., and Ishiwata, S., Stepwise motion of an actin filament over a small number of heavy meromyosin molecules is revealed in an *in vitro* motility assay, *J. Biochem. (Tokyo)*, 115, 644–647, 1994.

25. Miyata, H., Yoshikawa, H., Hakozaki, H., Suzuki, N., Furuno, T., Ikegami, A., Kinosita, K., Jr., Nishizaka, T., and Ishiwata, S., Mechanical measurements of single actomyosin motor force, *Biophys. J.*, 68, 286S–289S, 1995.

26. Veigel, C., Coluccio, L.M., Jontes, J.D., Sparrow, J.C., Milligan, R.A., and Molloy, J.E., The motor protein myosin-I produces its working stroke in two steps, *Nature*, 398, 530–533, 1999.

27. Kitamura, K., Tokunaga, M., Iwane, A.H., and Yanagida, T., A single myosin head moves along an actin filament with regular steps of 5.3 nanometres, *Nature*, 397, 129–134, 1999.

28. Kishino, A. and Yanagida, T., Force measurements by micromanipulation of a single actin filament by glass needles, *Nature*, 334, 74–76, 1988.

29. Kato, H., Nishizaka, T., Iga, T., Kinosita, K., Jr., and Ishiwata, S., Imaging of thermal activation of actomyosin motors, *Proc. Natl. Acad. Sci. USA*, 96, 9602–9606, 1999.

30. Shimamoto, Y., Microscopic Analysis of Inter-molecular Synchronization Observed in the Assembly of Molecular Motors, M.S. thesis, Waseda University, Tokyo, Japan, 2003.

4 Bacterial Flagellar Motor

Michio Homma and Toshiharu Yakushi

CONTENTS

INTRODUCTION

A *flagellum* (plural is *flagella*) is an organelle that bacteria require for movement. A flagellum has a filamentous and spiral structure whose diameter is about 20 nm. Its length is several times longer than the length of the cell body (Figure 4.1a). This filament is rotated as a screw and generates a propulsive force. It has a tubular structure composed of single protein subunits known as flagellins. The flagellin molecules are piled in a spiral manner (Figure 4.1b). A flagellar filament is too thin to observe with an ordinary optical microscope; it can be seen with a dark-field microscope using a very strong light source.

The antigenicity (H antigen) of flagellar filaments has been used for the classification of bacteria for many years. The polymerization reactions of flagellar filaments played an important role in forming the concept of self-assembly of the flagellin protein *in vivo*. The three-dimensional structure image can be constructed from the two-dimensional electron microscopy image because the filament has a simple repetitious helical three-dimensional structure. The correspondence between the structure and its physicochemical characteristics has been studied considerably and flagellin has been used as a model protein for elucidation of supermolecular characteristics.[1]

Filament growth takes place at the tip of the structure *in vivo*. It is thought that flagellin molecules are supplied through the central hollow of the filament. Moreover, when polymerization is carried out from the inside of the filament, the cap structure

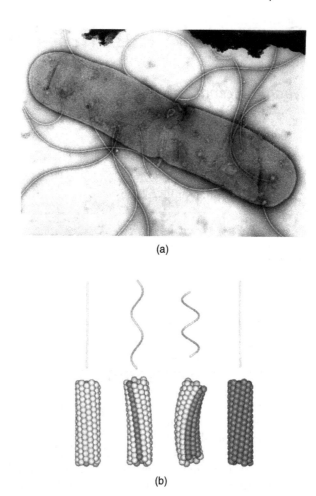

(a)

(b)

FIGURE 4.1 Cell body and flagella of *Salmonella*. (a) Osmotic shock treatment is carried out and cytoplasmic portion is removed. The basal part of the flagellum is made visible by the treatment. (b) Polymorphic structures of filaments. Left to right: L-type straight, normal, and curly, and R-type straight filaments. (Courtesy of K. Namba.)

made in a hook-associated protein 2 (HAP2) is required in the distal end of the filament. The three-dimensional structure of flagellin was clarified only recently.[2] This is a big step in aiding our understanding of how shape and flexibility are determined by the interactions among the domains of the flagellin molecule. It is proposed that the switch mechanism for the dynamic shape change of the filament has been proposed from the crystal structure and through simulation (Figure 4.1b).

The supramolecular complex structure, a motor part, is buried in a cell membrane with the basal body made from the rings and the rod structure that connects the rings (Figure 4.2). The hook structure is present between the basal body and the filament and has a length of about 50 nm. It is thought that the hook operates as a flexible joint to transmit the rotation force of the basal body. In order to form a

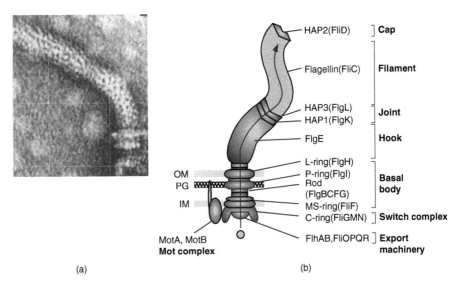

FIGURE 4.2 (a) Electron micrograph and (b) schematic diagram of flagellar structure of Gram-negative bacteria.

filament on a hook, hook-associated proteins (HAPs) are required.[3] The flagellar proteins exported outside the cells are guided by a specific flagellar export apparatus present under the basal body at the central hole of the flagellar structure. An essential motor function is handled by a motor (Mot) complex that carries out energy conversion of the inflow energy of ion and a switch complex that controls the direction of rotation of a motor. The Mot and switch complexes surround the basal body. The flagellar structure is shown in Figure 4.2b. The rotational movement made directly by flux of ion is very unique in a biological system. The flagella of the sperm of a eukaryotic organism are completely different from bacterial flagella; their propulsive force is made by whipping movement driven by adenosine triphosphate (ATP) as the energy source.

CHEMOTAXIS REGULATED BY DIRECTION OF FLAGELLAR ROTATION

In peritrichous flagella such as *Escherichia coli* and *Salmonella typhimurium*, cells can move forward (smooth swimming) when the filaments rotate counter-clockwise and tie up into a bundle. They tumble and cannot move when the filaments rotate clockwise and cannot form a bundle to serve as a screw (Figure 4.3a). Bacteria do not rotate flagella to move blindly. The direction of flagellar rotation is controlled by the stimulus from the external environment and the bacteria exhibit taxis behavior.

Figure 4.3b shows the outline of the signal transfer.[4,5] The special chemical sensing receptor (chemoreceptor) corresponding to each stimulus exists in a cell membrane. A chemical substance is bound to the chemoreceptor and the signals are transmitted to a switch complex by way of a phosphorylation cascade of cytoplasmic

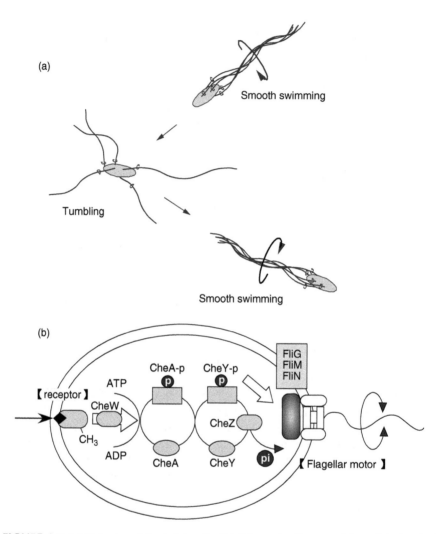

FIGURE 4.3 (a) Behavior of bacterial cells. (b) Schematic diagram of bacterial chemical sense and signal transfer. The chemoreceptor in a cell membrane binds with a chemotaxis substance or ligand. The signal is transmitted into a cell and transmitted further by carrying out phosphorylation of the Che protein. The phosphorylated CheY can bind to a protein of flagellar motor and the direction of the motor rotation is changed. Although the receptor and motor are shown separately, it is believed that they are near each other.

chemotaxis proteins. The binding of the phosphorylated protein changes the direction of the flagellar rotation. Under stimulus conditions, the *on* state of the signal is changed to the *off* state and the receptor will not respond or is adapted to the same amount of stimulation. The adaptation allows the receptor to stronger stimulations. The adaptation is caused by modification of the cytoplasmic portions of receptor proteins in which the several residues are methylated or demethylated.

VARIOUS FLAGELLAR SYSTEMS

The evidence for the flagellar system was mostly obtained from Gram-negative *E. coli* and *S. typhimurium* bacteria.[6] These bacteria have 5 to 10 peritrichous flagella. *Pseudomonas aeruginosa, Caulobacter crescentus*, and others contain one or a few flagella at their cell poles. *Vibrio parahaemolyticus* and *V. alginolyticus* have two different types (polar and lateral) flagella under certain conditions and H^+ or Na^+ ions serve as the energy source.[7] Most studies of the flagella of Gram-positive bacteria have used *Bacillus subtilis*.[8]

Although some differences were found in structures and proteins required for the functioning of flagella in different species, the fundamental compositions and structures discovered to date appear to be same. For that reason, the studies of *E. coli* and *S. typhimurium* presented in this chapter are discussed without distinguishing the species.

FLAGELLAR GENES

About 50 genes for the formation and the function of a flagellum have been identified and mapped on a chromosome (Figure 4.4). These genes are divided into three categories: a flagellum formation gene (*fla*), a motile gene (*mot*), and a chemotaxis gene (*che*).[6] The *fla* genes number about 40 and the homologous genes of *E. coli* and *S. typhimurium* have different names. In 1988, the gene names were unified and *flg, flh*, and *fli* are used to describe flagellar formations.[9] They correspond to the three regions of a chromosome.

In *S. typhimurium*, the genes for the flagellar phase variation were designated *flj*. When a gene mutation has a normal flagellar formation but the mutant cannot move, the gene is designated *mot*. Only two *mot* genes among the many flagellar genes have been identified. Six *che* genes responsible for bacterial sensing or taxis

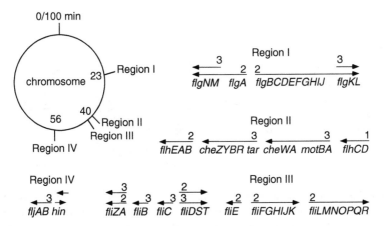

FIGURE 4.4 Flagellar-related genes of *Salmonella*. Arrows show the transcriptional directions and units. The numbers on arrows indicate transcriptional class in the flagella regulon.

have been identified. Several other receptor genes (*tar, tsr, trg,* etc.) responsible for the specific recognition of each ligand are thought to be flagellar genes.

FLAGELLAR FORMATION

A flagellum is fundamentally formed from the proximal end toward the distal tip (Figure 4.5). The MS ring composed of FliF is embedded into the cytoplasmic membrane and is thought to be the initiation of the flagellar formation. Although it is composed of a single type of protein, FliF takes a complicated form involving two ring structures in the MS ring.[10] Next, a ring-like structure called the switch complex or C ring consisting of FliG, FliM, and FliN proteins is constructed under the MS ring.[11]

Although the composition and the C ring structure observed by electron microscopy are still subject to argument, it is believed that FliG proteins are assembled on

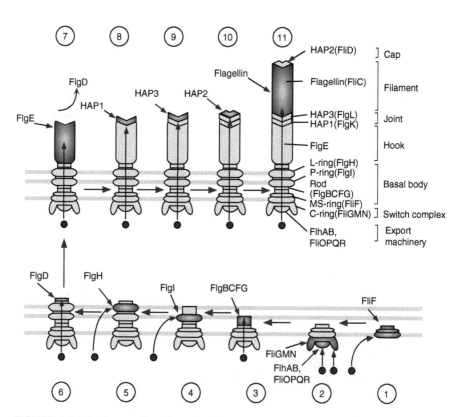

FIGURE 4.5 Morphogenesis of bacterial flagellum. The model is based on the assumption that the structure advances from a simple to a complicated form. Flagellar morphogenesis is thought to start by the formation of the MS ring structure and the proteins are attached to the structure in each of the steps.

the MS ring and FliM and FliN are the main components of the C ring.[12] The flagellar formation is stopped at the MS ring structure by a defect of the switch genes, so the switch complex is considered to be important for changing the direction of flagellar rotation and also to build the flagellar structure.[13] The FlgB, FlgC, FlgG, and FlgF components form a rod.[14] The growth of the rod probably stops when it encounters the obstacle of a peptidoglycan layer. FlgJ, which exerts a muramidase activity, opens a hole in the peptidoglycan layer, and rod formation proceeds.[15]

FlgI forms a P ring to the peptide glycan layer and FlgH forms an L ring to the outer membrane. The rod completes the formations of the ring structures. Unlike the flagellar specific secretory proteins, FlgH and FlgI have the signal peptides for a conventional Sec system that is the most common system for the protein secretion across the membrane. Once a rod is completed, the polymerization of the hook to the rod tip will start and FlgD, which is called hook cap protein and is necessary for polymerization, is located at the tip of the hook. During polymerization, the FlgE hook protein is inserted under the cap of FlgD. FlgD is released and replaced with FlgK when the hook is completed.[16]

FlgK, also known as HAP1, connects the hook and flagellar filament together with HAP3 (FlgL). The flagellar filament consists of flagellin (FliC) and is the largest part of the flagellum structure. The cap structure composed of HAP2 (FliD) is essential for *in vivo* polymerization of the flagellin monomer, although self-polymerization can be carried out *in vitro* without HAP2. Flagellin is polymerized under the cap structure of HAP2 as is the case with hook polymerization. The flagellin monomer is excreted into the culture medium of the HAP2 mutant because of the lack of polymerization. From the detailed structure of the HAP2 cap at the tip of the flagellar filament determined by an electron microscope, the model, the HAP2 cap rotating with the flagellin polymerization, is presented.[17]

FLAGELLAR-SPECIFIC TRANSPORT APPARATUS

Since most of the flagellar structure is located outside the cell membrane, many components must penetrate the membrane and a type of transport machinery serves as a motor. Most flagellum protein is carried by a flagellar-specific transport system in which the flagellar proteins do not have signal peptides recognized by the conventional Sec system.[18] A hollow structure inside the central part of the flagellar filament, hook, and rod serves as a channel.[19] The specific apparatus for the transport should be present at the entrance of the channel. The components have been proposed but the structure has not yet been detected (Figure 4.6).[20,21]

Substrates for the flagellar specific transport are flagellin (FliC), HAPs (FliD, FlgK, and FlgL), anti-sigma factor (FlgM), hook protein (FlgE), hook capping protein (FlgD), and rod proteins (FlgB, FlgC, FlgG, and FlgF). The substrates are divided into two classes: flagellin type and hook type. The chaperons (FlgN, FliT, FliS, or FliJ) recognize the substrates and guide them to the transport machinery. The transport machinery consists of six membrane proteins (FlhA, FlhB, FliO, FliP, FliQ, and FliR) and three cytoplasmic proteins (FliH, FliI, and FliJ).[22] FliI has a

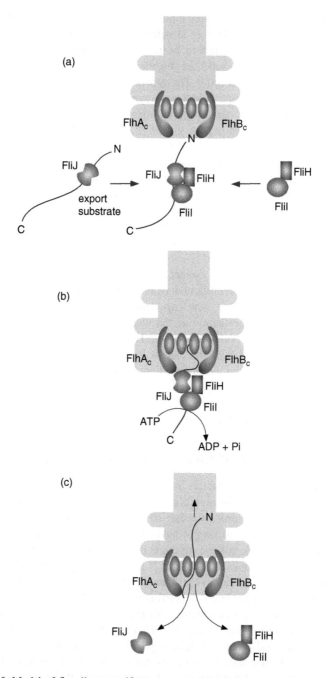

FIGURE 4.6 Model of flagellum specific transport. (a) A substrate interacts with a chaperon (FliJ) and the ATPase complex composed of FliI and FliH is further associated. (b) The ATPase complex interacts with the secretion machinery and pushes the substrate into the flagellar basal channel by using the energy of ATP. (c) After transport, soluble factors separate from the secretion machinery.

homogeny with the active site of the β-subunit of F_oF_1 ATPase, and ATPase activity is actually detected. It has been shown that FliH makes a complex with FliI and ATPase activity is controlled. A model indicates that the FliH–FliI complex interacts with FlhA and FlhB, and substrates are inserted into the channel of the flagellar basal body.[23] It is thought that FlhB is concerned with substrate recognition and works with FliK.[24,25] The flagellar secretion machinery is similar to the bacterial type III secretion system in which pathogen factors are transported.[26]

The type III substrates are secreted specifically using the N terminal signal or the 5′ end sequence of mRNA whose regions may be recognized by the chaperons.[27] FlgN, which is a specific chaperon, binds directly to FlgK (HAP1) and FlgL (HAP3) whose C terminal sequences are required for the interaction. It is thought that the degradation of the secretory proteins is prevented by the chaperon binding and that FlgN may have the role in translation control of secretory protein as a new function.[28] In the flagellar-specific secretion system, the substrates will have secretion signals in both protein and mRNA — like the other type III transport systems.

BASAL BODY PROTEINS

A flagellar basal body consists of ring structures corresponding to the outer membrane, the peptideglycan layer and the inner membrane, and a rod structure connecting the rings in the central part that acts as an axis (Figure 4.2). The flagellar filament functions as a screw and the basal body functions as a rotor as mentioned previously. It was speculated that ions flow between the M and S rings but this model has been criticized.

The flagellar structure is the biggest structure of the cell membrane. Basal body proteins do not have enzymatic activity. The cells during a logarithmic growth phase are treated with lysozyme to make spheroplasts and lysed by 1% Triton X-100. The lysate is treated with an alkali solution (pH 11) and the basal body is collected by centrifugation and purified further by $CsCl_2$ density gradient centrifugation. The basal body becomes pure enough for analysis of its protein composition. Each ring is made of a single protein. The M and S rings and rods are composed of FliF (65 kDa). The P ring consists of FlgI (38 kDa), and the L ring consists of FlgH (27 kDa).[29]

FlgI cannot build a ring in periplasmic space unless a disulfide bond is formed. The P and L rings are very stable and do not dissociate even under pH 2 and 7.5 M urea conditions.[30] The outsides of the rings are hydrophobic and they make aggregates without detergents. When FliF is overproduced in a cell, the FliF proteins assemble to the MS ring in the cytoplasmic membrane. The MS ring structure made by FliF also has a short rod structure in its center. A single type of protein forms three structurally discriminable domains.[31] The rod contains at least four proteins (FlgB, FlgC, FlgF, and FlgG). The rod assembly seems to require the coordination of the proteins and will not be formed even if one of them is missing. Although the hook is not assembled on the tip of the rod without an L or P ring, this defect is suppressed by overexpression of the hook protein. Consequently, the flagellum is constructed and can rotate without an L or P ring. It is thought that FlgD is required to build the hook at the tip of a rod. The number of subunits contained in the basal body was estimated based on the radioactive incorporation of methionine and cysteine. The basal body is a supramolecular complex of about 4300 kDa.

SWITCH COMPLEX

Many mutants for the flagellar formation (flagellar deficit or Fla⁻), were isolated. Among the genes, some mutations produce different phenotypes, a chemotaxis deficit (Che⁻) and a motility deficit (Mot⁻). The *fliG*, *fliM*, and *fliN* gene were identified and named as switch genes. They are considered to participate in flagellum construction, control of flagellar rotation direction, and energy conversion in rotational movement.[32] The suppressor mutations are isolated between the switch genes, and FliG, FliM, and FliN are thought to form a complex.[33]

A structure corresponding to the switch complex and also called the C ring can be observed by electron microscopy in the cytoplasmic side of the MS ring if flagellar basal bodies are isolated by a mild method.[12] Even if the FliG switch complex component fuses with FliF, the MS ring component, the motor is functional. The MS ring and the switch complex rotate together.

FliM seems to have the important role of controlling the direction. Many point mutations in FliM for the *che* phenotype are isolated. It has been shown that the phosphorylated CheY binds to FliM and changes the direction of the motor to the clockwise direction. The partial structures, the middle and C terminal domains of FliG from *Thermotoga maritima* thermophile, were determined at atomic resolution.[34] The functionally important charged residues are clustered along the ridges toward the outside of the FliG domain (Figure 4.7). It is proposed that the interactions of MotA and FliG are involved in the motor rotation and the charged residues (Arg90 and Glu98 in MotA and Lys264, Arg281, Arg288, Arg289, and Arg297 in FliG) contribute to the function.[35] A recent study of the sodium-driven motor indicates that the corresponding charges might not be important for torque generation.[36]

MOT PROTEINS

The motility-deficient mutants have complete flagella but cannot rotate. Essentially the gene that participates in motility is *motA* or *motB*. Some mutations of the switch genes (*fliG*, *fliM*, and *fliN*) produce the *mot* phenotype, as mentioned in the previous section.

The *motA* and *motB* genes encode 32-kDa and 34-kDa proteins, respectively. The MotA protein has four transmembrane segments and a large cytoplasmic loop and the MotB protein has a single transmembrane domain and a peptidoglycan-binding motif (Figure 4.7). It is thought that these Mot proteins have the role of changing the proton-motive force into the rotational movement. In the 1990s, the MotA and MotB complex was experimentally shown to have proton-conductive activity. The numbers of MotA and MotB molecules in an *E. coli* cell are estimated to be 600 ± 200 and 150 ± 70 copies, respectively.[37]

Many mutations isolated from *motA* and *motB* show the dominant phenotype. This evidence is consistent with the fact that some proteins are incorporated into the flagellar motor independently. When the *mot* genes, whose expressions are controlled under the inducible promoter, are introduced into the corresponding

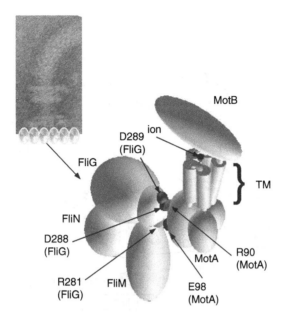

FIGURE 4.7 The switch and Mot complexes under the basal body. Models of the Mot complex composed of MotA and MotB and the switch complex composed of FliG, FliM, and FliN are presented from the assumption that each unit is composed of a single molecule of each component. The charged residues on FliG and MotA, which seem important for force generation, are indicated by the residue number near arrows. TM = transmembrane region.

mutant, the motility is soon recovered after the induction of the genes without cell division. The rotation speed of tethered cells fixed to a slide by flagella increases gradually after induction. The steps of the rotation speed are detected by the induction of motor protein.[38,39] It is thought that 8 to 16 independent torque generating units surround the basal body or the rotor. The 10 to 12 dots of a ring were observed by electron microscopy of a freeze fracture on the cytoplasmic face; the dots were lost in the *motA* or *motB* mutant.[40] The simplest explanation is that the particles are made of the motor proteins of MotA and MotB.

The activity of the motor proteins is measured as the ion (proton) flux that changes pH.[41] The membrane vesicle containing the MotA and MotB proteins is prepared in a 200-mM potassium ion solution and transferred to a low potassium ion (0.25-mM) solution. To produce a diffusion potential, valinomycin was added to the solution and pH changes of the solution were measured. The slowly swimming *motA* mutants were isolated and the mutations in the cytoplasmic domain were mapped. This suggests that the cytoplasmic domain influences the efficiency of energy conversion. Moreover, the proline residues located at the boundary of the transmembrane and cytoplasmic domains and the charged residues of arginine and glutamic acid located in the cytoplasmic domain residues have been shown to have important roles in energy conversion.[35,42]

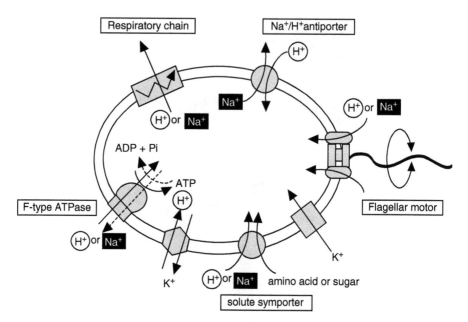

FIGURE 4.8 Major ion cycle of bacterial cell. To drive the flagellar motor, sodium-motive force can be generated by respiratory chain and Na^+/H^+ antiporter to drive flagellar motor in *Vibrio*. Proton-motive force can be generated by respiratory chain and F-type ATPase.

ION SPECIFICITY OF PROTON AND SODIUM TYPE MOTORS

Bacterial cells use the electrochemical potential of specific ions to maintain life. Protons and sodium serve as coupling ions in energy conversions (Figure 4.8). The most commonly studied bacteria, *E. coli*, *S. typhimurium*, and *B. subtilis*, have proton-driven flagella. *Vibrio* spp. (*V. alginolyticus*, *V. parahaemolyticus*, and *V. cholerae*) and alkalophilic *B. firmus* have sodium-driven flagella. The essential components are thought to be similar in the two systems because the structures of the basal bodies are similar.[43] The stator for the proton-driven system is composed of MotA and MotB and the stator for the sodium-driven motor is composed of PomA, PomB, MotX, and MotY.[7]

When the His_6–PomA/PomB complex is isolated by using β-octylglucoside in *V. alginolyticus,* the sodium ion uptake activity was detected in proteoliposomes reconstituted with the purified PomA/PomB complex. The ratio of PomA to PomB in the purified complex is estimated to be 2:1 from the intensity of the Coomassie blue staining. The estimated size of the complex by gel filtration assay is 175 kDa. This size corresponds to a complex of four PomA and two PomB molecules. It has been shown that PomA forms a stable homodimer and both halves of the dimer seem to function together to conduct sodium ions.[44,45]

The molar ratio of MotA to MotB was thought to be 1:1; an ion-conducting pore may form within the transmembrane region of each protein[46,47] but this assumption has not been supported by evidence. Cross-linking experiments suggest that MotB forms a dimer.[48] This suggests that the motor complex has a larger structure than previously assumed and we must isolate the motor complex in an intact state.

It has been reported that a hybrid motor made from the proton and sodium types is functional.[49] Components from *Rhodobacter sphaeroides* for the proton type and from *V. alginolyticus* for the sodium type motor were used because the A and B subunits of *R. sphaeroides* were found to be most similar to those of *V. alginolyticus*. A *pomA*-deficient *Vibrio* strain producing *R. sphaeroides* MotA can swim by using sodium ion flux. This suggests that A subunits do not determine ion specificity. B subunits were examined for ion recognition by using a chimeric protein named MomB, consisting of N-terminal regions of MotB and C-terminal regions of PomB.[50] With MotA, the chimera functioned as a sodium-driven motor component. Some of the different chimera, the junction sites of which are different in MotB and PomB, changed the specificities for Na^+ and Li^+. It was speculated that the differing ion specificities for rotation may correlate to ion size and these small differences may account for ion specificity changes. The periplasmic region of PomB proximal to the membrane may play a role in ion specificity or interaction with other sodium-motor proteins alters the ion size discrimination of the channel.

One report suggests that a $\Delta pomABmotXY$ strain of *V. cholerae* could swim by using *E. coli motAB* as a proton-driven motor.[51] This surprising result was confirmed in *V. alginolyticus*.[52] *E. coli motAB* does not require *motX* and *motY* for proton-driven rotation of *Vibrio* polar flagella. The chimeric proteins (PotB) consisting of the N-terminal extracellular domain of *Vibrio* PomB and C-terminal domain of *E. coli* MotB were constructed. One of the chimeric proteins can function with PomA in *Vibrio* as the stator of sodium-driven motor without *motX* or *motY*.[52] Furthermore, the H^+-driven motor of *E. coli* cells was converted to a Na^+-driven motor when the motor proteins, MotA/MotB, were only replaced with the PomA/PotB stator. This Na^+-driven motor of *E. coli* will be an excellent topic to study the mechanisms of ion selectivity, energy coupling, and force generation.

The ion selectivities of various chimeric and hybrid motors are shown in Figure 4.9. In the *Vibrio* polar flagellum, motors containing *E. coli* MotA/MotB function as proton motors (Figure 4.9a). The native sodium-driven motor of *V. alginolyticus* requires four proteins (PomA, PomB, MotX, and MotY) external to the basal body (Figure 4.9b). If the A subunit and the transmembrane region of the B subunit are derived from a proton-driven flagellum, the hybrid motor is sodium-driven, and both MotX and MotY are essential for its function (Figure 4.9d).

The reverse-type stator can function as a sodium-driven motor without MotX and MotY (Figure 4.9c). Thus, we have no clear candidate for coupling ion selection and the problem of the complexity of ion recognition. Without structural analysis, the mechanism of ion recognition or energy conversion will not be resolved.

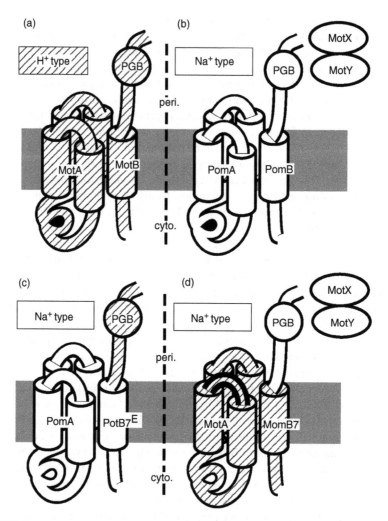

FIGURE 4.9 Hybrid and chimeric motors with the Na⁺- and the H⁺-driven components. The hatched and unhatched parts show regions of the H⁺-driven component (MotA or MotB) and the Na⁺-driven component (PomA or PomB), respectively. (See text for description of figure parts (a) through (d).) PGB = peptidoglycan binding region.

REFERENCES

1. Namba, K. and Vonderviszt, F., Molecular architecture of bacterial flagellum, *Quart. Rev. Biophys.*, 30, 1–60, 1997.
2. Samatey, F.A., Imada, K., Nagashima, S., Vonderviszt, F., Kumasaka, T., Yamamoto, M., and Namba, K., Structure of the bacterial flagellar protofilament and implications for a switch for supercoiling, *Nature*, 410, 331–337, 2001.

3. Homma, M., Kutsukake, K., Iino, T., and Yamaguchi, S., Hook-associated proteins essential for flagellar filament formation in *Salmonella typhimurium*, *J. Bacteriol.*, 157, 100–108, 1984.

4. Aizawa, S.I., Harwood, C.S., and Kadner, R.J., Signaling components in bacterial locomotion and sensory reception, *J. Bacteriol.*, 182, 1459–1471, 2000.

5. Manson, M.D., Armitage, J.P., Hoch, J.A., and MacNab, R.M., Bacterial locomotion and signal transduction, *J. Bacteriol.*, 180, 1009–1022, 1998.

6. Macnab, R., Flagella and motility, in *Escherica coli and Salmonella*, Neidhardt, F.C., Ed., American Society for Microbiology, Washington, D.C., pp.123–145, 1996.

7. Yorimitsu, T. and Homma, M., Na$^+$-driven flagellar motor of *Vibrio*, *Biochim. Biophys. Acta*, 1505, 82–93, 2001.

8. Ordal, G.W., Marquez-Magana, L., and Chamberlin, M., Motility and chemotaxis, in *Bacillus subtilis and Other Gram-Positive Bacteria: Biochemistry, Physiology, and Molecular Genetics*, Sonenshein, A.L., Hoch, J.A., and Losick, R., Eds., American Society for Microbiology, Washington, D.C., pp. 765–783, 1993.

9. Iino, T., Komeda, Y., Kutsukake, K., Macnab, R.M., Matsumura, P., Parkinson, J.S., Simon, M.I., and Yamaguchi, S., New unified nomenclature for the flagellar genes of *Escherichia coli* and *Salmonella typhimurium*, *Microbiol. Rev.*, 52, 533–535, 1988.

10. Ueno, T., Oosawa, K., and Aizawa, S.I., M-ring, S-ring and proximal rod of the flagellar basal body of *Salmonella typhimurium* are composed of subunits of a single protein, FliF, *J. Mol. Biol.*, 227, 672–677, 1992.

11. Kubori, T., Yamaguchi, S., and Aizawa, S., Assembly of the switch complex onto the MS ring complex of *Salmonella typhimurium* does not require any other flagellar proteins, *J. Bacteriol.*, 179, 813–817, 1997.

12. Francis, N.R., Sosinsky, G.E., Thomas, D., and Derosier, D.J., Isolation, characterization and structure of bacterial flagellar motors containing the switch complex, *J. Mol. Biol.*, 235, 1261–1270, 1994.

13. Kubori, T., Shimamoto, N., Yamaguchi, S., Namba, K., and Aizawa, S., Morphological pathway of flagellar assembly in *Salmonella typhimurium*, *J. Mol. Biol.*, 226, 433–446, 1992.

14. Homma, M., Kutsukake, K., Hasebe, M., Iino, T., and MacNab, R.M., FlgB, FlgC, FlgF and FlgG: a family of structurally related proteins in the flagellar basal body of *Salmonella typhimurium*, *J. Mol. Biol.*, 211, 465–477, 1990.

15. Nambu, T., Minamino, T., Macnab, R.M., and Kutsukake, K., Peptidoglycan-hydrolyzing activity of the FlgJ protein essential for flagellar rod formation in *Salmonella typhimurium*, *J. Bacteriol.*, 181, 1555–1561, 1999.

16. Ohnishi, K., Ohto, Y., Aizawa, S.I., MacNab, R.M., and Iino, T., FlgD is a scaffolding protein needed for flagellar hook assembly in *Salmonella typhimurium*, *J. Bacteriol.*, 176, 2272–2281, 1994.

17. Yonekura, K., Maki, S., Morgan, D.G., DeRosier, D.J., Vonderviszt, F., Imada, K., and Namba, K., The bacterial flagellar cap as the rotary promoter of flagellin self-assembly, *Science*, 290, 2148–2152, 2000.

18. Macnab, R.M., The bacterial flagellum: reversible rotary propellor and type III export apparatus, *J. Bacteriol.*, 181, 7149–7153, 1999.

19. Namba, K., Yamashita, I., and Vonderviszt, F., Structure of the core and central channel of bacterial flagella, *Nature* 342, 648–654, 1989.

20. Fan, F., Ohnishi, K., Francis, N.R., and Macnab, R.M., The FliP and FliR proteins of *Salmonella typhimurium*: putative components of the type III flagellar export apparatus are located in the flagellar basal body, *Mol. Microbiol.*, 26, 1035–1046, 1997.

21. Katayama, E., Shiraishi, T., Oosawa, K., Baba, N., and Aizawa, S., Geometry of the flagellar motor in the cytoplasmic membrane of *Salmonella typhimurium* as determined by stereo-photogrammetry of quick-freeze deep-etch replica images, *J. Mol. Biol.*, 255, 458–475, 1996.

22. Aizawa S.-I., Bacterial flagella and type III secretion, *FEMS Microbiol. Lett.*, 202, 157–164, 2001.

23. Minamino, T. and Macnab, R.M., FliH, a soluble component of the type III flagellar export apparatus of *Salmonella*, forms a complex with FliI and inhibits its ATPase activity, *Mol. Microbiol.*, 37, 1494–1503, 2000.

24. Kutsukake, K., Excretion of the anti-sigma factor through a flagellar substructure couples flagellar gene expression with flagellar assembly in *Salmonella typhimurium*, *Mol. Gen. Genet.*, 243, 605–612, 1994.

25. Williams, A.W., Yamaguchi, S., Togashi, F., Aizawa, S.-I., Kawagishi, I., and Macnab, R.M., Mutations in *fliK* and *flhB* affecting flagellar hook and filament assembly in *Salmonella typhimurium*, *J. Bacteriol.*, 178, 2960–2970, 1996.

26. Macnab, R.M., The bacterial flagellum: reversible rotary propellor and type III export apparatus, *J. Bacteriol.*, 181, 7149–7153, 1999.

27. Cheng, L.W. and Schneewind, O., Type III machines of Gram-negative bacteria: delivering the goods, *Trends Microbiol.*, 8, 214–220, 2000.

28. Karlinsey, J.E., Lonner, J., Brown, K.L., and Hughes, K.T., Translation/secretion coupling by type III secretion systems, *Cell*, 102, 487–497, 2000.

29. Aizawa, S., Dean, G.E., Jones, C.J., Macnab, R.M., and Yamaguchi, S., Purification and characterization of the flagellar hook–basal body complex of *Salmonella typhimurium*, *J. Bacteriol.*, 161, 836–849, 1985.

30. Akiba, T., Yoshimura, H., and Namba, K., Monolayer crystallization of flagellar L–P rings by sequential addition and depletion of lipid, *Science*, 252, 1544–1546, 1991.

31. Ueno, T., Oosawa, K., and Aizawa, S., Domain structures of the MS ring component protein (FliF) of the flagellar basal body of *Salmonella typhimurium*, *J. Mol. Biol.*, 236, 546–555, 1994.

32. Macnab, R., Flagellar switch, in *Two-Component Signal Transduction*, Hoch, J.A. and Silhavey, T.J., Eds., American Society for Microbiology, Washington, D.C., pp. 181–199, 1995.

33. Yamaguchi, S., Aizawa, S., Kihara, M., Isomura, M., Jones, C.J., and Macnab, R.M., Genetic evidence for a switchig and energy-transducing complex in the flagellar motor of *Salmonella typhimurium*, *J. Bacteriol.*, 168, 1172–1179, 1986.

34. Brown, P.N., Hill, C.P., and Blair, D.F., Crystal structure of the middle and C-terminal domains of the flagellar rotor protein FliG, *EMBO J.*, 21, 3225–3234, 2002.

35. Zhou, J.D., Lloyd, S.A., and Blair, D.F., Electrostatic interactions between rotor and stator in the bacterial flagellar motor, *Proc. Natl. Acad. Sci. USA*, 95, 6436–6441, 1998.

36. Yorimitsu, T., Sowa, Y., Ishijima, A., Yakushi, T., and Homma, M., The systematic substitutions around the conserved charged residues of the cytoplasmic loop of Na^+-driven flagellar motor component PomA, *J. Mol. Biol.*, 320, 403–413, 2002.

37. Wilson, M.L. and Macnab, R.M., Co-overproduction and localization of the *Escherichia coli* motility proteins MotA and MotB, *J. Bacteriol.*, 172, 3932–3939, 1990.

38. Ryu, W.S., Berry, R.M., and Berg, H.C., Torque-generating units of the flagellar motor of *Escherichia coli* have a high duty ratio, *Nature*, 403, 444–447, 2000.

39. Blair, D.F. and Berg, H.C., Restoration of torque in defective flagellar motors, *Science*, 242, 1678–1681, 1988.

40. Khan, S., Gene to ultrastructure: the case of the flagellar basal body, *J. Bacteriol.*, 175, 2169–2174, 1993.
41. Blair, D.F. and Berg, H.C., The MotA protein of *E. coli* is a proton-conducting component of the flagellar motor, *Cell*, 60, 439–449, 1990.
42. Braun, T.F., Poulson, S., Gully, J.B., Empey, J.C., Van, W.S., Putnam, A., and Blair, D.F., Function of proline residues of MotA in torque generation by the flagellar motor of *Escherichia coli*, *J. Bacteriol.*, 181, 3542–3551, 1999.
43. Bakkeva, L.E., Chumakov, K.M., Drachev, A.L., Metlina, A.L., and Skulachev, V.P., The sodium cycle. III. *Vibrio alginolyticus* resembles *Vibrio cholerae* and some other vibriones by flagellar motor and ribosomal 5S-RNA structures, *Biochim. Biopys. Acta*, 850, 466–472, 1986.
44. Sato, K. and Homma, M., Functional reconstitution of the Na^+-driven polar flagellar motor component of *Vibrio alginolyticus*, *J. Biol. Chem.*, 275, 5718–5722, 2000.
45. Sato, K. and Homma, M., Multimeric structure of PomA, the Na^+-driven polar flagellar motor component of *Vibrio alginolyticus*, *J. Biol. Chem.*, 275, 2023–2028, 2000.
46. Sharp, L.L., Zhou, J.D., and Blair, D.F., Tryptophan-scanning mutagenesis of MotB, an integral membrane protein essential for flagellar rotation in *Escherichia coli*, *Biochemistry*, 34, 9166–9171, 1995.
47. Sharp, L.L., Zhou, J.D., and Blair, D.F., Features of MotA proton channel structure revealed by tryptophan-scanning mutagenesis, *Proc. Natl. Acad. Sci. USA*, 92, 7946–7950, 1995.
48. Braun, T.F. and Blair, D.F., Targeted disulfide cross-linking of the MotB protein of *Escherichia coli*: evidence for two H^+ channels in the stator complex, *Biochemistry*, 40, 13051–13059, 2001.
49. Asai, Y., Kawagishi, I., Sockett, E., and Homma, M., Hybrid motor with the H^+- and Na^+-driven components can rotate *Vibrio* polar flagella by using sodium ions, *J. Bacteriol.*, 181, 6322–6338, 1999.
50. Asai, Y., Sockett, R.E., Kawagishi, I., and Homma, M., Coupling ion specificity of chimeras between H^+- and Na^+-driven motor proteins, MotB and PomB, in *Vibrio* polar flagella, *EMBO J.*, 19, 3639–3648, 2000.
51. Gosink, K.K. and Häse, C.C., Requirements for conversion of the Na^+-driven flagellar motor of *Vibrio cholerae* to the H^+-driven motor of *Escherichia coli*, *J. Bacteriol.*, 182, 4234–4240, 2000.
52. Asai, Y., Yakushi, T., Kawagishi, I., and Homma, M., Ion-coupling determinants of Na^+-driven and H^+-driven flagellar motors, *J. Mol. Biol.*, 327, 453–463, 2003.

5 Molecular Mechanisms of Cytoplasmic Streaming in Plant Cells

Teruo Shimmen and Etsuo Yokota

CONTENTS

INTRODUCTION

Cytoplasmic streaming is generally observed in plant cells. Unlike animal cells, plant cells cannot move because they are surrounded by rigid cell walls composed of polysaccharides. In general, plant cells are larger than animal cells because they elongate after cell division and develop large central vacuoles. To achieve cell activities, organelles and molecules must be effectively translocated within a cell. To accelerate intracellular translocation, plants evolved a mechanism of cytoplasmic streaming. The streaming modes vary among cell species and are classified into five types (Kamiya, 1959):

1. Agitation is the most poorly organized type of streaming. Small organelles move smoothly without turning aside over a stretch which is larger than that of Brownian motion. Agitation is generally observed in younger cells.
2. Circulation streaming is observed in cells having transvacuolar strands. In general, cytoplasm is localized at the peripheries of vacuolated cells.

In some cells, the cytoplasm penetrates the central vacuole, forming transvacuolar strands. Streaming occurs at the periphery and in the transvacuolar strands. Organization of transvacuolar strands is dynamic. It changes location, disappears, and reappears. The positions of streaming tracks and the velocities of streaming can change temporally and spatially within the same cell. Circulation is most commonly observed, for example, in epidermal cells of onion, stamen hair cells of *Tradescantia, Spirogyra*, etc.

3. Rotation. Streaming cytoplasm is limited to the periphery of a cell and streaming resembles a rotating belt. The direction and the velocity are almost constant. This streaming is observed in *Characeae, Elodea, Vallisneria*, etc.

4. Fountain streaming is an intermediate type between circulation and rotation. Cytoplasm streams acropetally or basipetally in a thick transvacuolar strand and in the opposite direction at the cell periphery. The most significant fountain streaming is observed in root hair cells of aquatic higher plants such as *Hydrocharis* or *Limnobium*. Cytoplasm streams acropetally at the cell periphery and basipetally in the transvacuolar strand. This is known as reverse fountain streaming.

5. Streaming along definite tracks. Cells have linear tracks at their peripheries and organelles move along these tracks. This streaming is observed in stalks of *Acetabularia, Codium, Bryopsis* and spolangiophores of *Phycomyces*.

MOTIVE FORCE GENERATED BY SLIDING

The direction and the velocity of streaming are very stable in characean cells that show rotational streaming. In addition, *Characeae* has large cylindrical cells with diameters of several hundred micrometers and lengths of several centimeters. All these characteristics favor the quantitative analysis of streaming.

The *Characeae* family contains six genera: *Chara, Nitella, Lamprothamnium, Nitellopsis, Lychnothamnus*, and *Tolypella*. Most species live in fresh water. However, *Lamprothamnium* can live in habitats with wide ranges of salt concentration: fresh, brackish, and sea water. For physiological studies, *Chara* and *Nitella* are generally used. *C. corallina* (*australis*) is most frequently used. Figure 5.1 shows the morphology of *C. corallina*. Morphologies are fundamentally the same for all characean species. Plants are anchored to the bottom of their habitat such as a pond, lake, rice field, sometimes even a small puddle. For anchoring, they develop rhizoids (not shown in Figure 5.1) that correspond to roots of higher plants. Between two nodes, one large internodal cell is intercalated. This node is composed of several nodal cells and several branchlets are extended.

Internodal cells are generally used for physiological experiments. In some *Chara* species such as *C. glubularis*, and *C. fibrosa*, internodal cells are surrounded by small cells. These species are not suitable for the study of streaming. Figure 5.1 also shows a longitudinal section of an internodal cell. Cells are surrounded by the cell walls — a characteristic of plant cells. The plasma membrane inside a cell wall is semipermeable and functionally separates the cell interior from the exterior. Just inside the plasma membrane is a very thin gel ectoplasm; a layer of chloroplasts is

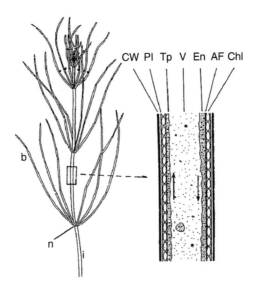

FIGURE 5.1 Morphology of *Chara corallina*. Left: whole plant (rhizoid is not shown); b = leaflet; n = node; i = internodal cell. Right: longitudinal section of an internodal cell; CW = cell wall; Pl = plasma membrane; Tp = tonoplast; V = vacuole; En = endoplasm; AF = bundle of actin filaments; Chl = chloroplast. Chloroplasts are emphasized and are much smaller.

attached to the gel ectoplasm. The sol endoplasm inside the chloroplast layer is actively streaming. Chloroplasts are emphasized in the figure. Although chloroplasts do not stream in internodal cells of *Characeae*, they stream together with endoplasmic organelles in other plants. The central part of the cell is occupied by a large vacuole surrounded by a tonoplast. Vacuolar sap containing various particles also streams, pulled by movement of endoplasm. The central vacuole occupies more than 90% of the total cell volume in matured internodal cells.

Professor N. Kamiya and his students extensively studied streaming in *Characeae* (cited in Kamiya, 1959, 1986) To elucidate the mechanism of motive force generation, identification of the site for the motive force generation is required. Kamiya and Kuroda (1956) succeeded in identification of the site by simply analyzing the velocity distribution in the cell. Young leaflet cells or internodal cells containing larger amounts of streaming endoplasm were used. Figure 5.2a shows velocity distribution in a young leaflet cell. Endoplasm streams to the opposite direction at both sides. The velocity gradient in the endoplasm is insignificant. The velocity in the vacuolar sap decreases inwardly and granules do not move at the central area.

A young leaflet cell was centrifuged and the streaming endoplasm was collected in the centrifugal end. A cell fragment lacking a vacuole was prepared by ligating the cell with a strip of thread. Velocity distribution in such a cell fragment is shown in Figure 5.2b. At both sides, the direction of the streaming is opposite and the velocity is largest at the peripheral region. The curve of velocity distribution shows a sigmoid shape with the point of inflexion at the long axis of the cell. Based on the above experiment and a model experiment, Kamiya and Kuroda (1956) concluded that "the interaction of organized gel surface and sol phase produces the

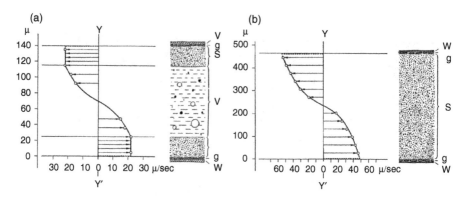

FIGURE 5.2 Distribution of streaming velocity in leaflet cells of *Nitella*. (a) Cell without centrifugation. (b) Vacuole-free cell prepared by centrifugation and following ligation. Part of the cell seen under microscope is shown on the right of each figure; v = vacuole; g = gel ectoplasm including chloroplasts; s = flowing endoplasm; w = cell wall. (From Kamiya, N. and Kuroda, K., *Bot. Mag. Tokyo*, 69, 554–554, 1956. With permission.)

shearing force which brings about the interfacial slippage." In other words, the motive force is generated by the active sliding of sol endoplasm along the surface of the stagnant gel layer (in this case, chloroplasts) — the sliding theory.

INVOLVEMENT OF ACTIN FILAMENT IN STREAMING

Identification of the site for motive force generation focused the target of the research to allow elucidation of the molecular mechanism. E. Kamitsubo and R. Nagai, two pupils of Professor N. Kamiya, carefully examined the inner surfaces of chloroplasts by optical and electron microscopy, respectively. They found cables or bundles composed of 50 to 100 microfilaments at the inner surfaces of the stagnant chloroplast layers (Figure 5.1, right) (Kamitsubo, 1966; Nagai and Rebhun, 1966).

Localization at the inner surfaces of chloroplast does not necessarily lead to a conclusion that the cables are involved in motive force generation. Kamitsubo (1972) solved this problem via an excellent experiment. He found that irradiation of a cell with a microbeam caused bleaching and swelling of chloroplasts. The chloroplasts were dislodged and carried away by streaming, thus leaving a "window" lacking chlorolasts and cables. Streaming of the window was disturbed, resulting in the accumulation of endoplasm. When the cell was kept for one to several days, cables were regenerated at the window. Streaming recovered concomitantly, suggesting that the cables are responsible for motive force generation.

To elucidate the molecular mechanism of streaming, the microfilament had to be identified. Probably, the diameter of the microfilaments, 5 nm (Nagai and Rebhun, 1966), evoked the idea of botanists that they were actin filaments. At present, actin filaments can be identified by binding of antibody or phallotoxin (Staiger and Schliwa, 1987). At that time, however, the heavy meromyosin method was the only way to identify actin filaments. When actin filaments were incubated in the absence

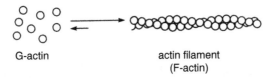

G-actin   actin filament
                              (F-actin)

FIGURE 5.3 Formation of filament by polymerization of monomer actin (G-actin).

of adenosine triphosphate (ATP), with heavy meromyosin obtained by partial pro-
teolysis of skeletal muscle myosin, they were decorated with arrowhead structures.
Adapting this method, microfilaments anchored at the inner surfaces of chloroplasts
were identified as actin filaments (Palevitz et al., 1974; Williamson, 1974; Palevitz
and Hepler, 1975; Kersey and Wessells, 1976; Kersey et al., 1976). Inhibition of
cytoplasmic streaming by treatment with cytochalasin, an actin filament-destabilizing
agent, indicated the involvement of actin filaments in motive force generation (Williamson, 1972; Bradley, 1973).

BUNDLING OF ACTIN FILAMENTS

After the discovery of plant actin filament in *Characeae*, it was also found in various
other plants (Staiger and Schliwa, 1987). A monomer of actin (globular actin or
G-actin) is a molecule of about 40 kDa. In the physiological milieu, molecules of
G-actin self-assemble to form a filamentous polymer (F-actin or actin filament;
Figure 5.3). Actin filament has a polarity: G-actin polymerizes at the plus (barbed)
end at a higher rate and at the minus (pointed) end at a lower rate. Actin filaments
are generally observed as bundles in plant cells.

Since actin filaments *per se* have no function of forming bundles, it is suggested
that actin bundling proteins will work in plant cells. We isolated an actin-binding
protein having a molecular mass of 135 kDa from pollen tubes of lily (*Lilium
longiflorum*) and found that it bundled actin filaments *in vitro* (Yokota et al., 1998).
The amino acid sequence deduced from the cDNA clone showed that this bundling
protein is plant villin (Vidali et al., 1999). Electron microscopy of actin bundles
formed *in vitro* showed that plant villin bundles actin filaments with uniform polarity
(Yokota and Shimmen, 1999). Electron and immunofluorescence microscopies
showed co-localization of villin with actin bundles in lily pollen tubes (Vidali et al.,
1999) and in root hair cells of *Hydrocharis* (Tominaga et al., 2000).

Experiments using root hair cells of *Hydrocharis* confirmed that plant villin
really works to form actin bundles in plant cells. Actin filaments in bundles had
uniform polarity, and microinjection of antibody against villin partially disintegrated
actin bundles in root hair cells (Tominaga et al., 2000). From lily pollen tubes,
another actin-bundling protein composed of a 115-kDa polypeptide was isolated
(Nakayasu et al., 1998). The 115-kDa bundling protein was also plant villin (Yokota
et al., 2003). Fimbrin, a member of the fimbrin/plastin family of actin filament
bundling or cross-linking proteins, was found to bind to arrays of fine actin filaments
in stamen hair cells of *Tadescantia* (Kovar et al., 2001). It is suggested that more
than one bundling protein is involved in bundle formation in plant cells.

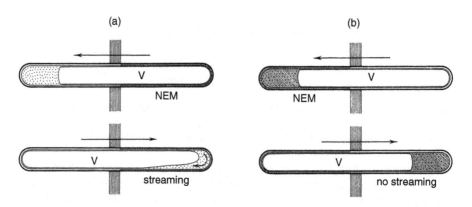

FIGURE 5.4 Differential treatment of gel endoplasm and flowing endoplasm with NEM. (a) Flowing endoplasm was collected at the centrifugal cell end and cell half depleted of endoplasm was treated with NEM (top). After washing NEM, endoplasm was transferred to the opposite cell end by centrifugation (bottom). (b) Flowing endoplasm was collected at the centrifugal cell end and the cell half containing endoplasm was treated with NEM (top). After washing NEM, endoplasm was transferred to the opposite cell end by centrifugation (bottom). (From Chen, J.C.W. and Kamiya, N., *Cell Struct. Funct.*, 1, 1–9, 1975. With permission.)

MYOSIN IS A MOTOR PROTEIN

Involvement of actin filaments inevitably evokes the idea that myosin is also involved in cytoplasmic streaming because the induction of contraction of skeletal muscle by sliding between actin filaments and myosin was established earlier (Bary, 1992). According to the sliding theory for cytoplasmic streaming proposed by Kamiya and Kuroda (1956), the motive force is generated by sliding of endoplasm along the surface of a stagnant chloroplast layer. Thus, it is suggested that myosin is contained in the flowing endoplasm. This possibility was supported by sophisticated experiments. Biochemical studies on skeletal muscle established that a sulfhydryl reagent (N-ethylmaleimide or NEM) irreversibly inhibits myosin but not actin (Sibata-Sekiya and Tonomura, 1975; Tonomura and Yoshimura, 1962; Yamaguchi et al., 1973).

Chen and Kamiya (1975) developed an elegant system to treat flowing endoplasm and gel ectoplasm by applying centrifugation to internodal cells of *Characeae* (Figure 5.4). After the streaming endoplasm was collected to one cell end, only the centripetal half of the cell was treated with NEM (Figure 5.4a, top). After removing NEM, the cell was centrifuged in the opposite direction to bring the endoplasm to the NEM-treated cell half. Streaming was observed (Figure 5.4a, bottom). In another experiment, the centrifugal cell half containing endoplasm was treated with NEM (Figure 5.4b, top). After washing, NEM-treated endoplasm was brought to the NEM-untreated cell end by centrifugation. In this case, streaming was not observed (Figure 5.4b, bottom). Thus, it was concluded that the NEM-sensitive component thought to be myosin is contained in the flowing endoplasm.

Although NEM has been used as an inhibitor of myosin (Liebe and Menzel, 1995; Liebe and Quader, 1994; McCurdy, 1999), this is not the case. NEM is only a membrane-permeable reagent that attacks SH-containing proteins. It has been reported that NEM also inhibits the activity of dynein (Michell and Warner, 1981; Cosson and Gibbons, 1978; Shimizu and Kimura, 1974).

Another useful method for studies on cytoplasmic streaming was developed by taking advantage of characean cells (Figure 5.5). Since internodal cells are large, both cell ends can be removed by cutting with scissors. Tazawa (1964) succeeded in introducing an artificial solution into the original vacuole by applying intracellular perfusion after cutting both cell ends of an internodal cell (Figure 5.5b). Since the tonoplast is a semipermeable membrane, chemical composition in the cytoplasm cannot be modified by vacuolar perfusion. When a Ca^{2+}-chelating agent (ethyleneg-lycol-bis-(beta-aminoethylether)N,N'-tetraacetic acid or EGTA) was added to the perfusion medium, the tonoplasts disintegrated (Figure 5.5c) (Williamson, 1975; Tazawa et al., 1976). This technique made it possible to modify the chemical composition of the original cytoplasmic space. This technique allowed unequivocal demonstration that ATP is a substrate of the putative motor protein involved in cytoplasmic streaming (Williamson, 1975; Tazawa et al., 1976). The ATP concentration for half maximum velocity (Michaelis constant) was found to be 0.06 to 0.08 mM (Shimmen, 1978). ADP, orthophosphate, pyrophosphate, and sulfate inhibited cytoplasmic streaming competitively with ATP (Shimmen, 1988a; Shimmen et al., 1990). Thus, this technique allows analysis of biochemical characteristics of the motor protein without biochemical purification.

Using intracellular perfusion technique, Williamson (1975) found an important phenomenon to speculate the localization of putative motor protein (myosin) in flowing endoplasm. Streaming organelles became anchored to actin cables upon depletion of ATP by perfusion with a medium lacking ATP, and they resumed movement upon addition of ATP. This tight binding of organelles in the absence of ATP recalls the cross bridge between actin filaments and myosins reported in skeletal muscle. Based on this observation, Williamson (1976) suggested that the motive force of cytoplasmic streaming is generated by sliding of myosin bound to organelles along actin filaments using the hydrolysis energy of ATP.

Shimmen and Tazawa (1982) also demonstrated binding of putative myosin with organelles by an experiment intended to reconstitute the streaming. They collected endoplasm from internodal cells of *Chara* and obtained an organelle fraction lacking soluble components by centrifugation. When this fraction was introduced into internodal cells of *Nitella* whose endoplasm had been removed, organelles moved along actin filaments, indicating that myosin is associated with organelles (Figure 5.5e) (Shimmen and Tazawa, 1982).

Association of myosin with organelles of pollen tubes was also demonstrated by the reconstitution experiment (Kohno and Shimmen, 1988a,b). Homogenate was prepared from pollen tubes of lily (*Lilium longiflorum*), in which active cytoplasmic streaming was also shown. When the homogenate was introduced into the internodal cells of *Characeae*, organelles moved along characean actin filaments (Figure 5.5e). This work not only showed association of myosin with organelles but also indicated that pollen tubes are suitable for biochemical isolation of myosin — a subject that will be dealt with later.

Ultrastructural studies were also carried out to determine the association of putative myosin and organelles. Nagai and Hayama (1979) found that protuberances

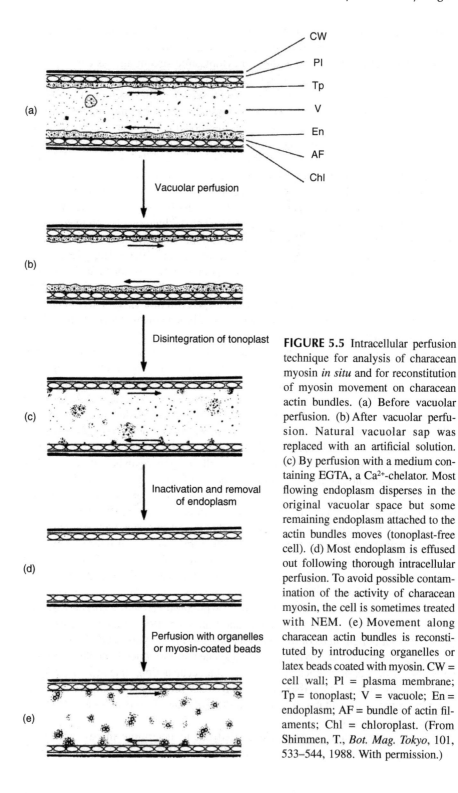

FIGURE 5.5 Intracellular perfusion technique for analysis of characean myosin *in situ* and for reconstitution of myosin movement on characean actin bundles. (a) Before vacuolar perfusion. (b) After vacuolar perfusion. Natural vacuolar sap was replaced with an artificial solution. (c) By perfusion with a medium containing EGTA, a Ca^{2+}-chelator. Most flowing endoplasm disperses in the original vacuolar space but some remaining endoplasm attached to the actin bundles moves (tonoplast-free cell). (d) Most endoplasm is effused out following thorough intracellular perfusion. To avoid possible contamination of the activity of characean myosin, the cell is sometimes treated with NEM. (e) Movement along characean actin bundles is reconstituted by introducing organelles or latex beads coated with myosin. CW = cell wall; Pl = plasma membrane; Tp = tonoplast; V = vacuole; En = endoplasm; AF = bundle of actin filaments; Chl = chloroplast. (From Shimmen, T., *Bot. Mag. Tokyo*, 101, 533–544, 1988. With permission.)

were present on organelles bound to the actin cables in the absence of ATP and that small globular bodies of 20 to 30 nm in diameter were associated with the protuberances. They suggested that these globular bodies act as functional units when endoplasmic organelles slide along the actin cables. Williamson (1979) found filaments associated with endoplasmic reticulum in the streaming cytoplasm and suggested that the filaments contained myosin. However, the chemical natures of these filaments (Williamson, 1979) and globular bodies (Nagai and Hayama, 1979) remain unidentified.

BIOCHEMICAL IDENTIFICATION OF MYOSIN

Isolation of myosin has been reported in various plants: *Nitella* (Kato and Tonomura, 1977), *Egeria* (Ohsuka and Inoue, 1979), tomato fruit (Vahey et al., 1982), and pea tendril (Ma et al., 1989). However, these works have not been reproduced. The most serious problem in isolating myosin has been the lack of a method to measure the myosin-specific activity in crude samples of plant cells. ATP hydrolysis activated by actin filaments (actin-activated ATPase) is myosin-specific. However, it will be difficult to discriminate the actin-activated ATPase from other ATPases in a crude sample.

Detection of myosin-specific activity in crude samples became possible after development of an *in vitro* motility assay (Kron and Spudich, 1986). Myosin molecules are attached to the surface of a cover glass and actin filaments are applied with ATP (Figure 5.6). Although actin filaments are supposed to slide on a glass surface by using the hydrolysis energy of ATP, it is impossible to observe a single actin filament with an optical microscope due to its small size. However, discovery of a mushroom toxin made it possible (Wieland and Faulstich, 1978).

Phalloidin, one of phallotoxins discovered from *Amanita phalloides,* binds to actin filament and stabilizes it (Cooper, 1987). When an actin filament is stained with phalloidin conjugated with fluorescent dye, it can be visualized with a fluorescence microscope equipped with an ultrasensitive video camera. Thus, it became possible to observe an actin filament moving on a glass surface coated with myosin (Figure 5.6). We introduced this method, known as the *in vitro* motility assay, in the study of plant myosin. When we applied fluorescently labeled actin filaments of skeletal muscle on a glass surface coated with a crude extract obtained from pollen tubes of lilies (*Lilium longiflorum*), they actively moved (Kohno et al., 1991). By monitoring the sliding activity, we succeeded in isolating plant myosin from pollen tubes of a higher plant, the lily (Kohno et al., 1992; Yokota and Shimmen, 1994).

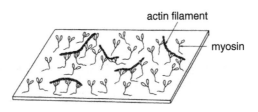

FIGURE 5.6 *In vitro* motility assay. Surface of cover glass is coated with myosin molecules and fluorescent actin filaments slide on the surface.

The molecular size of the heavy chain of the myosin was 170 kDa (170-kDa myosin). The velocity of actin filament translocation in motility assay was 7 μm/sec, which is close to the velocity of cytoplasmic streaming in living pollen tubes. This indicates that 170-kDa myosin is responsible for cytoplasmic streaming in pollen tubes (Yokota and Shimmen, 1994).

Based on the same strategy, plant myosins composed of 205 to 235 kDa heavy chains were isolated from *Chara corallina* algae (Yamamoto et al., 1994; Higashi-Fujime et al., 1995). We applied this method to tobacco-cultured BY-2 cells and found two myosins, a 175-kDa heavy chain and a 170-kDa myosin (Yokota et al., 1999b). Analysis using intact tobacco plants showed that vegetative organs (root, stem, and leaf) contain both types of myosin, but pollen tubes contain only 170-kDa myosin (Yokota et al., 1999b).

TYPES OF PLANT MYOSINS

At present, 18 classes of myosin have been reported in eukaryotes. Amino acid sequences deduced from analysis of cDNA clones showed that plant myosins (170-kDa myosin, 175-kDa myosin, and *Chara* myosin) belong to class XI and form dimers (Kashiyama et al., 2000; Morimatsu et al., 2000; Tominaga et al., 2003). Analysis with an electron microscope revealed that the plant myosin structure had two heads and a tail having with two small globular structures (Figure 5.7) (Yamamoto et al., 1995; Tominaga et al., 2003). It is suggested that the head region (N terminal of the heavy chain) is responsible for conversion of the chemical energy of ATP to the sliding movement and the tail globular region (C terminal) for binding to organelles.

Myosins are involved in various physiological activities, such as contraction and organelle transport. The tail region is responsible for expression of their physiological roles. The tail region of myosin II has a function of self-assembly to form bipolar thick filaments that generate the contraction force by sliding with actin filaments in muscle contraction, amoeba movement, and cytokinesis of animal cells (Bary, 1992). Myosin V also has globular bodies at the tail region and is responsible for organelle transport (Reck-Peterson et al., 2000). Plant myosin (myosin XI). also has globular structures and is responsible for organelle transport (Figure 5.7). Immunofluorescence microscopy revealed an association of plant myosin with organelles (Yokota et al., 1995a,b; Yokota et al., 2001).

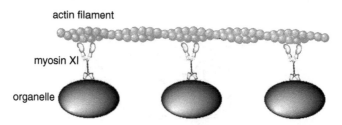

actin filament

myosin XI

organelle

FIGURE 5.7 Molecular structure of 175-kDa myosin of tobacco-cultured cell deduced from electron micrograph. (Original figure drawn by Hasimoto, K. and Tahara, H. With permission.)

Myosins have evolved not only at the tail region but also at the head region to express various physiological roles. Myosin II is involved in contraction of both skeletal and smooth muscles. However, the sliding velocity of skeletal muscle myosin is ten times higher than that of smooth muscle myosin. Interestingly, the velocity of characean myosin involved in cytoplasmic streaming is ten times higher than that of skeletal muscle myosin (Shimmen, 1988b). In addition to variations in velocity, it is becoming clear that the mechanochemical properties are different among myosins. Myosin V is a processive motor; this means that a single myosin molecule can support movement along an actin filament for longer distance (processivity). Kinetic analysis using 175-kDa myosin showed the that plant myosin responsible for cytoplasmic streaming is also a processive motor (Tominaga et al., 2003). Thus, myosin XI has evolved to perform a role of organelle transport in plant cells.

REGULATION OF CYTOPLASMIC STREAMING

Regulation mode of actin–myosin sliding in cytoplasmic streaming shows clear contrast with that in muscle contraction. Muscle cells are relaxed at the resting state and contract due to the start of actin–myosin sliding upon arrival of action potentials from motor neurons. On the other hand, actin–myosin sliding continues to generate the motive force of cytoplasmic streaming at the resting state in plant cells. It is reasonable to consider that cytoplasmic streaming is responsible for housekeeping work and intracellular transport. However, cytoplasmic streaming sometimes stops and we introduce two situations: *Characeae* and pollen tubes.

REGULATION IN CHARACEAE

At the resting state, the difference of electrical potential across the plasma membrane (membrane potential or E_m) sometime marks values more negative than -200 mV (inside negative). Upon mechanical or electrical stimulation, a characean cell generates an action potential as do muscles and nerves of animals (Shimmen, 1996). E_m quickly changes to the positive direction (depolarization) and returns to its original resting level (repolarization). Electrophysiological analyses have revealed that an action potential is generated by opening of two ion channels of the plasma membrane, Ca^{2+} and Cl^- channels (Shimmen et al., 1994). With a slight delay from the start of depolarization, cytoplasmic streaming quickly stops and gradually recovers to the original velocity (Hayama et al., 1979).

When Mg^{2+} or Ba^{2+} antagonists of Ca^{2+} were added to the external medium of *Nitella*, an action potential was generated by electrical stimulation but cytoplasmic streaming did not stop (Barry, 1968). It is supposed that Ca^{2+} flowing into the cytoplasm across the plasma membrane is responsible for stoppage of cytoplasmic streaming. Increases in Ca^{2+} influx and the concentration of free Ca^{2+} ion in the cytoplasm upon membrane excitation were demonstrated (Hayama et al., 1979; Williamson and Ashley 1982). Using a cell model whose plasma membrane had been permeabilized, it was demonstrated that cytoplasmic streaming is reversibly inhibited by 10^{-6} to 10^{-5} M Ca^{2+} (Tominaga et al., 1983), supporting the Ca^{2+}-hypothesis. Using inhibitors of protein kinase and phosphatase, it was suggested that cytoplasmic streaming is inhibited by inactivation of myosin activity via its phosphorylation, i.e., sliding activity of myosin is inhibited by its Ca^{2+}-dependent phosphorylation upon membrane excitation (Tominaga et al., 1987; Morimatsu et al., 2002). Association of Ca^{2+}-dependent protein kinase with actin cables (McCurdy and Harmon, 1992a) and Ca^{2+}-dependent phosphorylation of a putative myosin light chain (McCurdy and Harmon, 1992b) was reported. However, the light chain of myosin XI of *Chara* has not been identified yet.

REGULATION IN POLLEN TUBES

When a pollen grain arrives at the stigma of a pistil, it germinates to form a pollen tube that sends a sperm cell to an egg cell in an ovary. In the case of a lily plant, pollen tubes elongate to a length of about 10 cm within 60 h. Active cytoplasmic streaming is inevitable for this rapid growth of pollen tubes (Franke et al., 1972; Gibbon et al.,1999). At the tips of pollen tubes, large organelles are absent and only small vesicles are irregularly moving (clear zone) (Figure 5.8).

Streaming is reflected by organization of actin filaments. At the basal region, tremendous bundles of actin filaments run in a longitudinal direction that corresponds to the direction of cytoplasmic streaming. In the tip region, however, only a few thin bundles and short single actin filaments are arranged in random orientation (Miller et al.,1996; Lancelle et al., 1997). It has been suggested that such intracellular distribution of organelles and actin filaments is supported by intracellular gradients of free Ca^{2+}. There is a tip-focused gradient of Ca^{2+}, and the Ca^{2+} concentration at the tip has been estimated to be more than 3 μM (Pierson et al., 1994, 1996; Messerli and Robinson, 1997). When pollen tubes were treated with caffein, tip-focused Ca^{2+} gradient was diminished (Pierson et al., 1996), and tip growth stopped. In addition, bundles of actin filaments extended to the tip region and large organelles streamed into the tip region (Miller et al., 1996; Lancelle et al., 1997).

Thus, tip-focused Ca^{2+}-gradient seems to be responsible for organization of actin filaments and distribution of organelles. Our biochemical studies first shed light on

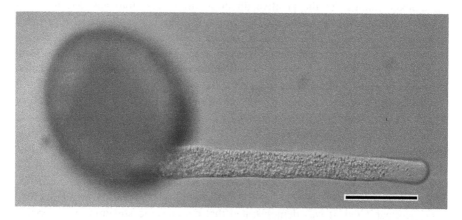

FIGURE 5.8 Morphology of pollen tube of lily (*Lilium longiflorum*). Bar represents 50 μm.

these relations. Although the activity of plant villin *per se* was insensitive to Ca^{2+}, it became Ca^{2+}-sensitive in the concomitant presence of calmodulin, a Ca^{2+}-binding protein. The bundling activity is inhibited by Ca^{2+} of μM order concentration (Yokota et al., 2000). Considering a Ca^{2+} concentration higher than 3 μM (Pierson et al., 1994, 1996; Messerli and Robinson, 1997), it is reasonable to suppose that formation of actin bundles by villin is inhibited at the tip region.

We found that the sliding activity of myosin XI of pollen tubes is inhibited by Ca^{2+} of μM order concentration and that myosin XI has calmodulin as a light chain. It seems that calmodulin is involved in Ca^{2+} regulation of the myosin activity (Yokota and Shimmen, 1999a). It is also suggested that myosin activity is inhibited at the tip region containing Ca^{2+} at high concentrations.

SECONDARY STREAMING

In most plants, cytoplasmic streaming continues in the absence of stimulation (primary streaming). In some aquatic higher plants, *Egeria* and *Vallisneria*, cytoplasmic streaming does not occur in the dark but it is activated upon illumination (secondary streaming). Streaming in these plants is also supported by the actin–myosin system (Ishigami and Nagai, 1980). Although involvement of Ca^{2+} has been suggested (Takagi and Nagai, 1986), the molecular mechanism of regulation by light remains undetermined.

REFERENCES

Barry, W.H. (1968), Coupling of excitation and cessation of cyclosis in *Nitella*: role of divalent cations, *J. Cell Physiol.*, 72, 153–160.

Bary, D. (1992), *Cell Movement*, Garland Publishing, New York.

Bradley, M.O. (1973), Microfilaments and cytoplasmic streaming: inhibition of streaming with cytochalasin, *J. Cell Sci.*, 12, 327–343.

Chen, J.C.W. and Kamiya, N. (1975), Localization of myosin in the internodal cell of *Nitella* as suggested by differential treatment with N-ethylmaleimide, *Cell Struct. Funct.*, 1, 1–9.

Cooper, J.A. (1987), Effects of cytochalasin and phalloidin on actin, *J. Cell Biol.*, 105, 1473–1478.

Cosson, M.P. and Gibbons, I.R. (1978), Properties of sea urchin sperm flagella in which bending waves have been preserved by pretreatment with mono- and bi-functional maleimide derivatives, *J. Cell Biol.*, 79, 286a.

Franke, W.W., Herth, W., van der Woude, W.J., and Morre, D.J. (1972), Tubular and filamentous structures in pollen tubes: possible involvement as guide elements in protoplasmic streaming and vectorial migration of secretory vesicle, *Planta*, 105, 317–341.

Gibbon, B.C., Kovar, D.R., and Staiger, C.J. (1999), Latrunculin B has different effects on pollen germination and tube growth, *Plant Cell*, 11, 2349–2363.

Hayama, T., Shimmen, T., and Tazawa, M. (1979). Participation of Ca^{2+} in cessation of cytoplasmic streaming induced by membrane excitation in *Characeae* internodal cells, *Protoplasma*, 99, 305–321.

Higashi-Fujime, S., Ishikawa, R., Iwasawa, H., Kagami, O., Kurimoto, E., Kohama, K., and Hozumi, T. (1995), The fastest actin-based motor protein from the green algae, *Chara*, and its distinct mode of interaction with actin, *FEBS Lett.*, 375, 151–154.

Ishigami, M. and Nagai, R. (1980), Motile apparatus in *Vallisneria* leaf cells. II. Effects of cytochalasin B and lead acetate on the rate and direction of streaming, *Cell Struct. Funct.*, 5, 13–20.

Kamitsubo, E. (1966), Motile protoplasmic fibrils in cells of Characeae. II. Linear fibrillar structure and its bearing on protoplasmic streaming, *Proc. Jpn. Acad.*, 42, 640–643.

Kamitsubo, E. (1972), A "window technique" for detailed observation of characean cytoplasmic streaming, *Exp. Cell Res.*, 74, 613–616.

Kamiya, N. (1959), Protoplasmic streaming, *Protoplasmatologia*, 8(3/a), Springer-Verlag, Vienna.

Kamiya, N. (1986), Cytoplasmic streaming in giant algal cells: a historical survey of experimental approaches, *Bot. Mag. Tokyo*, 99, 441–467.

Kamiya, N. and Kuroda, K. (1956), Velocity distribution of the protoplasamic streaming in *Nitella* cells, *Bot. Mag. Tokyo*, 69, 544–554.

Kashiyama, T., Kimura, N., Mimura, T., and Yamamoto, K. (2000), Cloning and characterization of a myosin from characean alga, the fastest motor protein in the world, *J. Biochem.*, 127, 1065–1070.

Kato, T. and Tonomura, Y. (1977), Identification of myosin in *Nitella flexilis*, *J. Biochem.*, 82, 777–782.

Kersey, Y.M., Hepler, P.K., Palevitz, B.A., and Wessells, N.K. (1976), Polarity of actin filaments in characean algae, *Proc. Natl. Acad. Sci. USA*, 73, 165–167.

Kersey, Y.M. and Wessells, N.K. (1976), Localization of actin filaments in internodal cells of characean algae, *J. Cell Biol.*, 68, 264–275.

Kohno, T., Ishikawa, R., Nagata, T., Kohama, K., and Shimmen, T. (1992), Partial purification of myosin from lily pollen tubes by monitoring with *in vitro* motility assay, *Protoplasma*, 170, 77–85.

Kohno, T., Okagaki, T., Kohama, K., and Shimmen, T. (1991), Pollen tube extract supports the movement of actin filaments *in vitro*, *Protoplasma*, 161, 75–77.

Kohno, T. and Shimmen, T. (1988a), Accelerated sliding of pollen tube organelles along Characeae actin bundles regulated by Ca^{2+}, *J. Cell Biol.*, 106, 1539–1543.

Kohno, T. and Shimmen, T. (1988b), Mechanism of Ca^{2+} inhibition of cytoplasmic streaming in lily pollen tubes, *J. Cell Sci.*, 91, 501–509.

Kovar, D.R., Gibbon, B.C., and McCurdy, D.W. (2001), Fluorescently-labeled fimbrin decorates a dynamic filament network in live plant cells, *Planta*, 213, 390–395.

Kron, S.J. and Spudich, J.A. (1986), Fluorescent actin filaments move on myosin fixed to a glass surface, *Proc. Natl. Acad. Sci. USA*, 83, 6272–6276.

Lancelle, S.A., Cresti, M., and Heper, P.K. (1997), Growth inhibition and recovery in freeze-substituted *Lilium longiflorum* pollen tubes: structural effects of caffein, *Protoplasma*, 196, 21–33.

Liebe, S. and Menzel, D. (1995), Actomyosin-based motility of endopasmic reticulum and chloroplasts in *Vallisneria* mesophyll cells, *Biol. Cell*, 85, 207–222.

Liebe, S. and Quader, H. (1994), Myosin in onion (*Allium cepa*) bulb scale epidermal cells: involvement in dynamics of organelles and endoplasmic reticulum, *Physiol. Scand.*, 90, 114–124.

Ma, Y.-Z. and Yen, L.-F. (1989), Actin and myosin in pea tendrils, *Plant Physiol.*, 89, 586–589.

McCurdy, D.W. (1999), Is 2,3-butanedione monoxime an effective inhibitor of myosin-based activities in plant cells? *Protoplasma*, 209, 120–125.

McCurdy, D.W. and Harmon, A.C. (1992a), Calcium-dependent protein kinase in the green alga *Chara, Planta*, 188, 54–61.

McCurdy, D.W. and Harmon, A.C. (1992b), Phosphorylation of a putative myosin light chain in *Chara* by calcium-dependent protein kinase, *Protoplasma*, 171, 85–88.

Messerli, M. and Robinson, K.R. (1997), Tip localized Ca²⁺ pulses are coincident with peak pulsatile growth rates in pollen tubes of *Lilium longiflorum, J. Cell Sci.*, 110, 1269–1278.

Miller, D.D., Lancelle, S.A., and Hepler, P.K. (1996), Actin microfilaments do not form a dense meshwork in *Lilium longiflorum* pollen tube tips, *Protoplasma*, 195, 123–132.

Mitchell, D.R. and Warner, F.D. (1981), Binding of dynein 21S ATPase to microtubules: effects of ionic conditions and substrate analogs, *J. Biol. Chem.*, 256, 12535–12544.

Morimatsu, M., Hasegawa, S., and Higashi-Fujime, S. (2002), Protein phosphorylation regulates actomyosin-driven vesicle movement in cell extracts isolated from the green algae, *Chara corallina, Cell Motil. Cytoskel.*, 53, 66–76.

Morimatsu, M., Nakamura, A., Sumiyosh, H., Sakabe, N., Taniguchi, H., Kohama, K., and Higashi-Fujime, S. (2000), The molecular structure of the fastest myosin from green algae, *Chara, Biochem. Biophys. Res. Commun.*, 270, 147–152.

Nakayasu, T., Yokota, E., and Shimmen, T. (1998), Purification of an actin-binding protein composed of 115-kDa polypeptide from pollen tubes of lily, *Biochem. Biophys. Res. Comm.*, 249, 61–65.

Ngagai, R. and Hayama, T. (1979), Ultrastructure of the endoplasmic factor responsible for cytoplasmic streaming in *Chara* internodal cells, *J. Cell Sci.*, 36, 121–136.

Nagai, R. and Rebhun, L.I. (1966), Cytoplasmic microfilaments in streaming *Nitella* cells, *J. Ultrastruct. Res.*, 14, 571–589.

Ohsuka, K. and Inoue, A. (1979), Identification of myosin in a flowering plant, *Egeria densa, J. Biochem.*, 85, 375–378.

Palevitz, B.A., Ash, J.F., and Hepler, P.K. (1974), Actin in the green alga, *Nitella, Proc. Natl. Acad. Sci. USA*, 71, 363–366.

Palevitz, B.A. and Hepler, P.K. (1975), Identification of actin *in situ* at the ectoplasm-endoplasm interface of *Nitella, J. Cell Biol.*, 65, 29–38.

Pierson, E.S., Miller, D.D., Callaham, D.A., Shipley, A.M., Rivers, B.A., Cresti, M., and Hepler, P.K. (1994), Pollen tube growth is coupled to the extracellular calcium ion flux and the intracellular calcium gradient: effect of BAPTA-type buffers and hypertonic media, *Plant Cell*, 6, 1815–1828.

Pierson, E.S., Miller, D.D., Callaham, D.A., van Aken, J., Hackett, G., and Hepler, P.K. (1996), Tip localized calcium entry fluctuates during pollen tube growth, *Dev. Biol.*, 174, 160–173.

Reck-Peterson, S.L., Provance, D.W., Jr., Moosker, M.S., and Mercer, J.A. (2000), Class V myosins, *Biochim. Biophys. Acta*, 1496, 36–51.

Shimizu, T. and Kimura, I. (1974), Effects of N-ethylmaleimide on dynein adenosine-triphosphatase activity and its recombining ability with outer fibers, *J. Biochem.*, 76, 1001–1008.

Shimmen, T. (1978), Dependency of cytoplasmic streaming on intracellular ATP and Mg²⁺ concentrations, *Cell Struct. Funct.*, 3, 113–121.

Shimmen, T. (1988a), Cytoplasmic streaming regulated by adenine nucleotides and inorganic phosphates in Characeae, *Protoplasma*, Suppl. 1, 3–9.

Shimmen, T. (1988b), Characean actin bundles as a tool for studying actomyosin-based motility, *Bot. Mag. Tokyo*, 101, 533–544.

Shimmen, T. (1996), Studies on mechano-perception in characean cells: development of a monitoring apparatus, *Plant Cell Physiol.*, 37, 591–597.

Shimmen, T. (1997), Studies on mechano-perception in characean cells: pharmacological analysis, *Plant Cell Physiol.*, 38, 139–148.

Shimmen, T., Kikuyama, M., Mimura, T., and Shimmen, T. (1994), Characean cells as a tool for studying electrophysiological characteristics of plant cells, *Cell Struct. Funct.*, 19, 263–278.

Shimmen, T. and Tazawa, M. (1982), Reconstitution of cytoplasmic streaming in Characeae, *Protoplasma*, 113, 127–131.

Shimmen, T., Xu, Y.-L., and Kohno, T. (1990), Inhibition of cytoplasmic streaming by sulfate in characean cells, *Protoplasma*, 158, 39–44.

Sibata-Sekiya, K. and Tonomura, Y. (1975), Desensitization of substrate inhibition of acto-H-meromysin ATPase by treatment of H-meromyosin with p-chloromercuribenzoate: relation between extent of desensitization and amount of bound-chloromerucribenzoate, *J. Biochem.*, 77, 543–557.

Staiger, C.J. and Schliwa, M. (1987), Actin localization and function in higher plants, *Protoplasma*, 141, 1–12.

Takagi, S. and Nagai, R. (1986), Intracellular concentration and cytoplasmic streaming in *Vallisneria* mesophyll cells, *Plant Cell Physiol.*, 27, 935–959.

Tazawa, M. (1964), Studies on *Nitella* having artificial cell sap. I. Replacement of the cell sap with artificial solutions, *Plant Cell Physiol.*, 5, 33–43.

Tazawa, M., Kikuyama, M., and Shimmen, T. (1976), Electric characteristics and cytoplasmic streaming of Characeae cells lacking tonoplasts, *Cell Struct. Funct.*, 1, 165–176.

Tominaga, M., Kojima, H., Yokota, E., Orii, H., Nakamori, R., Katayama, E., Anson, M., Shimmen, T., and Oiwa, K. (2003), Higher plant myosin XI moves processively on actin with 35 nm steps at high velocity, *EMBO J.*, 22, 1263–1272.

Tominaga, Y., Shimmen, T., and Tazawa, M. (1983), Control of cytoplasmic streaming by extracellular Ca^{2+} in permeabilized *Nitella* cells, *Protoplasma*, 116, 75–77.

Tominaga, Y., Wayne, R., Tung, H.Y.L., and Tazawa, M. (1987), Phosphorylation–dephosphorylation is involved in Ca^{2+}–controlled cytoplasmic streaming of characean cells, *Protoplasma*, 136, 161–169.

Tominaga, M., Yokota, E., Vidali, L., Sonobe, S., Hepler, P.K., and Shimmen, T. (2000), The role of plant villin in the organization of the actin cytoskeleton, cytoplasmic streaming and the architecture of the transvacuolar strand in root hair cells of *Hydrocharis*, *Planta*, 210, 836–843.

Tonomura, Y. and Yoshimura, J. (1962), Binding of p-chloromercuribenzoate to actin, *J. Biochem.*, 51, 259–266.

Vahey, M., Titus, M., Trautwein, R., and Scordilis, S. (1982), Tomato actin and myosin: contractile proteins from a higher plant, *Cell Motil.*, 2, 131–147.

Vidali, L., Yokota, E., Cheung, A.Y., Shimmen, T., and Hepler, P.K. (1999), The 135 kDa actin-bundling protein from *Lilium longiflorum* pollen is the plant homologue of villin, *Protoplasma*, 209, 283–291.

Wieland, T. and Faulstich, H. (1978), Amatoxins, phallotoxins, phalloidin, and antamanide: the biologically active components of poisonous *Amanita* mushrooms, *CRC Crit. Rev. Biochem.*, 5, 185–260.

Williamson, R.E. (1972), A light-microscope study of the action of cytochalasin B on the cells and isolated cytoplasm of the Characeae, *J. Cell Sci.*, 10, 811–819.

Williamson, R.E. (1974), Actin in the alga, *Chara corallina*, *Nature*, 248, 801–802.

Williamson, R.E. (1975), Cytoplasmic streaming in *Chara*: a cell model activated by ATP and inhibited by cytochalasin B, *J. Cell Sci.*, 17, 655–668.

Williamson, R.E. (1976), Cytoplasmic streaming in charecean algae, in *Transport and Transfer Processes in Plants*, Wardlaw, I.F. and Passioura, J.B., Eds., Academic Press, New York, pp. 51–58.

Williamson, R.E. (1979), Filaments associated with the endoplasmic reticulum in the streaming cytoplasm of *Chara corallina*, *Eur. J. Cell Biol.*, 20, 177–183.

Williamson, R.E. and Ashley, C.C. (1982), Free Ca^{2+} and cytoplasmic streaming in the alga *Chara*, *Nature*, 296, 647–651.

Yamaguchi, M., Nakamura, T., and Sekine, T. (1973), Studies on the fast reacting sulfihydryl group of skeletal myosin A: conversion of smooth muscle myosin type with N-ethyl-maleimide treatment, *Biochim. Biophys. Acta*, 328, 154–165.

Yamamoto, K., Kikuyama, M., Sutoh-Yamamoto, N., and Kamitsubo, E. (1994), Purification of actin based motor protein from *Chara corallina*, *Proc. Jpn. Acad. Ser. B*, 70, 175–180.

Yamamoto, K., Kikuyama, M., Sutoh-Yamamoto, N., Kamitsubo, E., and Katayama, E. (1995), Myosin from alga *Chara*: unique structure revealed by electron microscopy, *J. Mol. Biol.*, 254, 109–112.

Yokota, E. and Shimmen, T. (1994), Isolation and characterization of plant myosin from pollen tubes of lily, *Protoplasma*, 177, 153–162.

Yokota, E. and Shimmen, T. (1999), The 135-kDa actin-bundling protein from lily pollen tubes arranges F-actin into bundles with uniform polarity, *Planta*, 209, 264–266.

Yokota, E., McDonald, A.R., Liu, B., Shimmen, T., and Palevitz, B.A. (1995a), Localization of a 170 kDa myosin heavy chain in plant cells, *Protoplasma*, 185, 178–187.

Yokota, E., Mimura, T., and Shimmen, T. (1995b), Biochemical, immunochemical and immuno-histochemical identification of myosin heavy chains in cultured cells of *Catharanthus roseus*, *Plant Cell Physiol.*, 36, 1541–1547.

Yokota, E., Takahara, K., and Shimmen, T. (1998), Actin-bundling protein isolated from pollen tubes of lily: biochemical and immunocytochemical characterization, *Plant Physiol.*, 116, 1421–1429.

Yokota, E., Muto, S., and Shimmen, T. (1999a), Inhibitory regulation of higher-plant myosin by Ca^{2+} ions, *Plant Physiol.*, 119, 231–239.

Yokota, E., Yukawa, C., Muto, S., Sonobe, S., and Shimmen, T. (1999b), Biochemical and immunocytochemical characterization of two types of myosins in cultured tobacco bright yellow-2 cells, *Plant. Physiol.*, 121, 525–534.

Yokota, E., Muto, S., and Shimmen, T. (2000), Calcium-calmodulin suppresses the filamentous actin-binding activity of a 135-kilodalton actin-bundling protein isolated from lily pollen tubes, *Plant Physiol.*, 123, 645–654.

Yokota, E., Sonobe, S., Orii, F., Yuasa, T., Inada, S., and Shimmen, T. (2001), The type and the localization of 175-kDa myosin in tobacco cultured cells BY-2, *J. Plant Res.*, 114, 115–116.

Yokota, E., Vidali, L., Tominaga, M., Tahara, H., Orii, H., Morizane, Y., Hepler, P.K., and Shimmen, T. (2003), Plant 115-kDa actin–filament bundling protein, P-115-ABP, is a homologue of plant villin and is widely distributed in cells, *Plant Cell Physiol.*, 44, 1008–1099.

6 Natural Polymer Gels with Fast Responses

Namjin Baek and Kinam Park

CONTENTS

INTRODUCTION

Hydrogels that are sensitive to environmental stimuli have been extensively studied during the last two decades. Environmental stimuli include temperature, pH, light, electric signal, salt, organic solvent, and biomolecules such as glucose and proteins.[1-3] Although stimuli-sensitive hydrogels have potential applications in the fields of biomaterials and drug delivery systems, their use is limited because of slow responses to stimuli.[1] For purposes of practical applications, their response times must be faster than those of currently available systems.

Nature has developed a large number of well-organized polymeric systems composed of simple components: proteins, lipids, and carbohydrates. Some systems exhibit very fast responsiveness to external stimuli signals. It is believed that understanding the natural fast responsive systems is the first step in developing instantaneously responsive polymeric systems.

Examples of fast responsive natural systems are sol–gel transition in non-muscle cells,[4] contraction–relaxation of skeletal muscle cells,[5] rapid bending of *Mimosa* leaves,[4-6] contraction–expansion of spasmoneme in stalked protists,[7,8] and stopcocks in legume sieve tubes.[9] In these systems, the stimuli-induced responses are all reversible. Physiological significances, morphological characteristics, and possible mechanisms of these systems are reviewed here in order to explain them and apply them to artificial systems.

0-8493-1487-9/04/$0.00+$1.50
© 2004 by CRC Press LLC

EXAMPLES OF NATURAL SYSTEMS SHOWING FAST RESPONSES

MOVEMENT OF NONMUSCLE CELLS

To achieve movement, cells change their shapes and directions continuously, depending on signals they receive from their environment. Migrating cells are able to respond rapidly to environmental stimuli. Amoebae use cellular migration to find food; fibroblasts use it for wound healing; leukocytes utilize it in chemotactic responses to immune reactions. Pseudopods or lamellipods, which are dense networks of actin filaments, are extended over surfaces from the leading edges of free-living migrating *Amoeba proteus* cells and other cells such as fibroblasts and leukocytes.[5]

The actin filament network should be reversibly dismantled to allow protrusion and then reassembled to stabilize the extensions of pseudopods or lamellipods.[4] Thus, rapid sol–gel transitions of the actin filament network are required for the movement of many animal cells.

As shown in Figure 6.1, actin filament dynamics are regulated by WASp/Scar proteins and Arp2/3 complexes.[10,11] External stimuli signals are transmitted via receptors and multiple signal transduction pathways, and WASp/Scar proteins further integrate the signals. The defect in WASp results in Wiskott–Aldrich syndrome, a condition caused by the deficiencies in the actin cytoskeletons of platelets and leukocytes.

WASp/Scar proteins have multiple domains: (1) a WH2 domain that binds actin monomers, (2) an A domain that interacts with the ARPC3 subunit of the Arp2/3 complex, and (3) a proline-rich domain that binds profilin, an actin-binding protein. The C-terminal A domains of WASp/Scar proteins activate Arp2/3 complexes by interacting with ARPC3 subunits to promote nucleation of actin filaments using

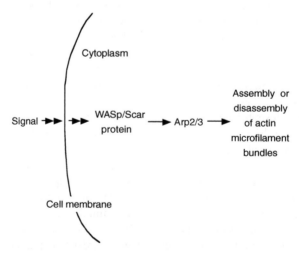

FIGURE 6.1 Transmission of extracellular signal for cell movement. Sensed signals induce assembly or disassembly of actin microfilament networks for gel–sol transitions in pseudopods and lamellipods of nonmuscle cells.

globular actin (G-actin) monomers. the Arp2/3 complex also promotes branching of actin filaments by interaction with them. Thereafter, the length of actin filaments (F-actins) increases as G-actins self-assemble at the ends of F-actins.[5] The elongation rate of an actin filament is 0.3 to 3 μm/sec.[10] In addition, with the help of actin-binding proteins such as fimbrin and α-actinin, parallel arrays of cross-linked actin filament bundles are also formed.[5]

The actin network disassembles by the action of gelsolin, a compound that has the functions of severing and capping actin filaments.[12] Severing is breaking an actin filament in two by weakening the noncovalent bonds between actin molecules within a filament; this is thought to be important for disassembling the actin network. The activity of gelsolin is regulated by Ca^{2+} and polyphosphoinositide 4,5-biphosphate (PIP_2). The molecular structure of gelsolin has been recently uncovered.[13] It has two Ca^{2+} binding sites shared with actin (type 1), and six Ca^{2+} binding sites wholly contained within gelsolin (type 2). Ca^{2+} binding to the type 2 sites facilitates the conformation change of gelsolin; thus, the severing function of gelsolin is activated. After severing, gelsolin remains attached to the filament as a cap. Detaching (uncapping) of gelsolin from filaments produces ends that can continue actin polymerization.

Hydrogels Prepared with Components of Cellular Motility

Formation of the actin filament network is a highly coordinated process using many proteins and factors. Efforts have been made to prepare gels using certain components involved in cellular and cytoplasmic movements. Nunnally et al. observed the formation of filamentous actin (F-actin) gel in the presence of filamin in vitro.[14] Polymerization of rabbit skeletal muscle actin was initiated by adjusting the KCl concentration to 50 mM. Filamin is a homodimer that holds two crossing actin filaments together,[5] thus working as a cross-linking point in the F-actin/filamin gel. The apparent viscosity of the gel is dependent on the concentration of filamin.

Gelsolin provided Ca^{2+} sensitivity to the F-actin/filamin hydrogel.[15] A hydrogel composed of F-actin was prepared in the presence of filamin and gelsolin. The addition of calcium inhibited gelation and also caused solation of existing gels. The gelation inhibitory activity of gelsolin was dependent on Ca^{2+} concentration (Figure 6.2). At 0.01 μM Ca^{2+}, gelsolin did not inhibit gelation of F-actin. Between 0.01 and 0.2 μM Ca^{2+}, gelsolin partially inhibited gelation. Gelation of F-actin was completely inhibited at >0.2 μM Ca^{2+}. Removal of free calcium by the addition of ethyleneglycoltetraacetate (EGTA) restored gelation properties of the mixture. Gelsolin, which has the capability to break actin filaments, is the key protein involved in this calcium-dependent gel–sol transition property. Although kinetics data were not presented, gelation or solation, depending on Ca^{2+} concentration, is expected to occur very fast since Ca^{2+} can diffuse quickly.

The presence of actinogelin also provided Ca^{2+}-sensitive solation of F-actin hydrogel,[16] similar to gelsolin-mediated F-actin solation, but did not require the presence of filamin to form a hydrogel. Solation of the F-actin gel was dependent on Ca^{2+} concentration, but the Ca^{2+} concentration for inhibiting gelation was about 10 times higher than that in gelsolin-mediated calcium sensitivity of the F-actin/filamin hydrogel. It is not clear how calcium binding induces the conformational

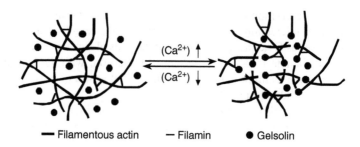

— Filamentous actin   — Filamin   ● Gelsolin

FIGURE 6.2 Ca^{2+}-sensitive gel–sol transition of filamentous actin (F-actin)/filamin hydrogel in the presence of gelsolin.

change in actinogelin that may lead to solation of the F-actin gel. Actinogelin belongs to the α-actinin superfamily of proteins because of similarity in amino acid composition, subunit and domain structures, and binding sites on actin.[17]

SKELETAL MUSCLE CELLS

Muscle is the best-understood and the most highly specialized example of actin-based motility.[5] Thus, we will briefly describe the mechanism of muscle contraction in this section. Skeletal muscle is composed of long thin muscle fibers, which are large single cells. Myofibrils, the contractile elements, fill the cytoplasms of those cells. Each myofibril consists of 2.2-μm long sarcomeres composed of thin actin filaments attached to Z-discs and thick myosin filaments.

When a signal is received from a motor nerve, the action potential in the muscle cell membrane is relayed and triggers the transient release of Ca^{2+} from the sarcoplasmic reticulum, and the cytoplasmic Ca^{2+} molecules are pumped back to the sarcoplasmic reticulum. The increase in cytosolic Ca^{2+} induces the sliding of thick myosin filaments toward thin actin filaments, which is the contraction of myofibrils. Energy obtained by ATP hydrolysis is used during the movement of myosin filaments. As soon as Ca^{2+} concentration returns to the normal level, the myofibrils relax. The process of myofibril contraction and relaxation occurs in less than 100 milliseconds (ms).

The instantaneous muscle contraction in response to a nerve signal is a combined result of energy-driven movements of myosin filaments within the sarcomere, the ability to control the transient release of Ca^{2+} into cytosols, and the highly coordinated behavior of many repeating units (sarcomeres).

SENSITIVE PLANTS: *MIMOSA PUDICA*

Although plants do not show dynamic responses to stimuli as animals do, rapid macroscopic movements of plants induced by localized mechanical stimuli are observed in *Mimosa pudica* and other insectivorous genera such as *Drosera, Dionaea, Aldrovanda,* and *Utricularia.*[18,19] Among those plants that show rapid stimuli-sensitive movements, *M. pudica* is the most studied. Figure 6.3 shows the general appearance of *M. pudica.*[6] The primary pulvinus is the joint between the stem and

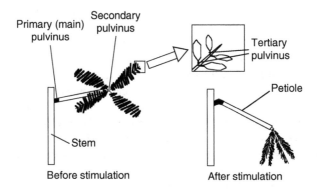

FIGURE 6.3 Parts of *Mimosa pudica* and its motor organs before and after stimulation.

petiole, and the secondary pulvinus is the junction between the petiole and a compound leaf. The tertiary pulvinus is the joint between the raiches and leaflets in a compound leaf. The pulvinus is the motor organ.

When mechanical stimuli are applied to *M. pudica* by hard shaking of the plant or a leaf, leaves show bending movements in pulvini, which are characterized by closing of leaflets, movement of four leaves together, and downward drooping of petioles.[6] The response to stimuli occurs within seconds, and the bent leaves recover slowly to their original status (about 30 min).

The mechanism of *M. pudica* bending has been studied by many researchers. The response of *M. pudica* to mechanical stimulation consists of three steps: (1) perception of stimulus, (2) transmission of the signal to the motor organ (pulvinus), and (3) induction of movement in motor cells.[20] No differentiated receptor tissue has yet to be found in *M. pudica*. Two action potentials are involved in bending of the primary pulvinus.[19] The signal perceived is transmitted via action potential from the stimulated site (petiole) to the motor organ (primary pulvinus). This petiolar action potential propagates through excitable cells in the vascular bundles at the rate of 2 to 3 cm/sec. Once petiolar action potential arrives at the primary pulvinus, it triggers a pulvinar action potential. In addition, the pulvinar action potential is induced after the stimulation. The leaf bending occurs 0.02 sec after the pulvinar action potential.[21]

It has been proposed that, upon action potential-induced Ca^{2+} release in motor cells, the rapid contraction of the cytoplasmic fibrillar network induces the expulsion of water and K^+ from cells.[19] Treatments with cytochalasin B and phalloidin, which affect actin filaments, inhibit the rapid bending movement of *M. pudica*,[22] suggesting that fibrils composed of microfilaments may be involved in the rapid leaf bending.

Sibaoka proposed that the pressure inside the motor cell, instead of the contraction of the fibrillar network, is the direct driving force.[19] Previous studies revealed that the rapid bending of the primary pulvinus is caused by loss of turgor pressure in the cells of the lower half. Upon stimulation of the pulvini, large effluxes of K^+ and Cl^- were observed in the excited cells. The migration of these ions resulted in loss of turgor pressure — a large positive internal pressure built up in the cells due to high contents of solutes. After rapid bending, the contents of K^+, Cl^-, and water in the lower half motor cells were decreased. The efflux of water was indicated by the presence of extracellular stained granular contents contained in the central vacuoles of the motor cells of the primary pulvinus before the rapid bending. The pressure inside the cells is supposed to be the driving force for the outward flow of vacuolar sap through pores in the membrane. The removal of water from the lower half motor cells resulted in a marked decrease in cell volume in the lower half cortex. The wall of the upper half cortex cells is three times thicker than that of the lower half of the primary pulvinus. Thus, the structural characteristic of the primary pulvinus plays an important role in rapid bending of *M. pudica* leaves.

Recent studies suggest that actin filaments may be disassembled before the water efflux. A gelsolin/fragmin family protein that can sever the actin microfilaments was identified in *M. pudica*.[23] Actin microfilaments were found in the cytoplasms of the motor cells[22] and actin filaments in the motor cells of the lower half pulvinus become more peripheral after bending.[24] The activity of gelsolin is regulated by the cytosolic concentration of Ca^{2+}.[12] The dependence of leaf bending movement on Ca^{2+} was also observed.[25] Treatments of excised leaves with 0.02 M lanthanum (La^{3+}), a Ca^{2+}-mimicking molecule that does not penetrate the plasma membrane, or ethylenediaminetetraacetate (EDTA) for 1.5 h inhibited rapid movements of the leaves.

The above results suggest that gelsolin activated by the increased cytoplasmic Ca^{2+} concentration upon stimulation may cut microfilaments into fragments during the leaf bending movement. This may result in easier collapse of the motor cells when turgor pressure is lost or it may increase the permeability of the plasma membrane.

Once leaves bend, the intracellular K^+ and Cl^- concentrations will be restored by the action of H^+/ATPase present in the plasma membranes of the motor cells of the pulvini.[26] K^+ and Cl^- ions are actively cotransported with H^+ by the enzyme; this will restore the turgor pressure in the lower half of the motor cells. Intracellular Ca^{2+} concentration is also likely to be reduced, which will be helpful in restoring the microfilaments in the cells. As a result, leaves will recover to the initial state before the stimulation.

SPASMONEME IN STALKED PROTISTS

Rapid stalk contraction is observed in stalked peritrichous ciliates of the family *Vorticellidae*, which includes *Vorticella convallaria*, *Zoothamnium geniculatum*, and *Carchesium polypinum*.[7] The contraction movement in this family is very unique, because it is dependent on Ca^{2+} but unlike skeletal muscle contraction does not require ATP as an energy source. Figure 6.4 is a schematic diagram of *Vorticella convallaria* showing contraction and extension of spasmoneme.

The cellular body of a vorticellid is normally attached to a solid support by a long slender stalk composed of spasmoneme, which is an intracellular contractile fibrous organelle, and a surrounding sheath.[7] The diameter of spasmoneme in *Vorticella*, which is a single cell organism, is about 1 μm,[7] and the length is about 100 μm.[27] Multicellular organisms, *Carchesium* and *Zoothamnium*, have main stalks of colonies with diameters of 10 and 30 μm, respectively. The main stalk length of *Zoothamnium* is larger than 1 mm.[7] The small branches to which single cells attach

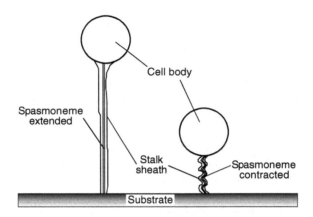

FIGURE 6.4 *Vorticella* attached to a substrate via stalk. Spasmoneme inside the stalk extends or contracts reversibly.

are smaller than 1 μm in diameter. Although a stalk is attached to a cellular body, it still contains cell cytoplasm. According to transmission electron microscopy, the stalk sheath of *V. convallaria* consists of a clearly defined outer layer and a less distinct inner layer.[28] When a stalked cell is exposed to harsh environmental conditions or damaged, it detaches from the stalk by violent twisting of the cell body relative to the stalk. The detached cell or telotroch moves around to find other places with suitable growth conditions.[29] Once the telotroch is attached to an appropriate surface, the stalk elongates.

Both the cell body and stalk of *Vorticella* contracted in response to being touched mechanically.[8] The touching of the cell body or stalk with a microneedle resulted in contractions of both. However, when a site between the stalk and the cell body was clamped, hitting the stalk did not induce a contraction, suggesting that the contraction that occurred upon hitting the stalk was through the transfer of a mechanical signal to the cell body. Thus, the cell body senses the initial signal, and the stalk contraction follows.

The cellular contraction and membrane depolarization of a single *V. convallaria* cell induced by a mechanical stimulus were simultaneously recorded using electrophysiological techniques.[30] The onset of membrane depolarization was observed 2.3 ms after the onset of cellular contraction. Thus, cellular contraction may trigger mechanosensitive ion channels in the cell membrane that produce membrane depolarization. Cytosolic Ca^{2+} is an important factor in stalk contraction. The extension and contraction of the stalks were repeated when the stalks were treated alternately with 0.01 and 1 μM of Ca^{2+} solutions.[31] Stalk contraction was dependent on Ca^{2+} concentration.

A mechanical stimulus applied to a cell body induced an increase in cytosolic Ca^{2+} concentration.[32] The onset of a transient cytosolic Ca^{2+} increase appeared 43 ms after stimulation in the absence of extracellular Ca^{2+} in the medium. Thus, a transient Ca^{2+} increase may be due to the release of Ca^{2+} from intracellular Ca^{2+} storage sites. The above results suggest that a mechanical stimulus triggers cellular contraction followed by membrane depolarization and a transient intracellular Ca^{2+} spike. The

Ca^{2+} spike induces the contraction of the stalk. The spontaneous contraction of the stalk was as fast as 8.8 cm/sec, according to microscopic images captured with a high-speed video system.[27] The stalk contraction takes only 9 ms,[27] while stalk extension takes several seconds.[7]

The contraction of the stalk in response to high Ca^{2+} concentration is entirely due to the contraction of spasmoneme. Spasmin, a member of a calcium-binding protein family, was isolated from the spasmoneme of *Carchesium polypinum*.[33] The presence of other proteins that can bind to spasmin was suggested because the combined mixture of spasmin and another fraction resulted in higher fluorescence of a fluorescent dye, 2-p-toluidinylnaphthalene-6-sulfonate (TNS). TNS fluorescence increases when the hydrophobicity of protein is increased by the binding of Ca^{2+} to spasmin.

The spasmin gene from *Vorticella* was also cloned and expressed in *E. coli*.[34] The electrophoretic mobility of the recombinant spasmin protein decreased in the presence of Ca^{2+}, which suggests that recombinant spasmin can bind Ca^{2+}. According to sequence comparison with centrin proteins that have Ca^{2+}-binding capability, spasmin from *Vorticella* was shown to have two Ca^{2+} binding sites.

Moriyama et al. measured the volume change of the main stalk spasmoneme from *Zoothamnium* under zero tension.[35] As shown in Figure 6.5, both the length and diameter of the spasmoneme decreased to about 50% of initial values. The volume of contracted spasmoneme was only 14% of the initial volume. By analyzing tension-extension curves and applying the rubber-like elasticity theory, it was found that the interchain cross-links of chains were not influenced by the addition or removal of Ca^{2+}. Since Ca^{2+} binding to spasmin increases the hydrophobicity of the spasmin-Ca^{2+} complex,[33] it may promote the hydrophobic interactions between spasmin-Ca^{2+} complexes in the spasmoneme. Considering the volume reduction of spasmoneme upon contraction and increasing hydrophobicity of spasmin upon binding to Ca^{2+}, the intramolecular folding and unfolding of spasmin in response to Ca^{2+} binding and detaching were suggested as the contractile and extension mechanisms of spasmoneme,[35] although the exact molecular mechanism is not clear yet. Possibly, folding and unfolding may occur in other proteins whose conformational changes are regulated by spasmin.[35]

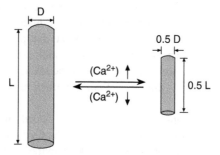

FIGURE 6.5 Reversible changes in dimensions of *Zoothamnium* spasmoneme upon changes in Ca^{2+} concentration. L = length; D = diameter.

STOPCOCKS IN LEGUME SIEVE TUBES

Very recently, a reversible rapid change of volume by a proteinaceous body was found in legume sieve tubes.[9] The long-distance transport of photoassimilated products in higher plants occurs through the sieve tubes, which are longitudinal arrays of sieve elements. Morphological change of phloem-specific protein (P-protein) crystalloids was studied in living sieve elements in the central veins of fully grown broad bean (*Vicia faba*) leaves. P-protein crystalloids are up to 30 μm long and 2 to 6 μm wide, and are located near the sieve plates on the lower ends of the sieve tube elements. Confocal laser scanning microscopy allowed visualization of the structures of undamaged sieve elements that are very sensitive to any kind of manipulation.[36] Sieve elements were stained by a fluorescent dye, 5(6)carboxyfluorescein diacetate.

It was suggested that a Ca^{2+} spike can cause crystalloid expansion.[9] Upon insertion of a micropipette (>2 μm in diameter) into a sieve element, the elongated crystalloid structure was transformed into a roundish plug that blocked the sieve element within a few seconds. Micropipette insertion may have caused leakage in the cell membrane, resulting in an increase in intracellular Ca^{2+} concentration. The incubation medium contained 10 mM Ca^{2+}. The expansion of the crystalloid was observed even in a Ca^{2+}-free medium and was due to endogenous Ca^{2+} that originated from the cell wall. However, the presence of Ca^{2+} chelators, EDTA or EGTA, at concentrations greater than 1 mM in a Ca^{2+}-free medium did not induce the expansion of P-protein crystalloids.

P-protein crystalloids can expand or contract reversibly, depending upon the Ca^{2+} concentration.[9] The addition of excess Ca^{2+} (12 mM) to chelator-containing media always induced rapid expansion of crystalloids. In addition, when the medium was changed to 10 mM Ca^{2+} or 10 mM EDTA, crystalloids instantly expanded or contracted (Figure 6.6).

Elongated crystalline P-proteins are found in Fabaceae, such as *Phaseolus vulgaris* and *Lupinus polyphyllos*. P-protein crystalloids from those organisms were shown

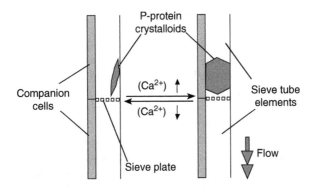

FIGURE 6.6 Longitudinal section of sieve tube element/companion cell complexes in *Vicia faba*. P-protein crystalloids in the sieve tubes are compressed or expanded, depending upon the concentration of calcium.

TABLE 6.1
Fast Responsive Biological Systems

Systems	Signal Mediator	Transition Induced	Response Time	Acting Components
Nonmuscle cell	Ca^{2+}	Solation/gelation	—	Actin microfilament
Skeletal muscle cell	Ca^{2+}	Contraction/relaxation	<0.1 sec	Actin, myosin bundles
Mimosa plant	Ca^{2+}	Folding/unfolding	<2 sec	Cortex cells
Vorticella stalk	Ca^{2+}	Contraction/extension	0.01 sec	Spasmin in spasmoneme
Legume sieve tubes	Ca^{2+}	Expansion/contraction	1–3 sec	P-protein crystalloids

to expand upon micropipette insertion. The expansion of crystalloids completely blocks the sieve tube, and this may prevent the loss of sieve tube contents in case of disturbance.[9] There is no information about how a change in Ca^{2+} concentration induces expansion or contraction of P-protein crystalloids. Further biochemical and structural characterization of P-protein crystalloids would help reveal the mechanism of reversible crystalloid expansion and contraction.

CONCLUDING REMARKS

Five different biological systems that show fast responsive transitions in response to stimuli signals were reviewed. The dimensions of the system and system components are the most important factors in fast responsiveness. As a system becomes smaller, a faster response is obtained. Some systems (sol–gel transition in nonmuscle cells, spasmoneme, P-protein crystalloids) are subcellular, which would enable them to show fast responses to signals. The responses occur within a few seconds after the Ca^{2+} signal. Even macrosystems, such as skeletal muscle cells and sensitive plants such as *Mimosa,* show fast responsiveness due to highly coordinated actions of many cells.

All the five systems reviewed here use Ca^{2+} as a signal-mediating molecule for the transition. It is notable that the same Ca^{2+} signal produces various kinds of responses (Table 6.1). For example, spasmoneme and P-protein crystalloids show opposite responses upon changes in Ca^{2+} concentrations. The production of different responses to the same signaling molecule is entirely due to differences in components of a system. Thus, it is very important in designing new artificial fast responsive systems to understand how the components work together.

Although we have a good understanding of the molecular mechanisms, the whole picture for many systems is not yet clear. Advances in molecular biological and other techniques will provide more detailed knowledge on the structural interactions of components involved in fast responses and help us understand the molecular mechanisms of natural fast responsive systems in the near future.

REFERENCES

1. Y. Qiu and K. Park, Environment-sensitive hydrogels for drug delivery, *Adv. Drug Delivery Rev.*, 54, 321–339, 2002.
2. A. Kikuchi and T. Okano, Pulsatile drug release control using hydrogels, *Adv. Drug Delivery Rev.*, 54, 53–77, 2002.
3. T. Miyata, T. Uragami, and K. Nakamae, Biomolecule-sensitive hydrogels, *Adv. Drug Delivery Rev.*, 54, 79–98, 2002.
4. J.F.V. Vincent, Actuating systems in biology, in *Polymer Sensors and Actuators*, Y. Osada and D.E. De Rossi, Eds., Springer-Verlag, New York, 2000, pp. 371–383.
5. B. Alberts, D. Bray, J. Lewis, M. Raff, K. Roberts, and J.D. Watson, *Molecular Biology of the Cell*, Garland Publishing, New York, 1994.
6. G. Roblin, *Mimosa pudica*: a model for the study of excitability in plants, *Biol. Rev.*, 54, 135–153, 1979.
7. W.B. Amos, Contraction and calcium binding in the Vorticellid ciliates, in *Molecules and Cell Movement*, S. Inoué and R.E. Stephens, Eds., Raven Press, New York, 1975, pp. 411–436.
8. K. Katoh and Y. Naitoh, A mechanosensory mechanism for evoking cellular contraction in *Vorticella*, *J. Exp. Biol.*, 168, 253–267, 1992.
9. M. Knoblauch, W.S. Peters, K. Ehlers, and A.J.E. van Bel, Reversible calcium-regulated stopcocks in legume sieve tubes, *Plant Cell*, 13, 1221–1230, 2001.
10. T.D. Pollard, L. Blanchoin, and R.D. Mullins, Molecular mechanisms controlling actin filament dynamics in nonmuscle cells, *Annu. Rev. Biophys. Biomol. Struct.*, 29, 545–576, 2000.
11. H.N. Higgs and T.D. Pollard, Regulation of actin filament network formation through Arp2/3 complex: activation by a diverse array of proteins, *Annu. Rev. Biochem.*, 70, 649–676, 2001.
12. H.Q. Sun, M. Yamamoto, M. Mejillano, and H.L. Yin, Gelsolin: a multifunctional actin regulatory protein, *J. Biol. Chem.*, 274, 33179–33182, 1999.
13. H. Choe, L.D. Burtnick, M. Mejillano, H.L. Yin, R.C. Robinson, and S. Choe, The calcium activation of gelsolin: insights from the 3 Å structure of the G4-G6/actin complex, *J. Mol. Biol.*, 324, 691–702, 2002.
14. M.H. Nunnally, L.D. Powell, and S.W. Craig, Reconstitution and regulation of actin gel–sol transformation with purified filamin and villin, *J. Biol. Chem.*, 256, 2083–2086, 1981.
15. H.L. Yin and T.P. Stossel, Control of cytoplasmic actin gel–sol transformation by gelsolin, a calcium-dependent regulatory protein, *Nature*, 281, 583–586, 1979.
16. N. Mimura and A. Asano, Ca^{2+}-sensitive gelation of actin filaments by a new protein factor, *Nature*, 282, 44–48, 1979.
17. S. Tsukita, N. Mimura, S. Tsukita, K. Khono, T. Ohtaki, T. Oshmia, H. Ishikawa, and A. Asano, Characteristic structures of actin gels induced with hepatic actinogelin or with chicken gizzard alpha-actinin: implication for their function, *Cell Motil. Cytoskeleton*, 10, 451–463, 1988.
18. M. Malone, Rapid, long-distance signal transmission in higher plants, in *Advances in Botanical Research*, Vol. 22, J.A. Callow, Ed., Academic Press, New York, 1996, pp. 163–228.
19. T. Sibaoka, Rapid plant movements triggered by action potentials, *Bot. Mag. Tokyo*, 104, 73–95, 1991.

20. T. Shimmen, Involvement of receptor potentials and action potentials in mechano-reception in plants, *Austr. J. Plant Physiol.,* 28, 567–576, 2001.

21. K. Oda and T. Abe, Action potential and rapid movement in the main pulvinus of *Mimosa pudica, Bot. Mag. Tokyo,* 85, 135–145, 1972.

22. P. Fleurat-Lessard, G. Roblin, J. Bonmort, and C. Besse, Effects of colchicine, vinblastine, cytochalasin B and phalloidin on the seismonastic movement of *Mimosa pudica* leaf and on motor cell ultrastructure, *J. Exp. Bot.,* 39, 209–221, 1988.

23. S. Yamashiro, K. Kameyama, N. Kanzawa, T. Tamiya, I. Mabuchi, and T. Tsuchiya, The gelsolin/fragmin family protein identified in the higher plant *Mimosa pudica, J. Biochem.,* 130, 243–249, 2001.

24. K. Kameyama, Y. Kishi, M. Yoshimura, N. Kanzawa, M. Sameshima, and T. Tsuchiya, Tyrosine phosphorylation in plant bending, *Nature,* 407, 37, 2000.

25. N.A. Campbell and W.W. Thomson, Effects of lanthanum and ethylenediaminetet-raacetate on leaf movements of *Mimosa, Plant Physiol.,* 60, 635–639, 1977.

26. P. Fleurat-Lessard, S. Bouché-Pillon, C. Leloup, and J.-L. Bonnemain, Distribution and activity of the plasma membrane H^+-ATPase in *Mimosa pudica* L. in relation to ionic fluxes and leaf movements, *Plant Physiol.,* 113, 747–754, 1997.

27. Y. Moriyama, S. Hiyama, and H. Asai, High-speed video cinematographic demonstration of stalk and zooid contraction of *Vorticella convallaria, Biophys. J.,* 74, 487–491, 1998.

28. R. Wibel, E.J. Vacchiano, J.J. Maciejewski, H.E.J. Buhse, and J. Clamp, The fine structure of the scopula-stalk region of *Vorticella convallaria, J. Biol. Chem.,* 44, 457–466, 1997.

29. E.J. Vacchiano, A. Dreisbach, D. Locascio, L. Castaneda, T. Vivian, and H.E.J. Buhse, Morphogenetic transitions and cytoskeletal elements of the stalked zooid and the telotroch stages in the peritrich ciliate *Vorticella convallaria, J. Protozool.,* 39, 101–106, 1992.

30. H. Shiono and Y. Naitoh, Cellular contraction precedes membrane depolarization in *Vorticella convallaria, J. Exp. Biol.,* 200, 2249–2261, 1997.

31. W.B. Amos, Reversible mechanochemical cycle in the contraction of *Vorticella, Nature,* 229, 127–128, 1971.

32. K. Katoh and M. Kikuyama, An all-or-nothing rise in cytosolic $[Ca^{2+}]$ in *Vorticella* sp., *J. Exp. Biol.,* 200, 35–40, 1997.

33. H. Asai, T. Ninomiya, R.-I. Kono, and Y. Moriyama, Spasmin and putative spasmin binding protein(s) isolated from solubilized spasmonemes, *J. Eukaryotic Microbiol.,* 45, 33–39, 1998.

34. J.J. Maciejewski, E.J. Vacchiano, S.M. McCutcheon, and H.E.J. Buhse, Cloning and expression of a cDNA encoding a *Vorticella convallaria* spasmin: an EF-hand calcium-binding protein, *J. Eukaryotic Microbiol.,* 46, 165–173, 1999.

35. Y. Moriyama, H. Okamoto, and H. Asai, Rubber-like elasticity and volume changes in the isolated spasmoneme of giant *Zoothamnium* sp. under Ca^{2+}-induced contraction, *Biophys. J.,* 76, 993–1000, 1999.

36. M. Knoblauch and A.J.E. van Bel, Sieve tubes in action. *Plant Cell,* 10, 35–50, 1998.

Section II

Theoretical Considerations

7 Kinetics of Smart Hydrogels

Nicholas A. Peppas

CONTENTS

HYDROGELS

It is well known that hydrogels are three-dimensional hydrophilic polymer networks able to imbibe large amounts of water.[1-2] The networks are composed of homopolymers or copolymers and are insoluble due to the presence of chemical or physical crosslinks. The physical crosslinks can be entanglements, crystallites,[3-8] or weak associations such as van der Waals forces or hydrogen bonds.[9-13] The crosslinks provide the network structure and physical integrity. Their thermodynamic compatibility with water allows the network to swell in aqueous media.[1,2,14-16]

Hydrogels can be classified as neutral or ionic, based on the natures of their side groups. Based on the physical structures of their networks, they can be amorphous, semicrystalline, hydrogen-bonded, or supermolecular structures or hydrocolloid aggregates.[1-13]

Another general category of hydrogels is composed of physiologically responsive hydrogels.[17] Their polymer complexes can be broken or their networks can be swollen as a result of changing external environment. These systems tend to show drastic changes in their swelling ratios as a result. Some of the factors affecting the swelling of physiologically responsive hydrogels include pH, ionic strength, temperature, and electromagnetic radiation.[17]

Environmentally sensitive hydrogels have the ability to respond to changes in their external environment. These polymers can exhibit dramatic changes in their swelling behavior, network structure, permeability, or mechanical strength in response to changes in the pH or ionic strength of the surrounding fluid or temperature. Other hydrogels have the ability to respond to applied magnetic fields. Additionally, some hydrogels can respond to changes in concentrations of glucose.[17] Because of their natures, these materials can be used in a wide variety of applications such as separation membranes, biosensors, artificial muscles, chemical valves, superabsorbents, and drug delivery devices.[17]

One particular class of physiologically responsive hydrogels is dependent on pH and ionic strength. Hydrogels that exhibit pH-dependent swelling behavior are swollen from ionic networks. These ionic networks contain either acidic or basic pendant groups.[18–29] As a result of the electrostatic repulsions, the uptake of water in the network will be increased.[18–29]

Ionic hydrogels are swollen polymer networks containing ionic moieties that show sudden or gradual changes in their dynamic and equilibrium swelling behaviors as a result of changing the external pH. Anionic materials contain pendant groups such as carboxylic acid or sulfonic acid. In these gels, ionization occurs when the pH of the environment is above the pK_a of the ionizable group.[18–32] As the degree of ionization increases (increased system pH), the number of fixed charges increases, resulting in increased electrostatic repulsions between the chains. This, in turn, results in an increased hydrophilicity of the network and greater swelling ratios. Conversely, cationic materials contain pendant groups such as amines.[25–35] These groups ionize in media at pH levels below the pK_b values of the ionizable species. Thus, in a low pH environment, ionization will increase, causing increased electrostatic repulsions. The hydrogel will become increasingly hydrophilic and will swell to an increased level

There are many advantages to using ionic materials over neutral networks. All ionic materials exhibit pH and ionic strength sensitivity. This characteristic can be exploited for applications in a wide variety of biomedical applications such as dental adhesives and restorations, controlled release devices, prodrugs and adjuvants, and biocompatible materials.[24] In addition, the swelling forces developed in these systems will be increased over the nonionic materials. This increase in swelling force is due to the localization of fixed charges on the pendant groups. As a result, anionic gels in media above their pK_a levels and cationic gels in media below their pK_b values reach degrees of swelling an order of magnitude higher than nonionic materials.

Here we discuss the fundamentals of the dynamic behavior of hydrogels due to changes in the surrounding environment. This is often known as the *kinetic behavior of gels* because the *kinetics* term is also used to describe dynamic transport processes.

SWELLING OF NEUTRAL HYDROGELS

It is well known that Flory and Rehner[14] developed the initial depiction of the swelling of crosslinked polymer gels using a Gaussian distribution of polymer chains. They developed a model to describe the equilibrium degree of crosslinked polymers postulating that the degree to which a polymer network swelled was governed by the elastic retractive forces of the polymer chains and the thermodynamic compatibility of the polymer and the water molecules. In terms of the free energy of the system, the total free energy change upon swelling can be described as:

$$\Delta G = \Delta G_{elastic} + \Delta G_{mix} \qquad (7.1)$$

where $\Delta G_{elastic}$ is the contribution due to the elastic retractive forces and ΔG_{mix} represents the thermodynamic compatibility of the polymer and the swelling agent.

Upon differentiation of Equation (7.1) with respect to the number of water molecules in the system at constant temperature (T) and pressure (P), an expression can be derived for the chemical potential change in the water in terms of the contributions due to swelling.

$$\mu_1 - \mu_{1,0} = \Delta\mu_{elastic} + \Delta\mu_{mix} \qquad (7.2)$$

where μ_1 is the chemical potential of the swelling agent within the gel and $\mu_{1,0}$ is the chemical potential of the pure fluid. At equilibrium, the chemical potential of the swelling agent inside and outside the gel must be equal; therefore, the elastic and mixing contributions to the chemical potential will balance one another at equilibrium.

The chemical potential change upon mixing can be determined from the heat of mixing and the entropy of mixing.[14–16] Using appropriate thermodynamic relationships, the chemical potential of mixing can be expressed as:

$$\Delta\mu_{mix} = RT\left(\ln(1-\upsilon_{2,s}) + \upsilon_{2,s} + \chi_1\upsilon_{2,s}\right) \qquad (7.3)$$

where $\upsilon_{2,s}$ is the volume fraction of the polymer in the gel and χ_1 is the polymer water interaction parameter.[14–16]

The elastic contribution to the chemical potential is determined from the statistical theory of rubber elasticity.[36] The elastic free energy depends on the number of polymer chains in the network and the linear expansion factor. For gels that are crosslinked in the absence of water, the elastic contribution to the chemical potential[14–16,36] is written as:

$$\Delta\mu_{elastic} = RT\left(\frac{V_1}{\upsilon \overline{M}_c}\right)\left(1 - \frac{2\overline{M}_c}{\overline{M}_n}\right)\left(\upsilon_{2,s}^{1/3} - \frac{\upsilon_{2,s}}{2}\right) \qquad (7.4)$$

where υ is the specific volume of the polymer, V_1 is the molar volume of the swelling agent, $\overline{M}_c$ is the molecular weight of the polymer chains between junction points, and $\overline{M}_n$ is the molecular weight of the polymer chains if no crosslinks had been introduced.

Equation (7.4) was developed for the case where the polymer chains had been crosslinked in the presence of the water. If they were, the elastic contributions must account for the volume fraction density of the chains during crosslinking.[3] For polymer gels crosslinked in the presence of water, the elastic contribution to the chemical potential is:

$$\Delta\mu_{elastic} = RT\left(\frac{V_1}{\upsilon\overline{M}_c}\right)\left(1 - \frac{2\overline{M}_c}{\overline{M}_n}\right)\upsilon_{2,r}\left(\left(\frac{\upsilon_{2,s}}{\upsilon_{2,r}}\right)^{1/3} - \frac{\upsilon_{2,s}}{2\upsilon_{2,r}}\right) \qquad (7.5)$$

where $\upsilon_{2,s}$ is the volume fraction of the polymer in the relaxed state. The relaxed state of the polymer is defined as occurring immediately after crosslinking of the polymer but prior to swelling or deswelling.

By combining Equations (7.3) and (7.4), the swelling behavior of neutral hydrogels crosslinked in the absence of water can be described by the following equation:

$$\frac{1}{\overline{M}_c} = \frac{2}{\overline{M}_n} - \frac{\left(\upsilon/V_1\right)\left[\ln(1-\upsilon_{2,s})+\upsilon_{2,s}+\chi_1\upsilon_{2,s}\right]}{\left(\upsilon_{2,s}^{1/3} - \dfrac{\upsilon_{2,s}}{2}\right)} \qquad (7.6)$$

For the case of gels prepared by crosslinking in the presence of water, the equation for the swelling of the polymer gel can be obtained by combining Equations (7.3) and (7.5) since the mixing contributions for both cases are the same. The swelling of networks crosslinked in the presence of water can then be written as:

$$\frac{1}{\overline{M}_c} = \frac{2}{\overline{M}_n} - \frac{\left(\upsilon/V_1\right)\left[\ln(1-\upsilon_{2,s})+\upsilon_{2,s}+\chi_1\upsilon_{2,s}\right]}{\upsilon_{2,r}\left(\left(\upsilon_{2,s}/\upsilon_{2,r}\right)^{1/3} - \left(\upsilon_{2,s}/2\upsilon_{2,r}\right)\right)} \qquad (7.7)$$

SWELLING OF IONIC HYDROGELS

Several factors affect the swelling of ionic hydrogels. Some of the major factors are the degree of ionization in the network, the ionization equilibrium, and the nature of the counterions. As the ionic content of a hydrogel is increased in response to environmental stimulus, increased repulsive forces develop and the network becomes more hydrophilic. The result is a more highly swollen network. Because of Donnan equilibrium, the chemical potential of the ions inside the gel must be equal to the chemical potential of the ions in the water outside the gel.

Ionization equilibrium is established in the form of a double layer of fixed charges on the pendant groups and counterions in the gel. Finally, the nature of counterions in the water will affect the swelling of the gel. As the valences of the counterions increase, they are more strongly attracted to the gel and will reduce the concentrations of ions needed in the gel to satisfy Donnan equilibrium conditions.

The swelling behavior of polyelectrolyte gels was initially described as a result of a balance between the elastic energy of the network and the osmotic pressure developed as a result of the ions. In electrolytic solutions, the osmotic pressure is associated with the development of a Donnan equilibrium. This pressure term is also affected by the fixed charges developed on the pendant chains.[18-29] The elastic term is described by the Flory expression derived from assumptions of Gaussian chain distributions.

Equations for the equilibrium swelling of ionic hydrogels were developed by equating three contributions to the free energy of the swollen gel. These contributions are due to mixing of the polymer and water, network elasticity, and ionic contributions. The general equation is given as:

$$\Delta G = \Delta G_{mix} + \Delta G_{el} + \Delta G_{ion} \tag{7.8}$$

In terms of the chemical potential, the difference between the chemical potential of the swelling agent inside the gel and outside the gel is:

$$\mu_1 - \mu_{1,0} = \Delta\mu_{elastic} + \Delta\mu_{mix} + \Delta\mu_{ion} \tag{7.9}$$

For weakly charged polyelectrolytes, the elastic contribution and mixing contributions will not differ from the case of nonionic gels. However, for highly ionizable materials there are ionization effects on the elastic and mixing terms.[26-29] As defined by this equation, at equilibrium the elastic, mixing, and ionic contributions to the chemical potential change must add up to zero.

The ionic term in Equation (7.9) is strongly dependent on the ionic strength and nature of the ions. Ricka and Tanaka[30] and Brannon-Peppas and Peppas[22,23] developed expressions to describe the ionic contributions to the swelling of polyelectrolytes. Assuming that the polymer networks under conditions of swelling behave similarly to dilute polymer solutions, the activity coefficient can be approximated as one and activities can be replaced with concentrations. The ionic term in Equation (7.9) becomes:

$$\Delta\mu_{ion} = RTV_1 \Delta c_{tot} \tag{7.10}$$

where Δc_{tot} is the difference in the total concentration of mobile ions within the gel.

The difference in the concentration of mobile ions is due to the fact that the charged polymer requires the same number of counterions to remain in the gel to achieve electroneutrality. The difference in the total ion concentration can then be calculated from the equilibrium condition for the salt.

Brannon-Peppas and Peppas[22,23] developed expressions for the ionic contributions to the swelling of polyelectrolytes for anionic and cationic materials. The ionic contribution for anionic networks is:

$$\Delta\mu_{ion} = \frac{RTV_1}{4I}\left(\frac{\upsilon_{2,s}^2}{\upsilon}\right)\left(\frac{K_a}{10^{-pH} + K_a}\right)^2 \tag{7.11}$$

For cationic networks, the ionic contribution is:

$$\Delta\mu_{ion} = \frac{RTV_1}{4I}\left(\frac{\upsilon_{2,s}^2}{\upsilon}\right)\left(\frac{K_b}{10^{pH-14} + K_a}\right)^2 \tag{7.12}$$

In these expressions, I is the ionic strength, K_a and K_b are the dissociation constants for the acid and base, respectively. It is significant to note that this expression has related the ionic contribution to the chemical potential to characteristics about the polymer/swelling agent that are readily determinable.

Equations (7.11) and (7.12) can be combined with the previous equations developed for nonionic networks. For the case of anionic polymer gels that were crosslinked in the presence of water, the equilibrium degree of swelling can be described by:

$$
\frac{V_1}{4I}\left(\frac{\upsilon_{2,s}^2}{\upsilon}\right)\left(\frac{K_a}{10^{-pH}+K_a}\right)^2 = \left(\ln(1-\upsilon_{2,s})+\upsilon_{2,s}+\chi_1\upsilon_{2,s}\right)+
$$
$$
\left(\frac{V_1}{\upsilon\overline{M}_c}\right)\left(1-\frac{2\overline{M}_c}{\overline{M}_n}\right)\upsilon_{2,r}\left(\left(\frac{\upsilon_{2,s}}{\upsilon_{2,r}}\right)^{1/3}-\frac{\upsilon_{2,s}}{2\upsilon_{2,r}}\right)
$$

(7.13)

For the cationic hydrogels prepared in the presence of water, the equilibrium degree of swelling is:

$$
\frac{V_1}{4I}\left(\frac{\upsilon_{2,s}^2}{\upsilon}\right)\left(\frac{K_b}{10^{pH-14}+K_a}\right)^2 = \left(\ln(1-\upsilon_{2,s})+\upsilon_{2,s}+\chi_1\upsilon_{2,s}\right)+
$$
$$
\left(\frac{V_1}{\upsilon\overline{M}_c}\right)\left(1-\frac{2\overline{M}_c}{\overline{M}_n}\right)\upsilon_{2,r}\left(\left(\frac{\upsilon_{2,s}}{\upsilon_{2,r}}\right)^{1/3}-\frac{\upsilon_{2,s}}{2\upsilon_{2,r}}\right)
$$

(7.14)

The abrupt change in swelling characteristics can be observed with hydrogels of various compositions. For example, Figure 7.1 indicates the swelling behavior of a gel made of poly(acrylic acid) grafted with chains of 200-mol weight poly(ethylene glycol) and swollen in water at 37°C. The figure shows the calculated values of M_c according to Equation (7.14). Such studies can be used to calculate the equivalent mesh sizes of the same networks by simple application of the Flory theory as indicated in Figure 7.2.

KINETICS OF SMART HYDROGELS

For many applications, the equilibrium swelling of the polyelectrolyte gels may not be the most important characteristic. For some applications, it is vital that the gel be able to exhibit fully reversible swelling and deswelling in response to pH changes or ionic strength. The rates at which a gel swells or collapses in response to changes in the environmental pH are vital in determining whether the gel is suitable for a given application.

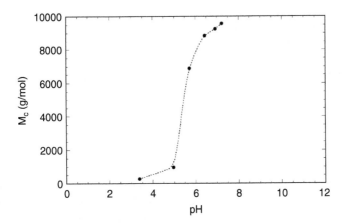

FIGURE 7.1 The effect of environmental pH on the molecular weight between crosslinks, M_c, calculated using Equation (7.14) for a polymer network of PAA-g-PEG2000.

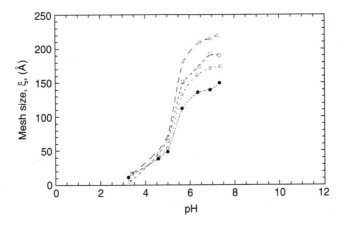

FIGURE 7.2 The effect of environmental pH on the mesh size, ξ_c, based on the values of M_c calculated using Equation (7.14) for PAA-g-PEG polymer networks with PEG grafts of molecular weights of 200, 400, 1000, and 2000.

Many researchers have studied the dynamic swelling of polyelectrolyte networks. The early work of Katchalsky[18–20] in the area of polyelectrolytes established the fact that the collapse and expansion of poly(methacrylic acid) gels occurred reversibly by simply adjusting the pH of the fluid. The group of Tanaka[21] performed significant work in this area as well and confirmed the reversible behavior of polyelectrolyte networks. Ohmine and Tanaka[31] also observed the sudden collapse of ionic networks in response to sudden changes in the ionic strength of the swelling media. Studies by Khare and Peppas[32] examined the swelling kinetics of poly(methacrylic acid) or poly(acrylic acid) with poly(hydroxyethyl methacrylate). They observed pH- and ionic strength-dependent swelling kinetics in these gels.

A model was developed by Brannon-Peppas and Peppas to describe the dynamic swelling of ionic hydrogels in response to ionic strength changes.[37] When an ionic gel swells in response to pH changes, there is a corresponding change in the volume or the length for one-dimensional transport. Based on the swelling, the strain in the gel, ε, can be calculated at any time during the swelling as:

$$\varepsilon = \frac{l - l_o}{l_o} \tag{7.15}$$

where l is the length at any time and l_o is the initial length.

In this analysis, it was assumed that the responses of the material (strain) to the inputs were additive and time-independent of the applied inputs. Therefore, the Boltzmann superposition principle can be invoked and the time-dependent strain in response to changes in environmental pH or ionic strength can be represented[37] by:

$$\varepsilon(t) = \int_0^t L(t - \tau) \frac{\partial I(\tau)}{\partial \tau} d\tau \tag{7.16}$$

where $\dfrac{\partial I(\tau)}{\partial \tau}$ is the change in pH or ionic strength and $L(t - \tau)$ is termed the ionic mechanochemical compliance and is a function of the polymer.

Assuming isotropic swelling in the hydrogel, the volume swelling ratio of the gel can be written as:

$$Q(t) = \frac{V_s(t)}{V_d} = \frac{l(t)^3}{l_o} = \left(1 + \varepsilon(t)\right)^3 \tag{7.17}$$

where $V_s(t)$ is the volume of the swollen gel at any time and V_d is the volume of the initially dry polymer. By combining Equations (7.16) and (7.17), the swelling of an ionic gel in response to ionic strength changes can be described by:

$$Q(t) = \left[1 + \int_0^t L(t - \tau) \frac{\partial I(\tau)}{\partial \tau} d\tau\right]^3 \tag{7.18}$$

Figure 7.3 shows an analysis of this behavior; data are presented for the equilibrium and dynamic responses of hydrogels swollen successively from one pH to another in order to determine the kernel of the previous equation.

ALTERNATIVE DYNAMIC ANALYSIS OF SWELLING

Water transport into polymeric hydrogels has been investigated over the past several decades, with several notable contributions made to the understanding of deviations from classical Fickian diffusion.[38–40] Due to the viscoelastic properties of polymers,

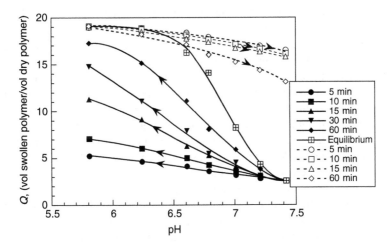

FIGURE 7.3 Results of experiments designed to derive the linear kernel function $L(t - \tau)$ of a hydrogel system. Hydrogel discs of polydiethylaminoethyl methacrylate-g-ethylene glycol PDEAEM-g-EG were pre-equilibrated and transferred from one pH to another and allowed to swell/deswell. The legend denotes the time between transfers.

which are enhanced by the presence of crosslinked networks, anomalous water diffusion can be observed. This behavior is bound by pure Fickian diffusion and Case II transport. Case II or constant rate transport has been observed for several polymer/water systems.[40]

Transport in all these physical situations can generally be reduced to three types of driving forces: a water concentration gradient, a polymer stress gradient, and osmotic forces. Osmotic behavior is observed as a result of the hydrophilicity of the polymer network; its magnitude is amplified when a hydrophilic solute is imbedded in the matrix such as in the case of swelling-controlled release devices.

As an important application, swelling-controlled release systems for drug delivery are based on the above principles by which an appropriate polymer can counterbalance normal Fickian diffusion by hindering the release of an embedded drug, leading to an extended period of drug delivery and possibly zero-order release.[41] The presence of a polymer network surrounding a drug or protein molecule has also been shown[42] to act as a stabilizer, maintaining biological activity until the solute is released.

Despite significant work to accurately model water transport in hydrogels,[43–46] simpler molecular models are needed. This can be done with the use of a diffusional Deborah (De) number, a measure of water motion relative to polymer relaxation; Sw relates water motion to solute release.

In nonswelling systems or where the relative relaxation time of a polymer is much shorter than the characteristic diffusion time for water transport, Fickian diffusion is observed, with water transport controlled by a concentration gradient. Once solvated, these polymers assume an equilibrium state almost immediately. In cases where polymer relaxation is the rate limiting step to water transport, Case II transport or time-independent diffusion is observed. However, in many systems, the water uptake mechanisms lead to transport behavior intermediate to Fickian and Case II transport, termed *anomalous transport*. Specific polymeric systems exhibiting the limiting cases of Fickian and Case II transport have been identified by Frisch et al.[45] and Thomas and Windle.[47]

Many experimental parameters can affect the kinetic swelling behavior of polymers. The effects of sample geometry on water uptake as described by the power law model have been investigated.[48,49] The effects of crosslinking density,[50] drug loading,[51] and copolymer composition[42] on swelling kinetics have also been determined experimentally. Recently, Colombo et al.[52] found a strong correlation between front motion and drug release kinetics. Case II drug release resulted when water and degradation fronts were synchronized.

There have been many investigations of diffusion in polymers, with results showing a range of transport behavior. In swelling polymer systems, stresses arising during the polymer swelling process have significant effects on water uptake behavior. Crazing phenomena have been noted in extreme systems; in other systems, these stresses can cause anomalous or Case II transport.[44]

Alfrey et al.[44] identified Case II transport with the existence of a sharp water front advancing at a constant velocity. Their results indicated that a polymer placed into a thermodynamically compatible water will swell and rearrange to accommodate the water, leading to anomalous and possibly Case II transport, while poor waters will be restricted to diffusion in the pore space inside the polymer, leading to Fickian transport. The rate of water uptake and compatibility of the polymer with a particular water leads to stresses occurring between the rubbery and glassy areas of the swelling polymer that were found to crack or craze in the presence of especially good waters.

Similarly, Hopfenberg and Frisch[39] showed how the type of transport observed for the same polymer/water pair can range from pure Fickian to Case II with variations in the temperature and water activity. The same group[45] also noted that two different waters had sharply different uptake characteristics in a glassy epoxy polymer. Benzene diffusion was observed to obey Case II transport, while methylene chloride diffusion into the same polymer was Fickian. By mixing the two waters, anomalous water uptake was observed, with the motion of the water front described by a linear combination of the two effects:

$$v = N_a k_a t^{1/2} + N_b k_b t \qquad (7.19)$$

where v is the front velocity, N_a and N_b represent the mole fraction of each water, and k_a and k_b are the uptake rate constants for pure liquid a or b.

Osmotic pressure is also an important factor in water uptake kinetics for polymer systems restrained by crosslinks.[48,53] These investigators utilized an osmotic pressure driving force to account for water uptake; however, they did not consider the increase in osmotic pressure for solute-loaded samples, which can be significant in a number of systems, leading to entirely different water uptake kinetics in the same polymeric material.

Gehrke et al.[54] investigated water uptake in poly(2-hydroxyethyl methacrylate), an important biomedical polymer used frequently in controlled drug delivery systems. They found that water uptake and front velocities were dependent on the square root of time, indicating Fickian transport. It was theorized that this was a result of the small sizes of water molecules relative to the pore space in the network thereby having no convective flux term. In cases where transport was facilitated by a concentration gradient and polymer relaxation occurred quickly, Fickian diffusion was expected.

Although less common, Super Case II transport has been reported to occur in certain polymer/water systems. Jacques et al.[55] observed an increase over the initial rate of n-hexane sorption into polystyrene and poly(phenylene oxide) as the polymer swelled. The sorption kinetics were seen to be strong functions of polymer composition, partial pressure (and therefore activity) of hexane, and temperature. The diameters of polystyrene spheres were also seen as major factors in swelling kinetics, with Case II diffusion occurring in larger diameter samples.[56]

There have been many experimental investigations to elucidate the state of a water (particularly water in polymer networks).[57-59] In hydrogels of certain compositions, water can bind with the polymer chains, creating a rigid area around the mesh that is not accessible to solute or water diffusion. This can greatly influence the type of transport observed, since the effective porosity of the material is decreased by bound water. Koda[57] determined that the velocity of ultrasonic waves was decreased markedly in polyelectrolyte hydrogels, indicating the presence of bound water.

The diffusional De number is expressed as a ratio between the characteristic polymer relaxation time and a characteristic diffusion time:

$$De = \frac{\lambda}{\theta} = \frac{\lambda D_{1,2}}{\left(\delta(t)\right)^2} = \frac{\text{Relaxation time}}{\text{Diffusion of solvent}} \tag{7.20}$$

where λ is the characteristic relaxation time for the polymer when subjected to swelling stresses and δ is the characteristic water diffusion time into a swelling sample.[60,61] The δ is defined as the square of the half thickness of a thin disc sample divided by the diffusion coefficient of water in the polymer ($\delta^2/D_{1,2}$). If either the relaxation time ($De \gg 1$) or water diffusion ($De \ll 1$) dominates the swelling process, the time dependence is Fickian; however, if De is on the order of 1, the two processes will occur on the same time scale, leading to anomalous transport behavior.

Wang et al.[46] developed an equation separating concentration gradient-dependent flux from stress relaxation:

$$\frac{\partial c}{\partial t} = \frac{\partial}{\partial x}\left[D(c,x,t)\frac{\partial c}{\partial x} - B(c,x,t)\, S\, c \right] \tag{7.21}$$

where D and B represent the diffusion coefficient and water mobility, respectively. S is a dimensionless variable similar to a De number, comparing the partial stress of the water to the total water uptake. Case II diffusion is observed when stress relaxation dominates.

Berens and Hopfenberg[62] also approached the problem by separating stress relaxation terms from diffusive flux:

$$M_t = M_{\infty,F}\left[1 - \frac{6}{\pi^2}\sum_{n=1}^{\infty}\frac{1}{n^2}\exp\left(-n^2 k_F t\right)\right] + \sum_i M_{\infty,i}\left[1 - \exp\left(-k_i t\right)\right] \qquad (7.22)$$

where $M_{\infty,F}$ is the equilibrium amount of sorption in the polymer before relaxation, k_F is a diffusional rate constant, $M_{\infty,i}$ represents the amount of water uptake during the ith relaxation process, and k_i is the corresponding relaxation rate constant. This model explicitly separated the diffusional and relaxation characteristics of water uptake. It was shown to fit experimental data, but many fitting parameters were necessary and it required information about a spectrum of relaxation processes.

CONCLUSIONS

In conclusion, several frameworks exist for the analysis of the kinetics of fast swelling of gels. Several recent theories from our laboratory[63–70] have indicated that it is possible to predict the exact swelling behavior of both neutral and ionic gels under various conditions. Such results can be used to analyze the behaviors of gels under various conditions. However, it must be noted that the exact analyses of such systems are significantly more complicated because of the presence of other thermodynamic components such as ions and small molecular weight compounds.

REFERENCES

1. N.A. Peppas and A.G. Mikos, Preparation methods and structure of hydrogels, in *Hydrogels in Medicine and Pharmacy*, Vol. 1, N.A. Peppas, Ed., CRC Press, Boca Raton, 1986, pp. 1–27.
2. L. Brannon-Peppas, Preparation and characterization of crosslinked hydrophilic networks, in *Absorbent Polymer Technology*, L. Brannon-Peppas and R.S. Harland, Eds., Elsevier, Amsterdam, 1990, pp. 45–66.
3. N.A. Peppas and E.W. Merrill, PVA hydrogels: reinforcement of radiation-crosslinked networks by crystallization, *J. Polym. Sci., Polym. Chem. Ed.*, 14, 441–457, 1976.
4. N.A. Peppas and E.W. Merrill, Differential scanning calorimetry of crystallized PVA hydrogels, *J. Appl. Polym. Sci.*, 20, 1457–1465, 1976.
5. N.A. Peppas, Hydrogels of polyvinyl alcohol and its copolymers, in *Hydrogels in Medicine and Pharmacy*, Vol. 2, N.A. Peppas, Ed., CRC Press, Boca Raton, 1986, pp. 1–48.
6. S.R. Stauffer and N.A. Peppas, Polyvinyl alcohol hydrogels prepared by freezing-thawing cyclic processing, *Polymer*, 33, 3932–3936, 1992.
7. A.S. Hickey and N.A. Peppas, Mesh size and diffusive characteristics of semicrystalline polyvinyl alcohol membranes prepared by freezing/thawing techniques, *J. Membr. Sci.*, 107, 229–237, 1995.
8. N.A. Peppas and N.K. Mongia, Ultrapure polyvinyl alcohol hydrogels with mucoadhesive drug delivery characteristics, *Eur. J. Pharm. Biopharm.*, 43, 51–58, 1997.

9. V.A. Kabanov and I.M. Papisov, Formation of complexes between complementary synthetic polymers and oligomers in dilute solution, *Vysokolmol. Soedin.*, A21, 243–281, 1979.

10. E.A. Bekturov and L.A. Bimendina, Interpolymer complexes, *Adv. Polym. Sci.*, 43, 100–147, 1981.

11. E. Tsuchida and K. Abe, Interactions between macromolecules in solution and inter-macromolecular complexes, *Adv. Polym. Sci.*, 45, 1–119, 1982.

12. J. Klier and N.A. Peppas, Structure and swelling behavior of polyethylene glycol/polymethacrylic acid complexes, in *Absorbent Polymer Technology*, L. Brannon-Peppas and R.S. Harland, Eds., Elsevier, Amsterdam, 1990, pp. 147–169.

13. C.L. Bell and N.A. Peppas, Biomedical membranes from hydrogels and interpolymer complexes, *Adv. Polym. Sci.*, 122, 125–175, 1995.

14. P.J. Flory and J. Rehner, Statistical mechanics of cross-linked polymer networks. II. Swelling, *J. Chem. Phys.*, 11, 521–526, 1943.

15. P.J. Flory, Statistical mechanics of swelling of network structures, *J. Chem. Phys.*, 18, 108–111, 1950.

16. P.J. Flory, *Principles of Polymer Chemistry*, Cornell University Press, Ithaca, NY, 1953.

17. N.A. Peppas, Physiologically responsive gels, *J. Bioact. Compat. Polym.*, 6, 241–246, 1991.

18. A. Katchalsky, Rapid swelling and deswelling of reversible gels of polymeric acids by ionization, *Experimentia*, 5, 319–320, 1949.

19. A. Katchalsky, S. Lifson, and H. Eisenberg, Equation of swelling for polyelectrolyte gels, *J. Polym. Sci.*, 7, 571–574, 1951.

20. A. Katchalsky and I. Michaeli, Polyelectrolyte gels in salt solution, *J. Polym. Sci.*, 15, 69–86, 1955.

21. T. Tanaka, Phase transition in gels and a single polymer, *Polymer,* 20, 1404–1412, 1979.

22. L. Brannon-Peppas and N.A. Peppas, The equilibrium swelling behavior of porous and non-porous hydrogels, in *Absorbent Polymer Technology*, L. Brannon-Peppas and R.S. Harland, Eds., Elsevier, Amsterdam, 1990, pp. 67–75.

23. L. Brannon-Peppas and N.A. Peppas, Equilibrium swelling behavior of pH-sensitive hydrogels, *Chem. Eng. Sci.*, 46, 715–722, 1991.

24. W. Oppermann, Swelling behavior and elastic properties of ionic hydrogels, in *Polyelectrolyte Gels: Properties, Properties, Preparation, and Applications,* R.S. Harland and R.K. Prud'homme, Eds., ACS Symposium Series No. 480, American Chemical Society, Washington, D.C., 1992, pp. 159–170.

25. A.B. Scranton, B. Rangarajan, and J. Klier, Biomedical applications of polyelectrolytes, *Adv. Polym. Sci*, 120, 1–54, 1995.

26. R. Skouri, F. Schoesseler, J.P. Munch, and S.J. Candau, Swelling and elastic properties of polyelectrolyte gels, *Macromolecules*, 28, 197–210, 1995.

27. M. Rubinstein, R.H. Colby, A.V. Dobrynin, and J.F. Joanny, Elastic modulus and equilibrium swelling of polyelectrolyte gels, *Macromolecules,* 29, 398–426, 1996.

28. U.P. Schroder and W. Opperman, Properties of polyelectrolyte gels, in *The Physical Properties of Polymeric Gels,* J.P. Cohen-Addad, Ed., John Wiley & Sons, New York, 1996, pp. 19–38.

29. E.Y. Kramarenko and A.R. Khoklov, Collapse of polyelectrolyte macromolecules revisited, *Macromolecules,* 30, 3383–3388, 1997.

30. J. Ricka and T. Tanaka, Swelling of ionic gels: quantitative performance of the Donnan theory, *Macromolecules,* 17, 2916–2921, 1984.

31. I. Ohmine and T. Tanaka, Salt effects on the phase transition of ionic gels, *J. Chem. Phys.*, 77, 5725–5729, 1992.
32. A.R. Khare and N.A. Peppas, Swelling/deswelling of anionic copolymer gels, *Biomaterials*, 16, 559–567, 1995.
33. B.A. Firestone and R.A. Siegel, Dynamic pH-dependent swelling of a hydrophobic polyelectrolyte gel, *Polym. Comm.*, 29, 204–208, 1988.
34. R.A. Siegel and B.A. Firestone, pH-Dependent equilbrium swelling properties of hydrophobic polyelectrolyte copolymer gels, *Macromolecules,* 21, 3254–3259, 1988.
35. J.M. Cornejo-Bravo and R.A. Siegel, Water vapor sorption behavior of copolymers of N,N-diethlyaminoethyl methacrylate and methyl methacrylate, *Biomaterials,* 17, 1187–1193, 1996.
36. P.J. Flory and J. Rehner, Statistical mechanics of cross-linked polymer networks. I. Rubberlike elasticity, *J. Chem. Phys.*, 11, 512–520, 1943.
37. L. Brannon-Peppas and N.A. Peppas, Time-dependent response of ionic polymer networks to pH and ionic strength changes, *Int. J. Pharm.*, 70, 53–57, 1991.
38. R.W. Korsmeyer, R. Gurny, E. Doelker, P. Buri, and N.A. Peppas, Mechanisms of solute release from porous hydrophilic polymers, *Intern. J. Pharm.*, 15, 25–35, 1983.
39. H.B. Hopfenberg and H.L. Frisch, Transport of organic micromolecules in amorphous polymers, *Polym. Lett.*, 7, 405–409, 1965.
40. T.K. Kwei, T.T. Wang, and H.M. Zupko, Diffusion in glassy polymers. V. Combination of Fickian and Case II mechanisms, *Macromolecules,* 5, 645–649, 1972.
41. G. Astarita and G.C. Sarti, A class of mathematical models for sorption of swelling waters in glassy polymers, *Polym. Eng. Sci.*, 18, 388–395, 1978.
42. N.M. Franson and N.A. Peppas, Influence of copolymer composition on non-Fickian water transport through glassy copolymers, *J. Appl. Polym. Sci.*, 28, 1299–1310, 1983.
43. J.C. Wu and N.A. Peppas, Modeling of water diffusion in glassy polymers with an integral sorption Deborah number, *J. Polym. Sci. Part B Polym. Phys.*, 31, 1503–1518, 1993.
44. T. Alfrey, Jr., E.F. Gurnee, and W.G. Lloyd, Diffusion in glassy polymers, *J. Polym. Sci. C,* 12, 249–261, 1966.
45. H.L. Frisch, T.T. Wang, and T.K. Kwei, Diffusion in glassy polymers II, *J. Polym. Sci. A2,* 7, 879–887, 1969.
46. T.T. Wang, T.K. Kwei, and H.L. Frisch, Diffusion in glassy polymers III, *J. Polym. Sci. A2,* 7, 2019–2028, 1969.
47. N.L. Thomas and A.H. Windle, Diffusion mechanics of the system PMMA–methanol, *Polymer,* 22, 627–639, 1981.
48. A. Peterlin, Diffusion with discontinuous swelling. V. Type II diffusion into sheets and spheres, *J. Polym. Sci. Polym. Phys.*, 17, 1741–1756, 1979.
49. P.L. Ritger and N.A. Peppas, Transport of waters in the macromolecular structure of coals. 7. Transport in thin coal sections, *Fuel,* 66, 1379–1388, 1987.
50. I. Orienti, E. Gianasi, V. Zecchi, and U. Conte, Release of ketoprofen from microspheres of poly2-hydroxyethyl methacrylate or poly2-hydroxyethyl methacrylate-co-b-methacryloyloxyethyl deoxycholate crosslinked with ethylene glycol dimethacrylate and tetraethylene glycol dimethacrylate, *Eur. J. Pharm. Biopharm.*, 41, 247–253, 1995.
51. G.W.R. Davidson III and N.A. Peppas, Solute and water diffusion in swellable copolymers versus relaxation controlled transport in phema-co-mma copolymers, *J. Control. Rel.*, 3, 243–258, 1986.
52. P. Colombo, R. Bettini, G. Massimo, P.L. Catellani, P. Santi, and N.A. Peppas, Drug diffusion front movement is important in drug release control from swellable matrix tablets, *J. Pharm. Sci.*, 84, 991–997, 1995.

53. A.H. Windle, Case II sorption, in *Polymer Permeability,* J. Comyn, Ed., Elsevier, London, 1985, pp. 75–118.
54. S.H. Gehrke, N. Vaid, and L. Uhden, Enhanced loading and activity retention of proteins in hydrogel delivery systems, *Proc. Int. Symp. Control. Rel. Bioact. Mater.,* 22, 145–146, 1995.
55. C.H.M. Jacques, H.B. Hopfenberg, and V. Stannett, Super Case II transport of organic vapors in glassy polymers, in *Polymer Permeability,* J. Comyn, Ed., Elsevier, Amsterdam, 1974, pp. 73–86.
56. D.J. Enscore, H.B. Hopfenberg, and V.T. Stannett, Effect of particle size on the mechanism controlling n-hexane sorption in glassy polystyrene microspheres, *Polymer,* 18, 793–800, 1977.
57. S. Koda, K. Yamashita, S. Iwai, and H. Nomura, Ultrasonic investigation of the states of water in hydrogels, *Polymer,* 35, 5626–5629, 1994.
58. H. Xu and J. Vij, Wide-band dielectric spectroscopy of hydrated polyhydroxyethyl methacrylate, *Polymer,* 35, 227–234, 1994.
59. W. Roorda, Review: do hydrogels contain different classes of water? *J. Biomater. Sci. Polym. Edn.,* 5, 383–395, 1994.
60. J.S. Vrentas, C.M. Jarzebski, and J.L. Duda, A Deborah number for diffusion in polymer–water systems, *AIChE J.,* 21, 894–901, 1975.
61. N.A. Peppas and N.M. Franson, The swelling interface number as a criterion for prediction of diffusional solute release mechanisms in swellable polymers, *J. Polym. Sci. Polym. Phys.,* 21, 983–997, 1983.
62. A.R. Berens and H.B. Hopfenberg, Diffusion and relaxation in glassy polymer powders. 2. Separation of diffusion and relaxation parameters, *Polymer,* 19, 489–496, 1978.
63. M.T. am Ende, D. Hariharan, and N.A. Peppas, Factors influencing drug and protein transport from ionic hydrogels, *Reactive Polym.,* 25, 127–137, 1995.
64. L. Brannon-Peppas and N.A. Peppas, Solute and water diffusion in swellable polymers. IX. The mechanisms of drug release from pH-sensitive swelling-controlled systems, *J. Control. Rel.,* 8, 267–274, 1989.
65. R.S. Harland and N.A. Peppas, Solute diffusion in swollen membranes. VII. Diffusion in semicrystalline networks, *Colloid Polym. Sci.,* 267, 2178–2225, 1989.
66. J. Klier and N.A. Peppas, Solute and water diffusion in swellable polymers. VIII. Influence of the swelling interface number on solute concentration profiles and release, *J. Control. Rel.,* 7, 61–68, 1988.
67. R.W. Korsmeyer, S.R. Lustig, and N.A. Peppas, Solute and water diffusion in swellable polymers. I. Mathematical modeling, *J. Polym. Sci. Polym. Phys.,* 24, 395–408, 1986.
68. S.R. Lustig and N.A. Peppas, Solute diffusion in swollen membranes. IX. Scaling laws for solute diffusion in gels, *J. Appl. Polym. Sci.,* 36, 735–747, 1988.
69. N.A. Peppas and C.T. Reinhart, Solute diffusion in swollen membranes. I. A new theory, *J. Membr. Sci.,* 15, 275–287, 1983.
70. C.T. Reinhart and N.A. Peppas, Solute diffusion in swollen membranes. II. Influence of crosslinking on diffusive properties, *J. Membr. Sci.,* 18, 227–239, 1984.

8 Polyelectrolyte Properties of Solutions and Gels

Hiroshi Frusawa and Kohzo Ito

CONTENTS

INTRODUCTION

A polyion is a linear chain (polymer) with ionizable groups on its backbone or side chain. Typical examples of a single polyion are biopolymers such as DNA, RNA, and proteins. Examples of synthesized polyions include polyacrylic acids, polystyrene sulfonates, and other compounds that are very useful industrially. Polyions are divided into two categories: when the polyions are crosslinked, they form gels localized macroscopically; otherwise they form solutions that are dispersed or segregated, depending on environmental conditions. Both types of polyelectrolytes have long been attractive subjects for many researchers.[1-8] For instance, polyelectrolyte gels have attracted much attention because of their volumetric responses to environments.[8]

We would like to focus on two characteristics of polyelectrolytes. One is the swelling of polyion chains, compared with nonionic chains. The like ions on the backbone of a polyion repel each other while counterions around the polyion shield the Coulombic repulsion. The competition between them determines the polyion conformation.[6] If the repulsion is dominant in dilute and salt-free solution, the polyion is stretched over some scale. On the other hand, if the repulsion is screened enough with excess amounts of added salts, the polyion shrinks down to a coiled form like neutral polymer chains. Accordingly, polyions take various forms from extended conformations to coiled ones by changing ionic environments.

The other feature is counterion condensation and fluctuation. A highly charged polyion yields a deep, steep valley of electrostatic potential in solution since many ionized groups are densely connected on the polymer backbone. As a result, some of counterions are bound to the polyion, which is called the Oosawa–Manning condensation.[1,2] The bound counterions then lose the activity and do not contribute to the conductivity. Instead, they yield large polarizability by fluctuating around the polyion. The low activity coefficient and large dielectric constant are also characteristics of polyelectrolytes, unlike the usual characteristics of electrolytes of microions.

The first part of this chapter mainly reviews our experiments that detected the counterion fluctuation and briefly discusses Oosawa–Manning condensation. Counterion fluctuation has been studied by electric relaxation spectroscopy techniques such as dielectric relaxation[3] and electric birefringence relaxation.[9] Electric relaxation spectroscopy reflects the dynamic properties of the polyion–counterion system that is highly sensitive to electric stimulus, and provides details of the Coulombic interaction between the bound counterions and the polyions. In the second part of this chapter, we treat polyion conformation. It has been theoretically analyzed in terms of electrostatic persistence length and experimentally studied by scattering techniques such as light scattering, small angle x-ray scattering, small angle neutron scattering, and dynamic light scattering. Special attention will be paid to recent theoretical work on chain conformations. Finally, the review ends with general conclusions and suggestions for future investigations.

COUNTERION FLUCTUATION

Oosawa–Manning Condensation

A charged polyion yields a deep valley of electrostatic potential in solution; most counterions are bound to the polyion. Accordingly, counterions in solution are separated into bound and free types. The free counterions contribute to the activity coefficient and conductivity. As the line charge density of the polyion increases, the fraction of the free counterions decreases with a deepening electrostatic valley. Oosawa[1] and Manning[2] independently proposed the counterion condensation theory that the number n_f of the free counterions per polyion is given independently of the line charge density e/d of the polyion by:

$$n_f = L/l_B \tag{8.1}$$

where the distance d between ionized groups on the polyion is less than the Bjerrum length,

$$l_B = e^2 / \left(4\pi\varepsilon_0\varepsilon_s k_B T\right) \tag{8.2}$$

where L is the contour length of the polyion, e the elementary charge, ε_0 the vacuum permittivity, ε_s the dielectric constant of water, and $k_B T$ the thermal energy. The Bjerrum length l_B is ca. 0.7 nm in water. The number n_t of the total counterions per polyion is given by $n_t = L/d$ proportional to the line charge density e/d. Therefore, the condensation theory predicts that the number n_b of the bound counterions increases with the line charge density e/d since n_f remains constant at $l_B > d$.

Most of counterions are bound to the polyion and do not contribute to the activity coefficient nor the conductivity at high line charge density. The validity of the condensation theory was supported by experiments related to osmotic pressure, conductivity, and other factors[2,6] and by calculation with the Poisson–Boltzmann equation.[10] See Deserno and Holm[11] and Levin.[12]

The condensation theory well explains the low activity coefficient of the linear polyelectrolyte solution by introducing bound counterions. Manning[2] assumed a two-phase model: the solution was separated into bound and free phases containing bound and free counterions, respectively, then evaluated the size of the bound phase. The size of the bound phase was ca. 1 nm in diameter around the polyion. This means that bound counterions are highly concentrated in the bound phase.

In contrast, Guéron et al.[10] numerically solved the Poisson–Boltzmann equation to determine the electrostatic potential profile and distribution of counterions around a polyion. The results indicated that no specific boundary separates the two phases in polyelectrolyte solution, and that if the bound phase is defined by having the electrostatic potential over $k_B T$ lower or higher than infinity away from the polyion, the size of the bound phase is close to the Debye–Hückel length κ^{-1} given by:

$$\kappa^2 = 4\pi l_B \left(2C_s + d C_p / l_B \right) \tag{8.3}$$

where C_s and C_p are the concentrations of added salts and counterions, respectively. The Debye–Hückel length κ^{-1} represents the screening lengths of Coulombic interactions among polyions and counterions. Since κ^{-1} characterizes the Coulombic interaction, it is regarded as one of the most important parameters in a polyelectrolyte solution. The terms within parentheses in Equation (8.3) correspond to the ionic environment, where the contribution of the free counterions is also taken into account. Accordingly, as the concentration C_s of added salts increases, the Debye–Hückel length decreases and the bound phase shrinks.

The calculation results of Guéron et al.[10] further indicated that tightly bound counterions are densely distributed in the vicinity of the polyion and their sizes and densities are almost independent of the ionic environments. This suggests that the bound counterions can be classified into tightly and loosely bound counterions. In contrast to the tightly bound counterions, the size and density of the loosely bound counterions are strongly affected by the ionic environment.

Finally, it should be stressed that the counterion condensation phenomenon, i.e., n_f independent of d, is derived from the two-dimensional electrostatic potential based on a quasi-cylindrical free volume occupied by a polyion.[1] This free volume is realized in the semidilute region of the polyelectrolyte solution without added salts, where polyions of extended forms are highly entangled. Accordingly, it is natural in dilute solution that n_f should depend on d even if the activity coefficient is similarly low.

DIELECTRIC RELAXATION

Bound counterions do not contribute to conductivity but instead yield large polarization. Therefore the dielectric relaxation spectroscopy for measuring the complex dielectric constant as a function of frequency directly gives us information on the dynamic behavior of bound counterions, i.e., on counterion fluctuation.[3] Since the bound counterions fluctuate within the bound phase, the dielectric relaxation of polyelectrolyte is closely related to the size of the bound phase.

In contrast, the static measurements such as direct current (DC) conductivity, osmotic pressure, and other factors reflect the activity coefficient, i.e., the fraction of free counterions regardless of the size of the bound phase. Consequently, the dynamic information on the bound counterions gives us the electrostatic potential profile in polyelectrolytes.

Solutions

Polyelectrolyte solutions with a small amount of added salt or no salt generally show two kinds of dielectric relaxation processes: low and high frequency types. Minakata and Imai[13] reported the first spectrum of the low and high frequency dielectric relaxations in 1972. As the measurable frequency range was extended to a few Hz[14] or 100 MHz,[15] the entire profiles of the low and high frequency relaxations were revealed.[3]

Low frequency dielectric relaxation was intensively studied experimentally and theoretically in the 1970s. The works were reviewed in detail by Mandel and Odijk.[3] The dielectric increment $\Delta\varepsilon_L$ and relaxation time τ_L of the low frequency relaxation strongly depend on the contour length L of a polyion, whereas the L dependence of $\Delta\varepsilon_L$ and τ_L varies in the exponent from two to three.[3,14] It was concluded from the strong L dependence of $\Delta\varepsilon_L$ and τ_L that the low frequency dielectric relaxation is ascribed to the fluctuation of the bound counterions along the polyion long axis or the rotation of the polyion with a permanent or quasi-permanent dipole moment. The experimental results also showed that $\Delta\varepsilon_L$ and τ_L are weakly dependent on the polymer concentration C_p.[15] It is difficult to measure low frequency dielectric relaxation with high accuracy since the DC conductivity is overwhelmingly larger than the polarizability in the low frequency range. As noted later, frequency-domain electric birefringence solves this problem and gives us detailed information on low frequency relaxation. The molecular mechanism of low-frequency relaxation will also be discussed.

Many theories were reported on dielectric relaxation due to counterion fluctuation.[3] Most of the theories from the 1970s were based on the two-phase model in which the bound counterions were confined in the bound phase[16,17] or sometimes exchanged with the free counterions in the free phase.[18] Then $\Delta\varepsilon_L$ and τ_L were proposed as proportional to the square of L in the confined case or to L in the exchangeable case, which is consistent with the experimental results. However, as noted earlier, the numerical calculation based on the Poisson–Boltzmann equation indicated no clear boundary between two phases. Consequently, the polarization due to the counterion fluctuation was numerically calculated in 1980s without the two-phase model by stricter theories by which the hydrodynamic Stokes equation, Poisson's equation, and conservation equations were satisfied simultaneously.[3,5,19]

Another important point in recent theories is that the complex dielectric constant ε^* is operationally defined from the complex conductivity σ^* by:

$$\sigma^* = \sigma(0) + i\omega\varepsilon_0\varepsilon^* \qquad (8.4)$$

where $\sigma(0)$ is the DC conductivity, ω the angular frequency of the applied sinusoidal electric field, and ε_0 the vacuum permittivity. This formalism is consistent with actual procedures of relaxation measurement for a conductive and dielectric system such as a polyelectrolyte solution because we experimentally obtain ε^* from the specific admittance proportional to σ^*. The complex conductivity σ^* directly reflects the counterion movement. The out-of-phase component of the counterion movement with respect to the external sinusoidal electric field is responsible for the electric polarization while the in-phase component causes DC conductivity. Thus, a counterion can contribute to polarization and conductivity at the same time.

Ito and Hayakawa[20] pointed out the significance of polyion mobility in estimating σ^*. Before that, the polyion was theoretically assumed to stand still and only the counterions were thought to fluctuate around the polyion. If the polyion is spherical latex, this assumption should be valid since the mass or frictional force of the polyion is much larger than those of counterions. However, it was experimentally seen that the linear polyion makes as large a contribution to DC conductivity as the counterions. Accordingly, the linear polyion movement and fluctuation strongly coupled with those of the bound counterions should yield conductivity and polarizability as substantially as counterions. The complex conductivity σ^*, complex dielectric constant ε^*, and the complex mobility U^* are closely related: they have dispersions in the same frequency region. In particular, σ^* is expected to be proportional to U^* in a polyelectrolyte solution without added salts. The validity of this theory along with the experimental results of high frequency dielectric relaxation will be discussed later in this chapter.

The molecular mechanism of high frequency dielectric relaxation has long been controversial: the Maxwell–Wagner effect, the bound counterion fluctuation along the polyion within the range of the correlation length,[3,21] the bound counterion fluctuation perpendicular to the polyion axis,[1,22–24] etc. The feature of the high frequency relaxation in the polyelectrolyte solution without added salts is a strong dependence on the monomer concentration C_m of polyions and independence of the polyion length L in contrast to the low frequency relaxation. As mentioned later in detail, the frequency-domain electric birefringence gave us information on direction of the counterion fluctuation responsible for the dielectric relaxation. The experimental results support the perpendicular model. Ito et al.[25] investigated high frequency relaxation in detail in wide concentrations ranging from dilute to semidilute and thereby clarified its molecular mechanism. They found a crossover behavior in the dielectric increment $\Delta\varepsilon_H$ and the relaxation time τ_H of high frequency relaxation in the dilute and semidilute regions. The C_m and L dependences of $\Delta\varepsilon_H$ and τ_H are summarized as:

$$\Delta\varepsilon_H \propto C_m^{1/3} L^{2/3}, \ \tau \propto C_m^{-2/3} L^{2/3} \ \text{(dilute)} \tag{8.5}$$

$$\Delta\varepsilon_H \propto C_m^0 L^0, \ \tau \propto C_m^{-1} L^0 \ \text{(semidilute)} \tag{8.6}$$

This crossover behavior is derived from a correlation length ξ that has the following C_m and L dependences:

$$\xi \propto C_m^{-1/3} L^{1/3} \ \text{(dilute)} \tag{8.7}$$

$$\xi \propto C_m^{-1} L^0 \ \text{(semidilute)} \tag{8.8}$$

It was concluded from these results that the high frequency relaxation in the dilute and semidilute region was attributed to the fluctuation of the loosely bound counterions within the range of the correlation length ξ, namely the average distance between polyions. The crossover concentration of the high frequency relaxation is nearly equal to that obtained by small angle x-ray scattering.[26] This shows the interesting feature that the dynamic measurement of high frequency relaxation is closely related to the static method of x-ray scattering, reflecting the structure in the polyelectrolyte solution. This is because the structure or arrangement of polyions yields the electrostatic potential profile in the solution while the fluctuation length of the counterion fluctuation is dominated by the potential profile.

The dependence of τ_H on the counterion species has recently been measured.[27] The τ_H was proportional to the intrinsic mobility μ_0 of the counterion. This is consistent with the interpretation of the molecular mechanism of high frequency relaxation since the counterions fluctuate with free mobility without specific binding to polyions. The coefficient represents an effective force constant loosely bound between the polyion and counterions.

The dependence of low frequency relaxation on the counterion species is quite different. On the other hand, the experimental results clearly showed an offset in the dependence of τ_H on μ_0. This offset, predicted by Ito and Hayakawa,[20] is ascribable to the polyion fluctuation strongly coupled with the bound counterions. The polyion mobility contributes to the polarizability as well as the DC conductivity. This supports the validity of the theory of Ito and Hayakawa.[20]

Gels

Gels are analogous to the above semidilute solutions in that polyions in both the systems are entangled with each other, although the polyions in gels are not uniformly dispersed as are those in solutions, but are localized in solution due to fixed crosslinks. Hence, dielectric relaxation spectroscopy is expected to enhance our knowledge of the Coulombic field in gels.

A highly charged network in a gel produces not only a strong Coulombic field around the backbone network, but also a Coulombic field at the gel boundary — in other words, a Coulombic potential difference between the inside and outside of the gel due to the localization of polyions constituting the gel. We expect two kinds of dielectric relaxation processes in gels. One process is due to the presence of a gel boundary that prevents counterions subject to the external electric field from passing through the gel. The counterions that are confined to the gel but mobile inside the gel contribute to the electric polarization. The relaxation time τ is determined by the diffusion time of counterions spreading over the inside of the gel and estimated as $\tau \cong L^2/2D$, where L is the linear dimension of the gel. If we use 1.0 cm as a typical value of L, we obtain a value more than 1.0×10 h for τ, which is too slow to detect experimentally. The other process is due to the Coulombic field around the charged network of gels and is expected to be observed in a high frequency range similar to semidilute solutions.

Indeed we could observe the high frequency (~MHz) dielectric relaxation which is ascribable to the diffusion process of counterions bound to a highly charged network.[28] From dielectric relaxation, we have found the following two properties of Coulombic field in gels. First, with increasing the salt concentration C_s, the Coulombic potential difference between the inside and outside of the gel estimated from the conductivity is saturated to an almost constant value after the initial sharp decrease. This is consistent with the result evaluated from the electrical neutrality condition inside the gel. Second, the C_s dependence of the relaxation time and the dielectric increment indicate that the number of counterions bound to the local

Coulombic potential around the network is independent of C_s, similarly to the results from solutions.

ELECTRIC BIREFRINGENCE RELAXATION

Dielectric relaxation spectroscopy is certainly a powerful tool for obtaining information on electric polarization. However, it is difficult to accurately measure the dielectric relaxation of electrically conductive systems such as a polyelectrolyte solution in a low frequency range because of high DC conductivity. In contrast, electric birefringence spectroscopy enables us to obtain the whole profile of low frequency dielectric relaxation in a polyelectrolyte solution even in a very low frequency range because the electric birefringence response due to electric polarization is an optical signal and hence not disturbed by conductivity.

Let us consider a rod-like molecule with optical and electrical anisotropy in solution. The polyion in the solution without added salts can be modeled as such a molecule. When the external electric field is applied, the dipole moment is induced on the molecule by the electrical anisotropy. Then the molecule is oriented to the applied electric field, which results in the birefringence of the solution. This is called the electric birefringence or Kerr's effect. The birefringence response Δn to the sinusoidal electric field with an amplitude small enough and an angular frequency of ω consists of DC (static) and 2ω (alternating current or AC) components, i.e., Δn_{dc} and $\Delta n_{2\omega}$, respectively. Hayakawa and Ookubo et al.[29-31] established frequency-domain electric birefringence (FEB) spectroscopy and revealed the physical meanings of these components in solutions of rod-like molecules with optical and electrical anisotropies.

The DC component Δn_{dc} gives us information on dielectric relaxation and the direction of polarization. The 2ω component $\Delta n_{2\omega}$ reflects the rotational relaxation of the polyion. Accordingly, FEB spectroscopy allows us to determine counterion fluctuation and polyion rotation separately and simultaneously. This means that we can determine whether a molecular mechanism of dielectric relaxation in a linear polyelectrolyte solution is a counterion fluctuation or a polyion rotation. The determination was controversial in studies of low frequency dielectric relaxation of linear polyelectrolyte solutions.[3] Furthermore, FEB spectroscopy enables us to measure dielectric relaxation in very low frequency ranges as mentioned above. These features indicate that FEB spectroscopy is superior to conventional dielectric relaxation spectroscopy. Incidentally, other electric birefringence methods with rectangular pulse fields[32-39] or offset sinusoidal fields[40,41] are widely used for investigation of the dynamics of rod-like molecules.

The low and high frequency dielectric relaxations in polyelectrolyte solutions without added salts were investigated in detail by FEB spectroscopy.[29,42] The FEB spectra clearly showed that the directions of these two relaxations were perpendicular to each other. The spectra confirmed that low frequency relaxation time strongly depended on the molecular weight or contour length L of the polyion while the high frequency relaxation time was nearly independent of L. These experimental results supported the molecular mechanism that low frequency relaxation was ascribed to counterion fluctuation along the polyion long axis while high frequency relaxation was due to counterion fluctuation perpendicular to the polyion axis.

The dependence of low frequency relaxation on counterion species was measured in detail by FEB spectroscopy.[27] The experimental results were quite different from the dependence of high frequency relaxation. Whereas the relaxation frequency f_H of high frequency relaxation was proportional to the free mobility μ_0 of the counterion species as mentioned earlier, the relaxation frequency f_L of low frequency relaxation is nearly independent of μ_0. The contrary tendency of f_H and f_L was also seen in the dependence on the neutralization ratio.[42] These results led to the conclusion that low frequency relaxation is ascribable to the counterion fluctuation of tightly bound counterions while high frequency relaxation is due to the fluctuation of loosely bound counterions.[27,42]

Electric birefringence is a useful technique to clarify the molecular mechanisms of polarization. However, the direction of polarization in a linear polyelectrolyte solution still involves some controversy. It was pointed out from determination of optical anisotropy by flow birefringence that low frequency relaxation should be the polarization perpendicular to the polyion long axis.[43–47] This conclusion is incompatible with the strong dependence of the low frequency relaxation on the molecular weight and the controversy has not been settled yet.[48]

Dynamic Light Scattering with Sinusoidal Electric Field

A new electric relaxation spectroscopy technique known as dynamic light scattering with sinusoidal electric field (DLS-SEF) has recently been developed to investigate polyion dynamics. The technique is strongly correlated with counterion fluctuation as noted earlier. This method was first proposed by Schmitz et al.[5,49] and finally established by Ito et al.[50–54] The apparatus was refined further by Mizuno et al.[55] who succeeded in detecting clear relaxation of colloidal mobility confined in membranes.

Ito et al. pointed out that light scattering under sinusoidal electric field does not obey stationary process but is periodically stationary. Hence the correlation function in DLS-SEF must be a two-variable function of the initial time and the time difference. Correspondingly, DLS-SEF gives us a two-dimensional power spectrum. Ito et al. developed a new correlator[51] to obtain the two-variable correlation function and a new spectrum analyzer[52] to measure the two-dimensional power spectrum based on an extended Wiener–Khinthcine theorem. These devices provided information on phase lag of the electrophoretic mobility to the external electric field for the first time. They determined the phase lag of the electrophoretic mobility of a polyelectrolyte solution.[53] Ito and Hayakawa[54] predicted the frequency dispersion of the apparent diffusion constant measured by DLS-SEF because of the strong coupling between the polyion and bound counterion. Thus, DLS-SEF has the potential to reveal information about counterion fluctuation through polyion dynamics.

CHAIN CONFORMATIONS

Polyions Considered

Polyionic chains can be classified in various ways based on certain characteristics of the constituent monomers. Nonionic properties include affinity with solvent (good or poor solvent?); backbone rigidity in the absence of charged groups (intrinsically flexible or rigid?). Ionic properties include signs of charges (polyelectrolytes or polyampholytes?); contour density of charged monomers along a chain (weakly or highly charged?); charge distribution along a chain (quenched or annealed?). Since the conformations strongly depend on all these factors, we will discuss them step by step.

Good or Poor Solvent?

We neglected the solvent effect (or considered the theta solvents), supposing that the chain configurations would be mainly determined by Coulomb interactions. Obviously the simplification is invalid for poor solvents. Recent theories and simulations predict the possibility of taking novel forms locally collapsed but stretched globally, the so-called necklace conformation.[56]

Intrinsically Flexible or Rigid?

In discussing the electrostatic contribution to the rigidity of chains, this grouping becomes significant. We consider both cases. The controversial problem is how to extend the classical theories developed by Odijk, Sklonick, and Fixman[57] for intrinsically rigid chains, to intrinsically flexible chains.

Polyelectrolytes or Polyampholytes?

This chapter restricts itself to the issues concerning polyelectrolytes carrying the same types of (cationic or anionic) groups, although some attention is also given to polyampholyte conformations as model materials of proteins.[58]

Weakly or Highly Charged?

This factor is also essential in considering the electrostatic contribution to chain conformations. We hence investigate the configurations for both cases.

Quenched or Annealed?

Typical examples of annealed polyions are weak polyacids or polybases in which the ionic groups dissociate depending on the pH. The charges along chains are not fixed; they can move by recombination and reassociation of H^+ ions. Such a degree of freedom is taken into account in some recent theories on conformations,[6] but the effect has not yet been elucidated experimentally and we will ignore this contribution and assume charged monomers to be fixed (or quenched).

To summarize, we will be concerned with quenched polyions in theta solvents over a variety of intrinsic rigidities and line charge densities. Since we neglect the solvent effect, the conformations of a backbone chain are determined by the competition of electrostatic interaction energy between charged groups and microions (counterions and added salts), and entropies due to both chain configurations and the translation of microions. In the absence of microions, it is expected that the long-range nature of electrostatic repulsion between charged groups can dominate over the cost of conformational entropy and hence the chains take stretched forms. As will be seen later, elaborate evaluations also support this speculation. The problem we would like to address is the role microions, especially counterions, play in chain conformations.

PRELIMINARY DISCUSSION WITHOUT COUNTERIONS

Consider here an intrinsically flexible and weakly charged chain. Let R be the size of a charged chain and N the polymerization degree. The elongation of a chain is represented by:

$$R \sim N \tag{8.9}$$

The scaling relation for the chain without microions (counterions and added salt) has been confirmed in three ways as follows.[6]

The primary approach is in line with Flory's approximation, a surprisingly successful evaluation in determining the sizes of neutral polymers. Let F be the free energy of a chain, which is written according to Flory's estimation as:

$$F \sim \left\{ \frac{R^2}{Nb^2} + \frac{(Nf)^2 l_B}{R^{d-2}} \right\} k_B T \tag{8.10}$$

omitting numerical factors. Here a is the monomer length, f is the fraction of charged monomers, l_B is the Bjerrum length defined as Equation (8.2), and d is the spatial dimension. Minimizing F with respect to R, we have $R \sim N^v$ ($v = 3/d$), confirming the linear relation (8.9) for $d = 3$. The second method is the renormalization group calculation that gives the exponent $v = 2/d - 2$ for $4 < d < 6$, different from Flory's result. Although no such calculation is available for $d = 3$, the result $v = 1$ for $d = 4$ somehow implies the stretching of chains in $d = 3$. Lastly, we would like to mention the variational methods, which also derive the linear relation $R \sim N$ with logarithmic correction in $d = 3$.

It is thus validated from various approaches that a charged chain in the absence of counterions takes an anisotropic form. Often misleading is the interpretation of $R \sim N$. The linear relation does not necessarily require a rod-like configuration in local scale. Rather, chains should keep Gaussian statistics in smaller scale where the electrostatic energy is lower than thermal energy and is a weak perturbation. The crossover length D is determined by the relation $(gf)^2 l_B/D \sim 1$, where g represents the number of monomers in a subunit called the electrostatic "blob." Figure 8.1 shows the present configuration locally Gaussian but globally stretched, i.e., a string of electrostatic blobs. In other words, conformation of an intrinsically flexible polyion in the absence of counterions is represented by a straight classical path with Gaussian fluctuation around it.

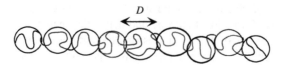

FIGURE 8.1 Blob picture of intrinsically flexible and weakly charged polyelectrolyte chain.

SCREENING EFFECTS ON CONFORMATIONS

Next consider the roles of microions in chain conformations. Historically, many models have been developed. Recent considerations, however, seem restricted to three contributions. For convenience of presenting them, let us first divide dissociated microions (counterions) into two types[1]: bound counterions that are localized around charged backbones and free counterions that are mobile in solution.

Using the ad hoc grouping we would like to list, first of all, the well-known contribution to reducing the sizes of the polyelectrolyte chains: the Debye–Hückel (DH) screening effect due to free counterions and added salt. The other contributions arise from bound counterions. Following the Oosawa–Manning condensation theory,[1,2] the bound counterions lead to the decrease of effective charge density σ along a chain: σ of a higher density is reduced to the value of $1/l_B z$, with z the bound counterion valence. In addition, recent theoretical attempts[59–64] suggest that bound-counterion fluctuation induces attraction between charged groups. In what follows, only the first DH screening effect will be seen in detail.

In the context of polyelectrolyte studies, the DH screening length κ^{-1} is operationally defined via assuming that the effective interaction between charged groups can be mimicked by the Yukawa-type function, i.e., $e^{-\kappa r}/r$, with r the distance between them. Since this type of screening arises from freely mobile microions, the screening length κ^{-1} is empirically expressed as $\kappa^2 = 4\pi l_B (2C_s + \alpha C_m)$, where C_m and C_s are the monomer and salt density, respectively, and α is a factor less than unity that takes into account the binding of counterions; $\alpha = d/l_B$ in a simple case such as Equation (8.3).

Due to such cut-off of the long-range Coulomb interaction, an infinitely long polyelectrolyte chain that will be the concern here takes isotropically swollen form in large scales, although for small separations the chains are still elongated due to the relevance of electrostatic repulsion. Thus comes into play the concept of the crossover length between the persistent (or rod-like) and isotopically swollen structure, i.e., persistence length l_p.

The dependence of l_p on the DH screening length κ^{-1} has been one of the central issues in theories, experiments, and computer simulations for more than two decades; nevertheless, no consensus has been reached, especially about intrinsically flexible polymers. A serious drawback seems to be the fact that *most experiments have not judged the theoretical predictions correctly or precisely*, as described below.

We point out two problems. One is the polymer density adopted in most experiments such as viscosity measurement, various scattering methods, etc. While few theories consider many chain effects on conformations, the experimental densities are too high to neglect the surrounded chain effect; the interchain interaction, however,

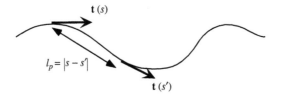

FIGURE 8.2 Persistence length in worm-like chain model.

favors the reduction of the persistence length so that chains can avoid each other.[65] Accordingly, most experimental results cannot be compared with theories in a straightforward manner.

Another experimental problem is associated with the modeling chains[66] when l_p is inferred from the obtained data. Most experimental analyses exploit the worm-like chain model (see Figure 8.2) in which l_p satisfies such a simple relation as:

$$\langle \mathbf{t}(0) \cdot \mathbf{t}(s) \rangle = \exp\left(-s/l_p\right) \tag{8.11}$$

with $t(s)$ the tangent vector of a monomer specified by the contour length s and the bracket representing an average. In fact, the conformations of intrinsically flexible polymers do not have worm-like forms except in special cases. More appropriate is the blob, as depicted in Figure 8.1. Most experimental estimations of persistence length are different quantities from those proposed by theories.

Apart from the above deficiencies, the experiments produced consistent results: linear or sublinear dependence on κ^{-1} as $l_e \sim \kappa^{-y}$ ($y \le 1$) for intrinsically flexible chains, and $l_e \sim \kappa^{-2}$ for intrinsically rigid chains like DNA, in correspondence with the classical result by Odijk, Skolnik, and Fixman (OSF).[57] The l_e represents the electrostatic contribution to the persistence length. These results are also in accord with recent computer simulations.[67] In spite of such coincidences, we would like to stress again that the above ambiguities of the evaluation still prevent the correct comparison of experimental, simulational, and theoretical results.

Considering the above problems, we then pursue only the consensus within theories. Let us first see the primary approach by OSF, because this suggests the theoretical difficulty in advance.[6,57] According to the OSF calculation, l_p varies by the contour length s. For small values of s, the electrostatic interactions are irrelevant and we have $l_p = l_0$, where l_0 is the intrinsic persistence length that characterizes the backbone rigidity in the absence of charged groups, whereas l_p is given for large s as:

$$l_p = l_0 + \frac{l_B}{4\kappa^2 A^2} \tag{8.12}$$

with A the contour distance between charges. That is, the chain flexibility varies on the crossover length scale s_c. The value s_c has been evaluated by the equality between the bare curvature energy due to the intrinsic rigidity and the electrostatic energy

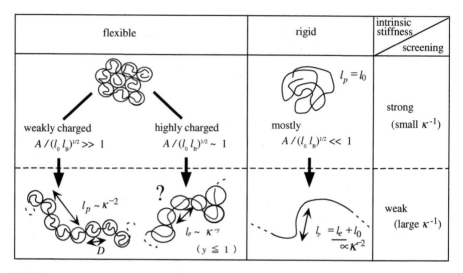

FIGURE 8.3 A schematic of both potential and entropy for a single polyion isolated.

due to the bend, giving $s_c \sim A(l_0/l_B)^{1/2}$.[6] The condition to validate the OSF calculation is hence written as:

$$\frac{s_c}{l_0} = \frac{A}{\left(l_0 l_B\right)^{1/2}} \ll 1 \qquad (8.13)$$

with the expression of s_c, because, in order that the OSF discussion holds, chains must be worm-like (or tangent vector fluctuations must be small) up to the scale s_c where the electrostatic interactions become relevant and can rigidify a chain.

The next question then arises. How is the evaluation of l_p to be modified when the Equation (8.13) condition is violated? Recent theoretical attempts have challenged this issue.

Figure 8.3 is a schematic acceptable to many theorists at present.[6,66] The columns are divided by intrinsic rigidity and the lines by the extent of DH screening.

More definite and simpler are intrinsically rigid polymers in which the Equation (8.13) condition holds for a large range of line charge density (or A). Figure 8.3 shows that charged chains with intrinsically large rigidities are always stiff even at small scales and take worm-like forms regardless of the DH screening effect. The increase of the DH screening length κ^{-1} only adds the electrostatic contribution to the intrinsic persistence length l_0 as represented by Equation (8.12).

Intrinsically flexible polymers, on the other hand, are to be further separated by contour charge density: weakly charged chains satisfying $A/(l_0 l_B)^{1/2} \gg 1$ and highly charged ones where $A/(l_0 l_B)^{1/2}$ always takes unity order, $A/(l_0 l_B)^{1/2} \sim 1$ due to counterion condensation. In the strong screening limit, both remain flexible and only relevant is the excluded volume effect modified by electrostatic interactions in some ways. With a decrease of DH screening, chains assume persistent forms at small length scales.

The persistent structures differ between weakly and highly charged chains. Plausible models of weakly charged chains are the coarse-grained worm-like polymers as the strings of electrostatic blobs (see Figure 8.1). In this case, persistence length is not defined by the contour length as Equation (8.11), but by the axial length of the coarse-grained semiflexible chain. Since the effective charge density along the axis becomes high, a similar result to the OSF method is expected to be recovered: $l_p \sim D + l_B/\kappa^2 D^2$. Note that the charge separation distance A in Equation (8.12) is replaced by the diameter of a blob D.

Most difficult are the last types of polymers with intrinsic flexibility and high contour charge density because their conformations are marginal between worm-like and blob-like forms. With less recognition of the difficulty, these types of polyelectrolytes have been investigated by many experiments and simulations.[6,7,66] Their results suggest weaker dependence on κ^{-1} than on results from OSF and the absence of a simple power law of κ^{-1}, which is also supported theoretically by some variational methods[6,66,68] and renormalization calculations.[69] The apparent coincidences, however, are to be put aside because comparisons of experiments, simulations, and theories have the above drawbacks, and also because the theories take little care about modeling of the intermediate range.

HISTORICAL MODELS OF SWELLING

Even with ample salt added, polyions still swell larger than neutral polymers. Historically, this has been attributed[70] to: (1) the translational entropy difference of microions between the inside and outside of the region occupied by a charged polymer in an averaged sense (the entropic origin),[71] (2) the averaged difference of the Coulomb potential between both sides (the potential difference origin),[72] and (3) the effective electrostatic interactions between charged groups (the electrostatic origin).[6,73–75]

In classical theories, it seems that the differences among these explanations is due to the distinct simplifications of the system generally including localized charges.[70] Recent theories also lack deliberate considerations about the ambiguity. Consequently, whether the equivalences among the above interpretations are true[6] remains undecided. Until now, three types of interpretations of the swelling of charged chains have existed.

Let us consider an isolated polyion with its occupied volume V. In high salt limits, both classical and modern treatments have converged to the completely identical explanation that the swelling of an intrinsically flexible polyion is due to the additional osmotic pressure Π_{ion} given by:

$$\Pi_{ion} = \frac{\left(f\bar{\rho}\right)^2}{4C_s} k_B T \tag{8.14}$$

where f is the fraction of charged monomers, $\bar{\rho}$ is the density of monomers smeared over the occupied region and is given as $\bar{\rho} \equiv n_m/V$ with the monomer number n_m, and C_s is the salt concentration. In what follows, we will see in detail how the above three approaches lead to the same result [Equation (8.14)].

Entropic Origin[71]

The entropic approach neglects the electrostatic energy mainly arising from the boundary of the occupied region. Consequently, we have:

$$\beta \overline{F}_{ion} \approx \sum_i n_i^{in} \ln \frac{n_i^{in}}{V} + \sum_i n_i^{out} \ln \frac{n_i^{out}}{U - V} \tag{8.15}$$

where n_i^{in} and n_i^{out} are the numbers of the ith microions inside and outside the region occupied by a charged chain and U is the system volume.

The ionic osmotic pressure Π_{ion}, given as $\Pi_{ion} \equiv -\partial F_{ion}/\partial V$, is obtained from Equation (8.15) as

$$\beta \Pi_{ion} = \sum_i \overline{c}_i^{in} - \sum_i \overline{c}_i^{out}$$

where $\overline{c}_i^{in} = n_i^{in}/V$ and $\overline{c}_i^{out} = n_i^{out}/(U - V)$. For simplicity, taking

$$\sum_i \overline{c}_i^{out} = 2C_s$$

(C_s: salt concentration), $\sum_i \overline{c}_i^{in}$ is represented as:

$$\sum_i \overline{c}_i^{in} = 2C_s \cosh \psi_D \tag{8.16}$$

in terms of the Coulomb potential difference ψ_D between the inside and outside of a chain, and the electrical neutrality condition inside the chain region reads:

$$f \overline{\rho} = 2C_s \sinh \psi_D \tag{8.17}$$

From Equation (8.16) and Equation (8.17), using the relation, $\cosh^2 x - \sinh^2 x = 1$, we get

$$\sum_i \overline{c}_i^{in} = \left\{ \left(f \overline{\rho} \right)^2 + 4C_s^2 \right\}^{1/2}$$

and thus obtain:

$$\beta \Pi_{ion} = \left(f^2 \overline{\rho}^2 + 4C_s^2 \right)^{1/2} - 2C_s \tag{8.18}$$

With fully added salt, i.e., $C_s \gg f\bar{\rho}$, Equation (8.18) is approximately rewritten as $\beta\Pi_{ion} \approx (f\bar{\rho})^2/4C_s$ in agreement with Equation (8.14).

Critical remarks: We point out one of the misleading points that the numbers of microions n_i^{in} and n_i^{out} are assumed to be independent of the occupied volume V; however they actually depend on V via the change of the averaged Coulombic potential ψ_D. Considering the dependence, the result becomes quite different.

Potential Difference Origin[72]

This approach starts with the following expression for the ionic free energy $\bar{F}_{ion}$:

$$\beta\bar{F}_{ion} = \int_0^1 \frac{d\lambda}{\lambda} \int d\mathbf{r} \, q_\lambda \bar{\psi}_\lambda + \sum_i n_i \ln\left(n_i/U\right) - n_i \qquad (8.19)$$

where λ is the parameter for the charging process ($0 \le \lambda \le 1$), the net charge density and the Coulombic potential, eq_λ and $\bar{\psi}_\lambda$, corresponding to λ are indicated by the subscript, N_i is the total number of the ith small ions, and the last term represents the entropy term of ideal small ions that are freely mobile throughout the system with its volume U.

In the approximation by Hermans, Overbeek, and Hill,[72] q_λ in Equation (8.19) is assumed to be $\lambda f\bar{\rho}$. This comes from the following speculation: since microions can be automatically supplied from the solvent while the backbone chain is being charged, the entropic change of microions is compensated by the change in the potential energy of microions as $z_i(\bar{\psi}_{\lambda_1} - \bar{\psi}_{\lambda_2}) + k_B T \ln(c_i^2/c_i^1) = 0$, where $c^2 = c_i^1 \exp\{-z_i (\bar{\psi}_2 - \bar{\psi}_1)\}$ and 1 and 2 denote steps of charging. Therefore, using $p = 2C_s/f\bar{\rho}$, we estimate $\bar{\psi}_\lambda$ from Equation (8.17) as $\bar{\psi}_\lambda = \sinh^{-1}(\lambda/p)$, so that $\bar{F}_{ion}$ given by Equation (8.19) is calculated as:

$$\beta\bar{F}_{ion} \approx f n_m\left(\sinh^{-1}(1/p) - \sqrt{p^2+1} + p\right) + \sum_i n_i \ln\left(n_i/U\right) - n_i \qquad (8.20)$$

giving Π_{ion} of the same form as Equation (8.14) in high salt solutions.

Critical remarks: The averaged potential $\bar{\psi}_\lambda$ is not an external field applied to microions, but a self-consistent potential determined from distribution of charged monomers and microions that is omitted in the above discussion of compensation. More explicitly, this approach includes the contradiction that the net charge density is assumed to be nonzero $eq_\lambda = e\lambda f\bar{\rho}$ although $\bar{\psi}_\lambda$ is estimated from the electrical neutrality condition.

Electrostatic Origin[6]

The Coulomb potential produced by charged monomers on the backbone chain would be small enough for the conventional DH approximation to hold. Suppose, in addition, that the microion contribution to ionic free energy is all incorporated into the screening effect. The electrostatic approach then identifies the ionic free energy $\bar{F}_{ion}$ with the effective interaction energy between charged groups:

$$\beta F_{ion} = \int d\mathbf{r} \int d\mathbf{r}' \frac{l_B f^2}{2} \rho(\mathbf{r}) \frac{e^{-\kappa|\mathbf{r}-\mathbf{r}'|}}{|\mathbf{r}-\mathbf{r}'|} \rho(\mathbf{r}') \qquad (8.21)$$

where $\rho(r)$ is the actual density of charged monomers and κ^{-1} is here given by $\kappa^2 = 8\pi l_B C_s$. Replacing $\rho(\mathbf{r})$ by the smeared value $\bar{\rho}$, Equation (8.21) simply reads:

$$\beta F_{ion} = \frac{f^2 \bar{\rho}^2}{2} \frac{4\pi l_B}{\kappa^2} V \qquad (8.22)$$

leading to the same osmotic pressure Π_{ion} as Equation (8.14).

Critical remarks: While the conventional DH approximation is relevant only around a single discrete point charge, Equation (8.22) uses the smeared density. The more essential problem is how to reconcile the discrete charge picture and the smeared models.

COUNTERION ROLE IN SWELLING: OUR VIEW

We have found an appropriate formalism to electrolytes with high charge asymmetry between counterions and polyions.[76] This leads to the following statement: *The ionic contribution to the swelling of polyions arises from the electrostatic origin (i.e., the DH interaction between charged groups on the chains) whether the polyion is crosslinked (gels) or not (solutions), and counterion entropy is irrelevant to the swelling.* The reason is presented below.

Outline of Deriving Our Formalism

Let us consider an isolated system with its volume U consisting of a polyion with the effectively occupied volume V and the surrounding reservoir. As a primary expression of the free energy of the total system, F, we start with the following path-integral form:

$$\exp(-\beta F) = \int D\mathbf{R}(s) \exp(-H_{ch} - H_{int}) \qquad (8.23)$$

where H_{ch} is the elastic energy of a Gaussian chain and the interaction energy H_{int} arises from the Coulombic interactions between charged groups and counterions. $\{\mathbf{R}(s)\}$ is the coordinate set of monomers specified by the arc length variables s.

We further perform the standard manipulation of mapping the positions of counterions onto the density field $c(\mathbf{r})$, so that the system free energy F is transformed to $\exp(-\beta F) = \int D\mathbf{R}(s) Dc \exp(-H_{ch} - H_{int-ent})$ with the Hamiltonian $H_{int-ent}$ including both the interaction energy and the translational entropy of the counterions (see

Frusawa and Hayakawa[75] for details). For the Coulombic form, it is more convenient to introduce the potential field $\psi(\mathbf{r})$ via the Hubbard–Stratonovich transformation. Finally, we obtain:[76]

$$\exp(-\beta F) = \int D\mathbf{R}(s)\, Dc\, D\psi\, \exp(-H_{ch} - H_{int-ent}) \qquad (8.24)$$

where $H_{int-ent}$ is rewritten as:

$$H_{int-ent} = \int d\mathbf{r}\, -\frac{|\nabla\psi|^2}{8\pi\, l_B} + \left[f\hat{\rho}(\mathbf{r}) + c(\mathbf{r})\right]\psi(\mathbf{r}) + \int d\mathbf{r}\, c(\mathbf{r})\ln c(\mathbf{r}) - c(\mathbf{r}) \quad (8.25)$$

and we define $\hat{\rho}(\mathbf{r}) = \int ds\, \delta[\mathbf{r} - \mathbf{R}(s)]$. The merit of the expression (8.25) is that this form separates two degrees of freedom, positions of both charged monomers and counterions. Such expression is relevant to asymmetric electrolytes as seen below.

Evaluating Free Energy

While in larger scale, a polyion is regarded as a localized sphere with high charges that absorbs many microions to maintain electrical neutrality, a charged monomer is expected locally to perturb the background potential so weakly that the Gaussian approximation may hold. To treat such different processes due to distinct coarse-graining scales in a unified way, we divide the system free energy into two parts: the free energy $\bar{F}$ in smearing charged monomers over the occupied region uniformly and the surplus contribution ΔF. They are written, respectively, as follows.

Let $\bar{\rho}$ be the smeared monomer density. From Equations (8.24) and (8.25) it follows that associated mean-field paths, $\psi^{mf}(\mathbf{r})$ and $c^{mf}(\mathbf{r})$, satisfy the following Poisson–Boltzmann equation: $\Delta\psi^{mf} = -4\pi l_B(f\bar{\rho} - c^{mf}(\mathbf{r}))$ and $c^{mf} \propto \exp(\psi^{mf}(\mathbf{r}))$, with which the mean-field free energy $\bar{F}_{mf}$ for smeared monomers is given as:

$$\beta\bar{F}_{mf} = \int d\mathbf{r}\, \frac{|\nabla\psi^{mf}|^2}{8\pi l_B} + \int d\mathbf{r}\, c^{mf}(\mathbf{r})\ln c^{mf}(\mathbf{r}) - c^{mf}(\mathbf{r}) \qquad (8.26)$$

in agreement with the conventional expression.

Let us then evaluate the translational entropy of counterions from exact transformations. A few mathematical manipulations[75] give:

$$\int d\mathbf{r}\, c^{mf}(\mathbf{r})\ln c^{mf}(\mathbf{r}) - fn_m\ln(fn_m/U) =$$
$$\frac{1}{8\pi l_B}\left[\int_0^1 d\lambda \int d\mathbf{r}\, \frac{2}{\lambda}|\nabla\psi_\lambda|^2 - \int d\mathbf{r}\, |\nabla\psi|^2\right] \qquad (8.27)$$

This relation reveals that the translational entropy of counterions is almost equal to that of the ideal system where counterions are mobile throughout the system. In

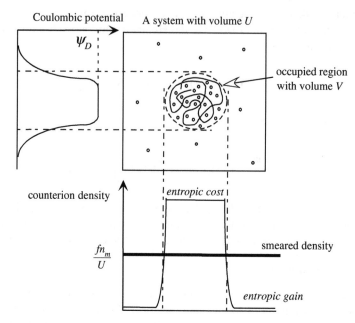

FIGURE 8.4 Persistence length dependencies for various types of polyions.

other words, the counterion entropy difference makes little contribution to the swelling of a polyion.

Can we give this novel picture an intuitive explanation? An affirmative answer can be obtained by looking at Figure 8.4. As shown in the figure, the entropic cost due to the gathering of counterions inside a charged chain reversely leads to the outside gain, merely because the density of the outside necessarily becomes lower when counterion density inside a polyion is higher than the ideal concentration fn_m/U. Therefore, summing up the entropic contributions of the two regions, the total is not so different from the ideal entropy, contrary to the speculation in "the entropy difference picture" where only the inside cost of counterion entropy is emphasized.

From the relation in Equation (8.27), the mean-field free energy for smeared monomers is approximately given by:

$$\beta \overline{F}_{mf} \approx \int d\mathbf{r} \frac{|\nabla \psi|^2}{8\pi l_B} + fn_m \ln\left(fn_m/U\right) - fn_m \qquad (8.28)$$

Considering further Gaussian fluctuations of microions around the mean-field value, we obtain the conventional DH correction term,[75] which this chapter skips for simplicity reasons.

Separating the smeared free energy $\overline{F}$ from F, the surplus free energy, $\Delta F = F - \overline{F}$, is obtained within the Gaussian approximation:[75]

$$\exp(-\beta\Delta F) = \int D\mathbf{R}(s)\exp(-H_{ch+\alpha})$$ (8.29)

and

$$H_{ch+\alpha} = -\frac{2\pi l_B}{\kappa_{in}^2}(f\bar{\rho})^2 V + \frac{l_B f^2}{2}\int ds\, ds'\,\frac{\exp(-\kappa_{in}|\mathbf{R}(s)-\mathbf{R}(s')|)}{|\mathbf{R}(s)-\mathbf{R}(s')|}$$ (8.30)

where V is the effective volume occupied by a chain, and κ_{in}^{-1} is the screening length determined by the counterion concentration inside. Note that the first term on the right side of Equation (8.30) comes out by construction in order to subtract the smeared DH interaction energy from the total. In the context of colloid study on mesoscopic structures, some attention has been recently paid to this term, the so-called volume term.[77]

What Our Result Suggests

Rearranging the results in the presence of salt, the system free energy F finally reads:

$$\beta F = \beta(F_{ion} + F_{irr})$$ (8.31)

$$\beta F_{ion} = \int d\mathbf{r}\,\frac{|\nabla\psi|^2}{8\pi l_B} - \beta\ln\left[\int D\mathbf{R}(s)\exp\left(-\frac{l_B f^2}{2}\int ds\int ds\,\frac{e^{-\kappa_{in}|\mathbf{R}(s)-\mathbf{R}(s')|}}{|\mathbf{R}(s)-\mathbf{R}(s')|}\right)\right]$$ (8.32)

$$\beta F_{irr} = -\frac{2\pi l_B}{\kappa_{in}^2}(f\bar{\rho})^2 V + \sum_i n_i \ln(n_i/U) - n_i$$ (8.33)

with the subscripts *ion* and *irr* denoting, respectively, an ionically relevant term to the swelling of polyelectrolyte chains and an irrelevant term. We group the first term on the right side of Equation (8.33) as an irrelevant term because the osmotic pressure Π_{irr} produced by this term plays no significant role, especially in the weakly screening regime. Since we have $\kappa_{in}^2 = 4\pi l_B\{(f\bar{\rho})^2 + 4C_s^2\}^{1/2}$, the derivative of F_{irr} with respect to V yields:

$$\beta\Pi_{irr} = -\frac{f\bar{\rho}}{2}\left(\frac{2C_s}{f\bar{\rho}}\right)^2\left\{1+\left(\frac{2C_s}{f\bar{\rho}}\right)^2\right\}^{-3/2}$$ (8.34)

indicating that Π_{irr} vanishes with little added salt (i.e., $2C_s/f\bar{\rho} \ll 1$) although Π_{irr} converges to the conventional Donnan form [Equation (8.14)] with the opposite sign, i.e., $\beta\Pi_{irr} \approx -(f\bar{\rho})^2/4C_s$ in the case of fully added salt satisfying $2C_s/f\bar{\rho} \ll 1$.

We thus arrive at the following conclusion. The ionic swelling of a polyelectrolyte chain mainly arises from the screened repulsion between charges on the backbones (i.e., electrostatic origin). It is also elucidated that all of the theories have omitted two additional terms. The first is the interfacial energy due to the presence of electric double layer at the boundary between the inside and outside of a charged chain; it is not trivial whether this contribution is negligible or not in the order of a single polymer. The second is the subtraction of the smeared DH interaction energy [the first term on the right side of Equation (8.33)], which is indispensable for avoiding double count of the electrostatic energy for smeared distibution of charged monomers and reveals that the smeared energy discussed in the electrostatic origin section is to be canceled in correct counting.

Application to Other Systems

The above formulation of a single polyion is applicable not only to polyelectrolyte gels (a crosslinked polyion), but also to various systems in which some charges are localized in a subregion while others are freely mobile throughout the system such as star-branched polyelectrolyte chains, polyelectrolyte brushes whose chains are attached to planar solid surfaces, and Donnan membrane systems consisting of both an outside and inside to which some charges are confined. These examples are depicted in Figure 8.5.

For star-branched polyelectrolyte chains and grafted polyelectrolyte layers, theories have been mainly developed based on the electrostatic picture that the effective electrostatic repulsion between charged groups stretches chains, although the osmotic picture is also exploited in the simplest approximation.[6] For charged gels and the Donnan membrane systems, on the other hand, the osmotic explanation seems to be well accepted[8,78] although some utilize the electrostatic picture.[74,75]

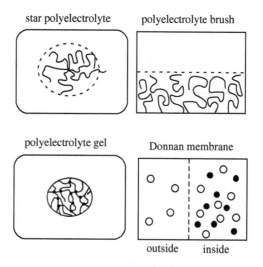

FIGURE 8.5 Systems similar to an isolated polyion system.

In other words, these systems have allowed two interpretations (osmotic and electrostatic) to coexist along with the theories of single polyions. However, similar discussions lead to the conclusion that all the present systems are described by the electrostatic interaction picture with two supplements: the addition of interfacial energy due to the electric double layer and subtraction of the DH interaction energy for smeared distribution of charged monomers.

CONCLUDING REMARKS

Physical properties of neutral polymers such as the entanglement effect and scaling relation have been investigated intensively and understood well for three decades.[4,79] In contrast, polyelectrolyte solutions and gels have created various controversies, partly because it is not easy to control ionic strength with high accuracy and the results vary from time to time due to small amounts of ionic impurities.

Beyond the experimental ambiguity and theoretic difficulties, we have reached some basic understanding of a single polyion as described in this article; however many chain effects are still mysterious. For example, polyelectrolyte solutions even in good solvent have been reported to form huge heterogeneities or domains by small angle neutron scattering and dynamic light scattering.[80–82] Moreover, microphase separation in poor solvents has been observed recently.[83,84] In forming mesoscopic structures, counterion fluctuation should play some roles. It is thus expected that new experiments will be developed to reveal the relationship between counterion fluctuation and heterogeneities and produce advanced theories.

REFERENCES

1. Oosawa, F., *Polyelectrolytes*, Marcel Dekker, New York, 1971.
2. Manning, G.S., Limiting laws and counterion condensation in polyelectrolyte solutions I., *J. Chem. Phys.*, 51, 924, 1969.
3. Mandel, M. and Odijk, T., Dielectric properties of polyelectrolyte solutions, *Ann. Rev. Phys. Chem.* 35, 75, 1984.
4. Grosberg, A.Y. and Khokhlov, A.R., *Statistical Physics of Macromolecules,* AIP Press, New York, 1994.
5. Schmitz, K.S., *An Introduction to Dynamic Light Scattering by Macromolecules,* Academic Press, San Diego, 1990.
6. Barrat, J.-L. and Joanny, J.-F., Theory of polyelectrolyte solutions, *Adv. Chem. Phys.,* 94, 1, 1997.
7. Holm, C., Kekicheff, P., and Podgornik, R., Eds., *Electrostatic Effects in Soft Matter and Biophysics,* Kluwer Academic, London, 2001.
8. Dusek, K., Responsive gels: volume phase transitions, *Adv. Polym. Sci.,* 109, 1993.
9. O'Konski, C.T. and Krause, S., *Molecular Electro-Optics*, Plenum, New York, 1976.
10. Guéron, M. and Weisbuch, G., Polyelectrolyte theory, *Biopolymers*, 19, 353, 1980; *J. Phys. Chem.*, 83, 1991, 1979.
11. Deserno, M. and Holm, C., Cell model and Poisson–Boltzmann theory, in *Electrostatic Effects in Soft Matter and Biophysics*, Kluwer Academic, London, 2001, 27.
12. Levin, Y., Electrostatic correlations: from biology to plasma, *Rep. Prog. Phys.*, 65, 1577, 2002.

13. Minakata, A. and Imai, N., Dielectric properties of polyelectrolytes, *Biopolymers*, 11, 329, 1972.

14. Sakamoto, M., Kanda, H., Hayakawa, R., and Wada, Y., Dielectric relaxation of DNA in aqueous solutions, *Biopolymers*, 15, 879, 1976.

15. van der Tow, F. and Mandel, M., Dielectric increment and dielectric dispersion of solutions containing simple charged linear macromolecules. II. Experimental results with synthetic polyelectrolytes, *Biophys. Chem.*, 2, 231, 1974.

16. Mandel, M., The electric polarization of rod-like, charged macromolecules, *Mol. Phys.*, 4, 489, 1961.

17. Oosawa, F., Counterion fluctuation and dielectric dispersion in linear polyelectrolytes, *Biopolymers*, 9, 677, 1970.

18. van Dijk, W., van der Touwand, F., and Mandel, M., Influence of counterion exchange on the induced dipole moment and its relaxation for a rodlike polyion, *Macromolecules*, 14, 792, 1981; Model estimate for the relaxation time of the counterion distribution in the radial direction around a rodlike, charged macromolecule, *Macromolecules*, 14, 1554, 1981.

19. Fixman, M. and Jagannathan, S., Spherical macroions in strong fields, *Macromolecules*, 16, 685, 1983.

20. Ito, K. and Hayakawa, R., Theory on the relation between the dielectric relaxation and the polyion mobility relaxation in polyelectrolyte solutions, *Macromolecules*, 24, 3857, 1991.

21. Odijk, T., Possible scaling relations for semidilute polyelectrolyte solutions, *Macromolecules*, 12, 688, 1979.

22. Minakata, A., Dielectric dispersions of polyelectrolytes due to ion fluctuation, *Ann. N.Y. Acad. Sci.*, 303, 107, 1977.

23. Imai, N. and Sasaki, S., Dielectric increment in polyion solutions due to the distortion of counterion distribution, *Biophys. Chem.*, 11, 361, 1980.

24. Cametti, C. and Di Biasio, A., Counterion residence time and counterion radial diffusion in rodlike polyelectrolyte solutions, *Macromolecules*, 20, 1579, 1987.

25. Ito, K., Yagi, A., Ookubo, N., and Hayakawa, R., Crossover behavior in high frequency dielectric relaxation of linear polyions in dilute and semidilute solutions, *Macromolecules*, 23, 857, 1990.

26. Nishida, K., Kaji, K., and Kanaya, T., Improved phase diagram of polyelectrolyte solutions, *J. Chem. Phys.*, 115, 8217, 2001; High concentration crossovers of polyelectrolyte solutions, *ibid.*, 114, 8671, 2001.

27. Nagamine, Y., Ito, K., and Hayakawa, R., Low and high frequency relaxations in linear polyelectrolyte solutions with different counter-ion species, *Colloids Surfaces* A, 148, 149, 1999.

28. Frusawa, H., Ito, K., and Hayakawa, R., High frequency dielectric relaxation of polyelectrolyte gels, *Phys. Rev. E*, 55, 7283, 1997.

29. Ookubo, N., Hirai, Y., Ito, K., and Hayakawa, R., Anisotropic counterion polarizations and their dynamics in aqueous polyelectrolytes as studied by frequency-domain electric birefringence relaxation spectroscopy, *Macromolecules*, 22, 1359, 1989.

30. Hayakawa, R., Electric birefrringence relaxation spectroscopy, *Polym. Prep. Jpn.*, 33, 1796, 1981.

31. Hosokawa, K., Shimomura, T., Frusawa, H., Kimura, Y., Ito, K., and Hayakawa, R., Two-dimensional spectroscopy of electric birefringence relaxation in frequency domain: measurement method for second-order nonlinear after-effect function, *J. Chem. Phys.*, 110, 4101, 1999.

32. Elias, J.G. and Eden, D., Transient electric birefringence study of the persistence length and electrical polarizability of restriction fragments of DNA, *Macromolecules*, 14, 410, 1981.

33. Tricot, M. and Houssier, C., Electrooptical studies on sodium poly(styrenesulfonate). 1. Electric polarizability and orientation function from electric birefringence measurements, *Macromolecules*, 15, 854, 1982.

34. Szabo, A., Haleem, M., and Eden, D., Theory of the transient electric birefringence of rod-like polyions: coupling of rotational and counterion dynamics, *J. Chem. Phys.*, 85, 7472, 1986.

35. Ookubo, N., Teraoka, I., and Hayakawa, R., Low frequency dynamics of counterions polarization in aqueous polyelectrolyte as studied by electric birefringence relaxation method, *Ferroelectrics*, 86, 19, 1988.

36. Degiorgio, V., Bellini, T., Piazza, R., Mantegazza, F., and Goldstein, R.E., Stretched-exponential relaxation of electric birefringence in polymer solutions, *Phys. Rev. Lett.*, 64, 1043, 1990.

37. Degiorgio, V., Mantegazza, F., and Piazza, R., Transient electric birefringence measurement of the persistence length of sodium polystyrene sulfonate, *Europhys. Lett.*, 15, 75, 1991.

38. Krämer, U. and Hoffmann, H., Electric birefringence measurements in aqueous polyelectrolyte solutions, *Macromolecules*, 24, 256, 1991.

39. Coffey, W.T., Déjardin, J.-L., Kalmykov, Y.P., and Titov, S.V., Nonlinear dielectric relaxation and dynamic Kerr effect in a strong dc electric field suddenly switched on: exact solutions for the three-dimensional rotational diffusion model, *Phys. Rev. E*, 54, 6462, 1996.

40. Déjardin, J.-L., *Dynamic Kerr Effect*, World Scientific, Singapore, 1995.

41. Déjardin, J.-L., Déjardin, P.-M., and Kalmykov, Y.P., Analytical solutions for the dynamic Kerr effect: linear response of polar and polarizable molecules to a weak ac electric field superimposed on a strong dc bias field, *J. Chem. Phys.*, 107, 508, 1997.

42. Nagamine, Y., Ito, K., and Hayakawa, R., Low and high frequency electric birefringence relaxations in linear polyelectrolyte solutions, *Langmuir*, 15, 4135, 1999.

43. Kramer, H., Deggelmann, M., Graf, C., Hagenbüchle, M., Johner, C., and Weber, R., Electric birefringence measurements in aqueous fd virus solutions, *Macromolecules*, 25, 4325, 1992.

44. Kramer, H., Graf, C., Hagenbüchle, M., Johner, C., Martin, C., Schwind, P., and Weber, R., Electro-optic effects of aqueous fd-virus suspensions at very low ionic-strength, *J. Phys. II* (France), 4, 1061, 1994.

45. Johner, C., Kramer, H., Batzil, S., Graf, C., Hagenbüchle, M., Martin, C., and Weber, R., Static light scattering and electric birefringence experiments on saltfree solutions of poly(styrenesulfonate), *J. Phys. II* (France), 4, 1571, 1994.

46. Johner, C., Kramer, H., Martin, C., Biegel, J., Deike, R., and Weber, R., Characterization of poly(styrenesulfonate) at minimum ionic strength by electric and magnetic birefringence experiments, *J. Phys. II* (France), 5, 721, 1995.

47. Cates, M.E., The anomalous Kerr effect: implication for polyelectrolyte structure, *J. Phys. II* (France), 2, 1109, 1992.

48. Lachenmayer, K. and Oppermann, W.J., Electric birefringence of dilute aqueous solutions of poly(p-phenylene) polyelectrolytes, *J. Chem. Phys.*, 116, 392, 2002.

49. Schmitz, K.S., Quasielastic light scattering by biopolymers, *Chem. Phys. Lett.*, 63, 259, 1979.

50. Imaeda, T., Kimura, Y., Ito, K., and Hayakawa, R., New formulation for data analysis in the quasielastic light scattering with the sinusoidal electric field and its application to the spherical polyions in aqueous solutions, *J. Chem. Phys.*, 100, 950, 1994.

51. Ito, K., Ooi, S., Nishi, N., Kimura, Y., and Hayakawa, R., New measurement method of the autocorrelation function in the quasielastic light scattering with the sinusoidal electric field, *J. Chem. Phys.*, 100, 6098, 1994.

52. Ito, K., Ooi, S., Kimura, Y., and Hayakawa, R., New measurement method for the quasielastic light scattering with the sinusoidal electric field by use of an extended Wiener–Khinchin theorem, *J. Chem. Phys.*, 101, 4463, 1994.

53. Ito, K., Maruyama, Y., Hiroyasu, N., and Hayakawa, R., Dynamic light scattering in a periodically stationary system, *Langmuir*, 15, 4139, 1999.

54. Ito, K. and Hayakawa, R., Quasi-elastic light scattering with the sinusoidal electric field: new measurement methods and frequency dispersion of the electrophoretic mobility and diffusion constant of polyions, *Colloids Surface A*, 148, 135, 1999.

55. Mizuno, D., Kimura, Y., and Hayakawa, R., Electrophoretic microrheology in a dilute lamellar phase of a nonionic surfactant, *Phys. Rev. Lett.*, 87, 088104, 2001.

56. Dobrynin, A.V., Rubinstein, M., and Obukhov, S.P., Cascade of transitions of polyelectrolytes in poor solvents, *Macromolecules*, 29, 2974, 1996; Micka, U., Holm, C., and Kremer, K., Strongly charged, flexible polyelectrolytes in poor solvents: molecular dynamics simulations, *Langmuir*, 15, 4033, 1999.

57. Odijk, T.J., Polyelectrolytes near the rod limit, *J. Polym. Sci. Polym. Phys. Ed.*, 15, 477, 1977; Skolnick, J. and Fixman, M., Electrostatic persistence length of a wormlike polyelectrolyte, *Macromolecules*, 10, 944, 1977.

58. Everaers, R., Johner, A. and Joanny, J.-F., Polyampholytes: from single chains to solutions, *Macromolecules*, 30, 8478, 1997.

59. Soils, F.J. and Olvera de La Cruz, M., Collapse of flexible polyelectrolytes in multivalent salt solutions, *J. Chem. Phys.*, 112, 2030, 2000.

60. Nguyen, T.T., Rouzina, I., and Shklovskii, B.I., Negative electrostatic contribution to the bending rigidity of charged membranes and polyelectrolytes screened by multivalent counterions, *Phys. Rev. E*, 60, 7032, 1999.

61. Golestanian, R., Kardar, M., and Liverpool, T.B., Collapse of stiff polyelectrolytes due to counterion fluctuations, *Phys. Rev. Lett.*, 82, 4456, 1999.

62. Brilliantov, N.V., Kuznetsov, D.V., and Klein, R., Chain collapse and counterion condensation in dilute polyelectrolyte solutions, *Phys. Rev. Lett.*, 81, 1433, 1998.

63. Schiessel, H. and Pincus, P., Counterion-condensation-induced collapse of highly charged polyelectrolytes, *Macromolecules*, 31, 7953, 1998.

64. Ariel, G. and Andelman, D., Persistence length of a strongly charged rodlike polyelectrolyte in the presence of salt, *Phys. Rev. E*, 67, 011805, 2003.

65. Witten, T.A. and Pincus, P., Structure and viscosity of interpenetrating polyelectrolyte chains, *Europhys. Lett.*, 3, 315, 1987.

66. Netz, R.R. and Orland, H., Variational theory for a single polyelectrolyte chain, *Eur. Phys. J. B*, 8, 81, 1999.

67. Micka, U. and Kremer, K., Persistence length of the Debye–Hückel model of weakly charged flexible polyelectrolyte chains, *Phys. Rev. E*, 54, 2653, 1996.

68. Ha, B.-Y. and Thirumalai, D., Persistence length of flexible polyelectrolyte chains, *J. Chem. Phys.*, 110, 7533, 1999.

69. Liverpool, T.B. and Stapper, M., Renormalization group analysis of weakly charged polyelectrolytes, *Eur. Phys. J. E*, 5, 359, 2001.

70. Rice, S.A. and Nagasawa, M., *Polyelectrolyte Solutions*, Academic Press, New York, 1961; Marcus, R.A., Calculation of thermodynamic properties of polyelectrolytes, *J. Chem. Phys.*, 23, 1057, 1955.

71. Flory, P.J., Molecular configuration of polyelectrolytes, *J. Chem. Phys.*, 21, 162, 1953.

72. Hermans, J.J. and Overbeek, T.T.G., The dimensions of charged long chain molecules in solutions containing electrolytes, *Rec. Trav. Chim.*, 67, 761, 1948; Hill, T.L., Some statistical mechanical models of elastic polyelectrolytes and proteins, *J. Chem. Phys.*, 20, 1259, 1952.

73. Katchalsky, A. and Lifson, S., The electrostatic free energy of polyelectrolyte solutions, *J. Polym. Sci.*, 11, 409, 1953.

74. Muthukumar, M., Polyelectrolyte gels: replica theory, in *Molecular Basis of Polymer Networks*, Baumgartner, A. and Picot, C.E. Eds., Springer-Verlag, Berlin, 1989, 28; Wilder, J. and Vilgis, T.A., Elasticity in strongly interacting soft solids: a polyelectrolyte network, *Phys. Rev. E*, 57, 6865, 1998; Vilgis, T.A. and Wilder, J., Polyelectrolyte networks: elasticity, swelling, and the violation of the Flory–Rehner hypothesis, *J., Comput. Theor. Polym. Sci.*, 8, 61, 1998.

75. Frusawa, H. and Hayakawa, R., Swelling mechanism unique to charged gels, *Phys. Rev. E*, 58, 6145, 1998.

76. Frusawa, H. and Hayakawa, R., Generalizing Debye–Hückel theory in terms of density functional integral, *Phys. Rev. E*, 61, R6079, 2000; Field theoretical representation of the Hohenberg–Kohn free energy, *ibid.*, 60, R5048, 1999.

77. von Grunberg, H.H., van Roij, R., and Klein, G., Gas–liquid phase coexistence in colloidal suspensions? *Europhys. Lett.*, 55, 580, 2001; Schmitz, K.S., Volume-term theories of phase separation in colloidal systems and long-range attractive tail in the pair potential between colloidal particles, *Phys. Rev. E*, 63, 011503, 2000.

78. Shneider, S. and Linse, P., Swelling of crosslinked polyelectrolyte gels, *Eur. Phys. J. E*, 8, 457, 2002.

79. Doi, M. and Edwards, S.F., *The Theory of Polymer Dynamics*, Oxford Science Publications, Oxford, 1986.

80. Ermi, E.D. and Amis, E.J., Influence of backbone solvation on small angle neutron scattering from polyelectrolyte solutions, *Macromolecules*, 30, 6937, 1997; Domain structures in low ionic strength polyelectrolyte solutions, *ibid.*, 31, 7378, 1998.

81. Sedlak, M., What can be seen by static and dynamic light scattering in polyelectrolyte solutions and mixtures? *Langmuir*, 15, 4045, 1999.

82. Ito, K., Yoshida, H., and Ise, N., Void structure in colloidal dispersions, *Science*, 263, 66, 1994.

83. Braun, O., Boue, F., and Candau, F., Microphase separation in weakly charged hydrophobic polyelectrolytes, *Eur. Phys. J. E*, 7, 141, 2002.

84. Shibayama, M. and Tanaka, T., Small-angle neutron scattering study on weakly charged poly(N-isopropyl acrylamide-co-acrylic acid) copolymer solutions, *J. Chem. Phys.*, 102, 9392, 1995.

9 Kinetics in Cyclic Hydrogel Systems

Ryo Yoshida

CONTENTS

INTRODUCTION

Over the last two decades, many researchers have developed stimuli-responsive polymer gels that change volume abruptly in response to changes in their surroundings, for example, changes in solvent composition, temperature, pH, and supply of electric field, as described in other chapters. Their ability to swell and deswell according to conditions makes them interesting propositions for use in new intelligent materials. In particular, applications to biomedical fields, e.g., as actuators

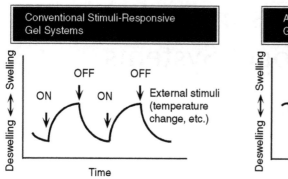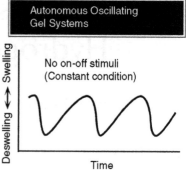

FIGURE 9.1 Stimuli-responsive systems and autonomous oscillating systems.

(artificial muscles), biosensors, and self-regulating drug delivery systems and for purification of chemical or bioactive agents, cell culture, and on–off regulation of enzymatic reactions, have been extensively studied.[1,2] One of the strategies of these applications is to develop biomimetic material systems with stimuli-responding functions, i.e., systems whose materials sense environmental changes and tale action. For these systems, the on–off switching of external stimuli is essential to instigate the action of the gel. Upon switching, the gels provide only one unique action: swelling or deswelling.

This stimuli-responding behavior is a temporary action toward an equilibrium state. In contrast, many physiological phenomena in human bodies continue their own native cyclic changes. These phenomena exist over a wide range from cellular to body level, as represented by cell cycle, cyclic reaction in glycolysis, pulsatile secretion of hormones, pulsatile potential of nerve cells, brain wave, heartbeat, peristaltic motion in digestive tract, and human biorhythm. If such self-oscillation can be achieved for gels, possibilities for new biomimetic intelligent materials that exhibit autonomous rhythmical motion would emerge.

In this chapter, new design concepts for cyclic gel systems that exhibit spontaneous and autonomous periodic swelling–deswelling changes under constant condition without on–off switching of external stimuli will be introduced (Figure 9.1). The studies attempted so far can be classified into two categories: (1) construction of oscillating systems by using conventional stimuli-responsive gels and (2) design of new-type gels to generate spontaneous mechanical oscillation. In both cases, nonlinear dynamics of chemical reactions and material characteristics of gel as open systems play important roles.

OSCILLATING SYSTEMS USING STIMULI-RESPONSIVE GELS

COUPLING SYSTEMS WITH pH-OSCILLATING REACTIONS

In order to achieve oscillating systems of polymer gels, several ideas have been devised by utilizing conventional stimuli-responsive gels. One method is to couple the pH-responsive gels to pH-oscillating reactions. As typical reactions to produce nonlinear chemical dynamics, several pH-oscillating systems have been reported by many researchers. In general, two main composite processes are needed: (1) autocatalytic production of H^+ (positive feedback) and (2) consumption of H^+ (negative feedback). For the mixed Landolt reaction (iodate–sulfite–thiosulfate system) discovered by Rabai and Beck,[3,4] the following simplified model (called the alternator) is presented.

$$A + Y + X \rightarrow 2X + P_2$$

$$A + B + X \rightarrow P_1$$

$$A + B \rightarrow Y$$

In this model, A corresponds to iodate, B to thiosulfate, Y to hydrogen sulfite, X to hydrogen ion, P_1 to tetrathionate, and P_2 to sulfate. The alternator is closely related to the Lotka model[5] often used to characterize predator–prey interactions. The first reaction is an autocatalytic H^+ production, the second is a H^+ consumption step, and the third regenerates the reactant Y that serves as the source of X. In order to construct pH-oscillating systems, a continuous-flow stirred tank reactor (CSTR) is often used because the third process can be replaced by the input flow in a CSTR. Therefore only two processes are necessary to construct an oscillatory reaction in a CSTR.

Yoshida et al.[6,7] demonstrated a mechanical oscillating system of pH-responsive poly(N-isopropylacrylamide(NIPAAm)-co-acrylic acid-co-butyl methacrylate) gels by coupling with a pH-oscillating reaction (hydrogen peroxide–hydrogen sulfite–hexacyanoferrate (II) system).[8] The main subprocesses are the oxidation of hydrogen sulfite ions by hydrogen peroxide and the oxidation of hexacyanoferrate (II) ions by hydrogen peroxide as follows:

$$HSO_3^- + H_2O_2 \rightarrow SO_4^{2-} + H_2O + H^+$$

$$2Fe(CN)_6^{4-} + H_2O_2 + 2H^+ \rightarrow 2Fe(CN)_6^{3-} + 2H_2O$$

Premixed solutions of sulfuric acid, sodium sulfite, and potassium hexacyanoferrate (II) trihydrate, and pure hydrogen peroxide solution, respectively, were continuously supplied to the CSTR with a high performance liquid chromatography (HPLC) pump at a constant flow rate (Figure 9.2). In the CSTR, hydrogen sulfite ions are oxidized by hydrogen peroxide and produce hydrogen ions, while hexacyanoferrate (II) ions are oxidized by hydrogen peroxide with consumption of hydrogen ions. The production and consumption of hydrogen ions occur at comparable rates that generate pH oscillations in the reactor with constant amplitude and period.[8] The amplitude and period depend on feed concentration, flow rate, and temperature.[9] At 22°C, the pH oscillates with a period of 8 min and at pH amplitudes between 4.7 and 6.9. In the CSTR, the gels demonstrate rhythmic swelling and deswelling changes synchronized with the pH oscillation (Figure 9.3).

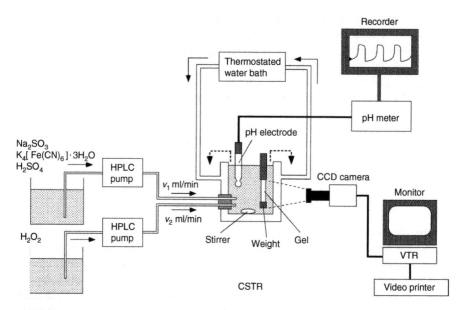

FIGURE 9.2 Continuous monitoring system for oscillations in medium pH and gel length in a CSTR.

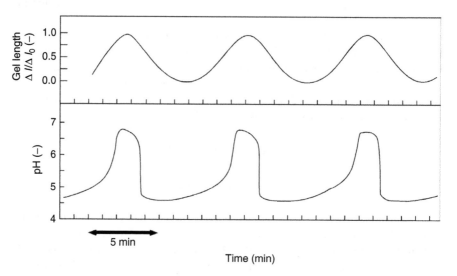

FIGURE 9.3 Oscillations in poly(NIPAAm-co-AAc-co-BMA) gel length and pH in an oscillating CSTR.

In contrast to the observed asymmetric pulsatile pattern for pH changes, the gel oscillating profiles are symmetric, similar to trigonometric functions. The oscillating patterns of pH-sensitive gels in pH-oscillating reactions have been theoretically analyzed by considering the characteristic response times for gels and external pH changes.[7] The theoretical curve provides symmetric pulsatile patterns and closely simulates the observed experimental oscillating profiles with good agreement for times exhibiting minima and maxima in gel length. This system has the characteristics that the oscillating output is generated by constant input (constant flow of solution), and the period and amplitude of the gel oscillation can be controlled by changing one parameter such as concentration of the solution, the flow rate, etc.

Crook et al.[10] constructed cyclic gel systems by coupling a pH-sensitive poly(methacrylic acid) (PMAA) gel with a Landolt pH-oscillator base on a bromate–sulfite–ferrocyanide reaction. The main processes are the oxidation of sulfite by bromate and the oxidation of ferrocyanide by bromate as follows.

$$BrO_3^- + 3HSO_3^- + H^+ \rightarrow Br^- + 3SO_4^{2-} + 4H^+$$

$$BrO_3^- + 6Fe(CN)_6^{4-} + 6H^+ \rightarrow Br^- + 6Fe(CN)_6^{3-} + 3H_2O$$

This system has advantages of reliable oscillation at room temperature and a large pH range; it stays at pH extremes for approximately equal time to allow the gel to change conformation. The pH oscillates with a period of 20 min and a pH range of $3.1 \leq 7.0$ at room temperature. In CSTR, PMAA gel particles of submillimeter size exhibited periodic swelling–deswelling changes following pH oscillation.

Several studies to apply such a gel oscillator to controlled drug release systems have been attempted. In the research field of drug delivery systems (DDS), many types of modulated systems in response to external signals of disease have been devised by utilizing stimuli-responsive gels; e.g., glucose-responsive insulin delivery, temperature-responsive antipyretic delivery, etc. As another category of modulated delivery different from stimuli-responsive systems, delivery systems that automatically release drugs in periodic pulses have attracted great interest from the standpoint of chronopharmacotherapy. The efficacy of certain hormones significantly increases if the hormones are administered in pulses rather than at a constant (zero-order release) rate. The significance of administering drugs in a preprogrammed pulsatile manner has been pointed out for a number of hormones that exhibit rhythmic secretion patterns, cell-cycle specific chemotherapeutic agents for cancer treatment, and drugs that exhibit tolerance or circadian variation in efficacy or toxicity.

Giannos et al.[11,12] designed and constructed oscillatory drug release systems by coupling the mixed Landoldt pH oscillator with membrane diffusion. The diffusion of benzoic acid (BzA) and nicotine across an ethylene vinyl acetate (EVAc) membrane from donor solutions containing the mixed Landolt reaction was investigated. By changing the pH of a solution, a drug may be rendered charged or uncharged relative to the pK_a value of the drug. Only the uncharged form of a drug can penetrate across lipophilic membranes, so a periodic delivery profile may be obtained by oscillating the pH of the donor solution. As a result of experiment, however, oscillations of the flux were limited to once or twice because (1) the ionizable drug has a buffer capacity that results in damping of the oscillations in pH, (2) the oscillators are extremely sensitive to initial conditions, and (3) the desired frequency and amplitude are not always possible. These limitations made observation of multiple pulses difficult.

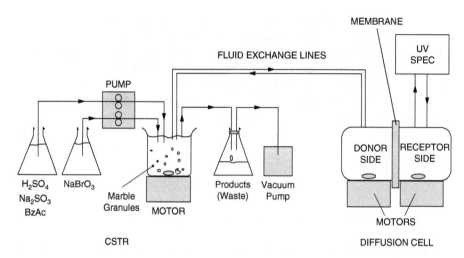

FIGURE 9.4 CSTR/diffusion cell set-up, with rapid fluid exchange between the CSTR and the donor side of the diffusion cell. (From Misra, G.P. and Siegel, R.A., *J. Controlled Release*, 79, 293, 2002. With permission.)

In order to produce pH oscillations of lengthened periodicity, Misra and Siegel[13,14] utilized the pH oscillator based on the bromate–sulfite–marble reaction presented by Rabai and Hanasaki (RH).[15] The proposed simple mechanism for the RH oscillator involves the following three relatively slow reactions.

$$3HSO_3^- + BrO_3^- \rightarrow 3SO_4^{2-} + Br^- + 3H^+$$

$$3H_2SO_3 + BrO_3^- \rightarrow 3SO_4^{2-} + Br^- + 6H^+$$

$$H^+ + CaCO_3 \rightarrow Ca^{2+} + HCO_3^-$$

In this reaction, solid granular or lumpy marble is used for removal of H^+ from an aqueous reaction mixture of sulfur (IV)–bromate ion. The $CaCO_3$ content of marble reacts with H^+ when the pH is low. As shown in Figure 9.4, the reactants were pumped into a beaker (CSTR) through two separate lines and removed by aspiration to maintain a constant volume. In one reservoir of reactants, benzoic acid (BzA) is contained as a model acidic drug. The reacting solution in the CSTR was circulated into the donor side of the diffusion cell and returned to the CSTR. The donor side was separated from the receptor side by a lipophilic (hydrophobic) ethylene–vinyl acetate copolymer (EVAc) membrane. In the CSTR (and donor cell), the pH oscillated between 6.5 to 7.0 and 3.2 with a 1-h period. Accompanying the pH oscillation, multiple and periodic pulses of drug flux across the membrane were observed when the concentration of drug was sufficiently low (Figure 9.5).

COUPLING SYSTEMS WITH ENZYMATIC REACTIONS

Another method of designing autonomous cyclic systems utilizes an enzymatic reaction. Siegel and Pitt[16] mathematically designed a new pulsating system to provide

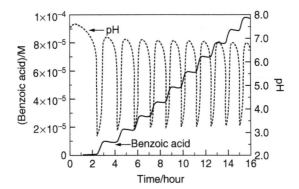

FIGURE 9.5 Time course of pH in CSTR (dashed line) and accumulation of benzoic acid in the receptor side of the diffusion cell (solid line). (From Misra, G.P. and Siegel, R.A., *J. Controlled Release*, 79, 293, 2002. With permission.)

periodic drug release by coupling enzyme reaction and pH-responsive gels (Figure 9.6). They devised a chamber containing a drug and an enzyme (glucose oxidase) separated from the exterior by a semipermeable membrane (a pH-sensitive hydrogel based on acrylic acid). The substrate (glucose) is present externally at constant concentration [S*] and diffuses into the chamber through the membrane to give the concentration of internal substrate [S]. In the chamber, gluconic acid is produced by the enzyme reaction, which results in increasing proton concentration [P].

The membrane permeability to the substrate K(t) is lowered with the pH decrease, and the drug release from the chamber is also decreased. The reduced permeability leads to a drop in [S], followed by a decrease in [P]. Due to the decreasing [P], the lowered K(t) rises up to the initial value and the cycle is repeated as long as [S*] remains constant. As a result, the drug is released from the chamber in a pulsatile manner. By selecting adequate parameters, the simulated system continues oscillating behavior. In addition, it has been demonstrated experimentally and theoretically that pH hysteresis is present in glucose permeability of poly(NIPAAm-co-MAA) gel, and the hysteresis is a crucial feature of the pulsating system.[17–20]

They realized self-oscillatory release of gonadotropin-releasing hormone (GnRH) through the poly(NIPAAm-co-MAA) membrane in the presence of a constant level of glucose.[21] The membranes were mounted in a water-jacketed, side-by-side diffusion cell (Figure 9.7). Saline containing a constant concentration of glucose flows through Cell I and the pH is clamped at 7.0 using pH-Stat. Cell II initially contains glucose-free saline solution, a piece of marble, small particles of polyacrylamide gel containing enzymes (glucose oxidase and catalase), and labeled GnRH. The marble acts as a shunt for eliminating H+.

Oscillations were followed by continuously recording the pH in Cell II and measuring the concentration of the released model drug in Cell I. GnRH was released in short, repetitive pulses over 1 week (Figure 9.8). Regardless of the large volume of Cell II, pH swings were accelerated but kept in range by increasing glucose concentration and introducing marble. Methods to maintain rhythmic behavior under more realistic physiological conditions have also been investigated.[22]

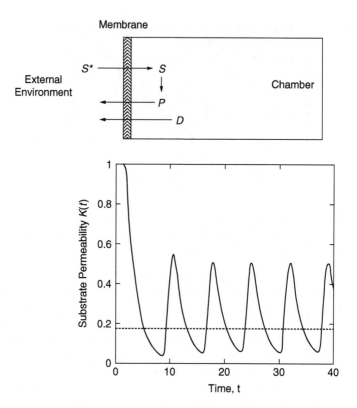

FIGURE 9.6 Oscillatory drug release system and numerical simulation of oscillating behavior in the system. (From Siegel, R.A. and Pitt, C.F., *J. Controlled Release*, 33, 173, 1995. With permission.)

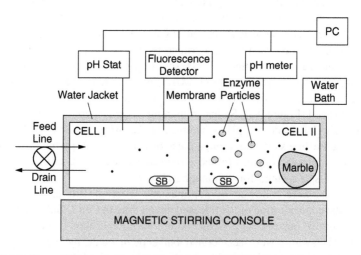

FIGURE 9.7 Test cell for rhythmic pulsatile delivery of GnRH. (From Misra, G.P. and Siegel, R.A., *J. Controlled Release*, 81, 1, 2002. With permission.)

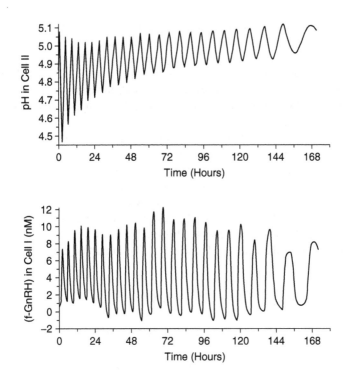

FIGURE 9.8 Time course of oscillations of pH in Cell II (top). Corresponding time course of concentration of f-GnRH in Cell I (bottom). (From Misra, G.P. and Siegel, R.A., *J. Controlled Release*, 81, 1, 2002. With permission.)

AUTONOMOUS OSCILLATING SYSTEMS: SELF-OSCILLATING GELS

DESIGN OF SELF-OSCILLATING GELS

Oscillating Chemical Reactions: Belousov–Zhabotinsky Reaction

As mentioned above, cyclic gel systems (periodic swelling–deswelling changes of gels soaked in an autonomous pH-oscillating solution in a CSTR and an oscillatory drug release system utilizing gel membrane coupled with pH-oscillating or enzymatic reaction) have been studied. However, gels that provide mechanical oscillation without external control in a closed solution have not been developed yet.

The Belousov–Zhabotinsky (BZ) reaction[23-25] is well known for exhibiting temporal and spatial oscillating phenomena with periodic redox changes of the catalysts in a closed solution. The reaction was discovered by B.P. Belousov who sought an inorganic analog of the Krebs or TCA (tricarboxylic acid) cycle — a key metabolic process in which citric acid is an intermediate — and then modified by A.M. Zhabotinsky. The overall process of the BZ reaction is the oxidation of an organic substrate such as citric or malonic acid (MA) by an oxidizing agent (bromate) in the presence of metal catalyst under acidic conditions. Metal ions or a metal complex with high redox potential (1.0 to 1.4 V/SHE), such as cerium ion, ferroin, or ruthenium tris(2,2′-bipyridine) (Ru(bpy)$_3$) are widely used as catalysts. In the course of the reaction, the catalyst ion periodically changes its charge number to oscillate between the oxidized and reduced states for several hours, as long as the substrate exists. When the solution is homogeneously stirred, the color of the solution periodically changes, like a neon sign, based on the redox changes of the metal catalyst. When the solution is placed under stationary conditions as a thin film, concentric or spiral wave patterns develop in the solution. The wave of oxidized state propagating in the medium at a constant speed is called the *chemical wave*.

The BZ reaction has a cyclic reaction network similar to the TCA cycle. The oscillation mechanism has been explained primarily by models composed of three cyclic subprocesses (the FKN or Field–Körös–Noyes mechanism):[26] the consumption of bromide ion (Br⁻) (Process A), autocatalytic reaction of bromous acid (HBrO$_2$) with oxidation of the catalyst (Process B), and an organic reaction accompanying reduction of the catalyst (Process C). The important steps in each process are as follows:

Process A: $BrO_3^- + 2Br^- + 3H^+ \rightarrow 3HOBr$

Process B: $BrO_3^- + HBrO_2 + 2M_{red} + 3H^+ \rightarrow 2HBrO_2 + 2M_{ox} + H_2O$

Process C: $2M_{ox} + MA + BrMA \rightarrow f\,Br^- + 2M_{red} + $ other products

The stoichiometric factor f represents the number of bromide ions produced as two M_{ox} ions (oxidized metal ions) are reduced. To mathematically express the FKN scheme, the Oregonator model has widely been employed.[27] This is frequently written in the form:

$$A + Y \rightarrow X + P$$

$$X + Y \rightarrow 2P$$

$$A + X \rightarrow 2X + 2Z$$

$$2X \rightarrow A + P$$

$$B + Z \rightarrow 1/2\,fY$$

where $A = BrO_3^-$, $B = $ all oxidizable organic species, $P = HOBr$, $X = HBrO_2$ (activator), $Y = Br^-$(inhibitor), and $Z = M_{ox}$.

The concentrations of the major reactants A and B are treated as constants. The rate equations for the intermediate species X, Y, and Z can be derived from the model. Thus, we can numerically simulate the aspects of the BZ reaction. The mechanisms lead to several phenomena such as such as oscillations and excitability, traveling reaction fronts, target patterns, spiral and scroll waves, bifurcation and chaos, etc. These phenomena are related to important processes in biology. The

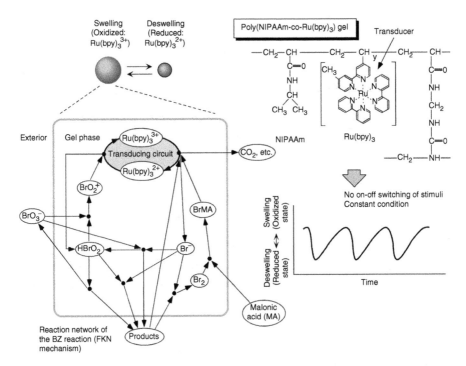

FIGURE 9.9 Self-oscillation of poly(NIPAAm-co-Ru(bpy)₃) gel coupled with Belousov–Zhabotinsky reaction.

significance of the BZ reaction has been recognized as a chemical model for understanding some aspects of biological phenomena such as glycolytic oscillations or biorhythms,[28] cardiac fibrillation,[29] self-organization of amoeba cells,[30] pattern formation on animal skin,[31,32] and visual pattern processing on the retina.[33]

Preparation of Poly(NIPAAm-co-Ru(bpy)₃) Gel Undergoing Redox Changes

Yoshida et al. attempted to convert the chemical oscillation of the BZ reaction to the mechanical changes of gels and generate an autonomic swelling–deswelling oscillation under nonoscillatory outer conditions.[34–43] The gel has a cyclic reaction network and generates periodic mechanical energy from the chemical energy of the BZ reaction (Figure 9.9).

While hydrogels have been used as BZ reaction media in order to suppress hydrodynamic convection and immobilize catalysts,[44] Yoshida et al. utilize a gel in which the BZ reaction causes periodic redox changes within the polymer network. In conventional stimuli-responsive gels, gels in which enzymes are immobilized by physical entrapping in the networks have been prepared to convert chemical change to mechanical work.[45] These gels undergo volume phase transition by addition of a substrate. In these systems, gels act as immobilization supports and swelling or deswelling is induced only when environmental chemical change occurs. In our

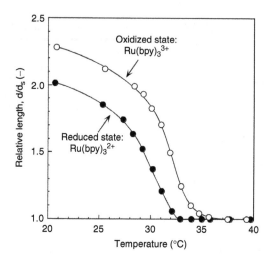

FIGURE 9.10 Temperature dependence of normalized length for poly(NIPAAm-co-Ru(bpy)$_3$) gel under oxidizing and reducing conditions. The normalization was performed by use of the original gel length determined at 45°C.

novel gel, however, the polymer networks undergo reactions and spontaneously create their periodic motions without environmental changes.

A copolymer gel that consists of NIPAAm and ruthenium (II) tris(2,2'-bipyridine) (Ru(bpy)$_3$) was prepared. Ru(bpy)$_3$, acting as a catalyst for the BZ reaction, is pendent to the polymer chains of NIPAAm. Homopolymer gels of NIPAAm have thermosensitivity and undergo an abrupt volume collapse (phase transition) when heated at around 32°C.[46,47] The oxidation of the Ru(bpy)$_3$ moiety caused an increase in the swelling degree of the gel and a rise in the transition temperature (Figure 9.10). These characteristics may be interpreted by considering an increase in hydrophilicity of the polymer chains due to the oxidation of Ru (II) to Ru (III) in the Ru(bpy)$_3$ moiety. As a result, we may expect that our gel undergoes a cyclic swelling–deswelling alteration when the Ru(bpy)$_3$ moiety is periodically oxidized and reduced under constant temperature.

Swelling–Deswelling Oscillation of Gel with Periodic Redox Changes

Self-Oscillation of Miniature Bulk Gel

The miniature cubic poly(NIPAAm-co-Ru(bpy)$_3$) gel (with a length of about 0.5 mm) was immersed into an aqueous solution containing MA, sodium NaBrO$_3$, and HNO$_3$ at a constant temperature (20°C). This outer solution contained the reactants of the BZ reaction with the exception of the catalyst and the redox oscillation did not take place in this solution. However, as it penetrated into the gel, the BZ reaction was induced within the gel by the Ru(bpy)$_3$ copolymerized as a catalyst on the polymer

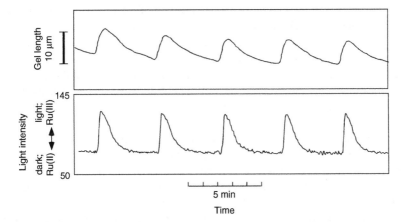

FIGURE 9.11 Swelling–deswelling oscillation at 20°C (top). Periodic redox changes of miniature cubic poly(NIPAAm-co-Ru(bpy)$_3$) gel (bottom). Transmitted light intensity is expressed as an 8-bit grayscale value. Outer solution: [MA] = 62.5 mM; [NaBrO$_3$] = 84 mM; [HNO$_3$] = 0.6 M.

chains. Under reaction, the Ru(bpy)$_3$ in the gel network periodically changed from reduced to oxidized states.

In the miniature gel whose size is smaller than the wavelength of chemical wave (typically several millimeters), the redox change of the ruthenium catalyst can be regarded to occur homogeneously without pattern formation. The oscillation behavior was observed under a microscope. Color changes of the gel accompanying the redox oscillations (orange: reduced state, light green: oxidized state) were converted to 8-bit grayscale changes (dark: reduced, light: oxidized) by image processing. Due to the redox oscillation of the immobilized Ru(bpy)$_3$, mechanical swelling–deswelling oscillation of the gel autonomously occurred over the same period as for redox oscillation (Figure 9.11). The volume change was isotropic and the gel beat as a whole, like a heart muscle cell. The chemical and mechanical oscillations were synchronized without a phase difference (i.e., the gel exhibited swelling during the oxidized state and deswelling during the reduced state).

Control of Oscillation Period and Amplitude

In order to enhance the amplitude of swelling–deswelling oscillations of the gel, it was attempted to change the period and amplitude of the redox oscillation by varying the initial concentration of substrates. It is a general tendency for the oscillation period to increase with a decrease in concentration of substrates.

For a bulk solution consisting of MA, NaBrO$_3$, HNO$_3$, and Ru(bpy)$_3$Cl$_2$, the following empirical relations between the period (T[s]) and initial molar concentration of substrates was obtained: T = 2.97 [MA]$^{-0.414}$[NaBrO$_3$]$^{-0.796}$[HNO$_3$]$^{-0.743}$. For the self-oscillating gel, the empirical relation was different from that of the bulk solution system as follows : T = 60.3 [MA]$^{-0.155}$[NaBrO$_3$]$^{-0.436}$[HNO$_3$]$^{0.469}$. The reasons may be:

1. In the case of the miniature gel, the dilution of intermediates from the gel into the surrounding aqueous phase must be more remarkable. The dilution effect, especially that for the activator ($HBrO_2$), leads to an increase in the period of chemical oscillations.
2. The concentration changes of substrates or products within the gel phase resulting from the swelling–deswelling oscillations may have some effects on the chemical oscillations (i.e., feedback effects).

The variation in chemical oscillation leads to a change in the swelling–deswelling oscillation, i.e., the swelling–deswelling amplitude (change in gel length, Δd) increases with increases in the period and amplitude of the redox changes. Empirically, the relation between Δd [μm] and the substrate concentrations was expressed as $\Delta d = 2.38[MA]^{0.392}[NaBrO_3]^{0.059}[HNO_3]^{0.764}$. It is apparent that the swelling–deswelling amplitude of the gel is controllable by changing the initial concentrations of substrates. The swelling–deswelling amplitude with ca. 20% to the initial gel size was obtained as a maximum value maximum value.[40] It is worth noting that the waveform of redox changes deformed to rectangular shape during a plateau period when the amplitude of swelling–deswelling oscillation increased (Figure 9.12). From this result, it is supposed that an energy transformation from chemical to mechanical change and a feedback mechanism from mechanical to chemical change act in the synchronization process.

As an inherent behavior of the BZ reaction, the abrupt transition from steady (nonoscillating) to oscillating state occurs with a change in a controlling parameter

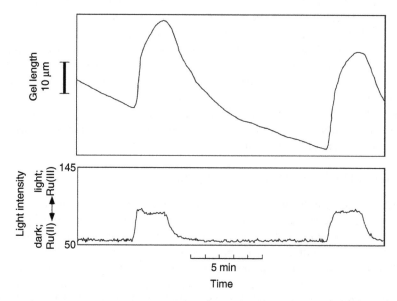

FIGURE 9.12 Swelling–deswelling oscillation at 20°C (top). Periodic redox changes of miniature cubic poly(NIPAAm-co-Ru(bpy)3) gel (bottom). Transmitted light intensity is expressed as an 8-bit grayscale value. Outer solution: [MA] = 62.5 mM; [NaBrO$_3$] = 84 mM; [HNO$_3$] = 0.894 M.

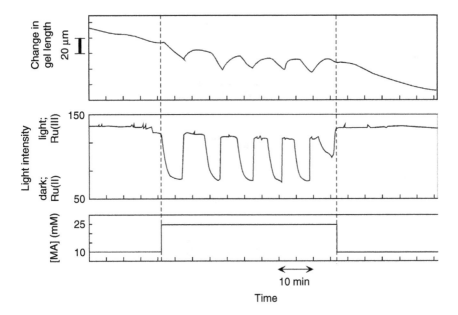

FIGURE 9.13 Change in oscillating behavior of gel in response to stepwise concentration changes of MA between 10 mM and 25 mM (others: [NaBrO$_3$] = 84 mM, [HNO$_3$] = 0.3 M, 20°C).

such as chemical composition. This change is termed *bifurcation*. It is expected that the rhythmic motion of the gel can be controlled by changing substrate concentration during oscillation. For example, if MA is switched between the concentration regions of steady state and oscillating state, on–off control of the beating would be possible.[43]

Figure 9.13 shows the oscillating behavior of the gel when a stepwise change in MA was repeated between lower concentration (10 mM) in steady state and higher concentration (25 mM) in oscillating state. At MA = 10 mM, the redox oscillation did not occur and consequently the gel exhibited no swelling–deswelling changes. Then the concentration was quickly increased to 25 mM. Immediately after increasing concentration, the gel started self-beating. The beating stopped again as soon as the concentration was decreased back to the initial value. In these ways, reversible on–off regulation of self-beating triggered by MA was successfully achieved. Since certain organic acids (e.g., citric acid) can serve as substrates for the BZ reaction, the same regulation of beating is possible by using those organic acids instead of MA. Since the gel has thermosensitivity due to the NIPAAm component, the beating rhythm can be also controlled by temperature.

SELF-OSCILLATING BEHAVIORS WITH PROPAGATION OF CHEMICAL WAVES

Peristaltic Motions of Rectangular Gels

Figure 9.14 shows a rectangular piece of the gel (ca. 1 mm × 1 mm × 20 mm) immersed in an aqueous solution containing the three reactants of the BZ reaction. The chemical waves propagate in the gel at a constant speed in the direction of the

Chemical wave   Rectangular poly (NIPAAm-
(oxidized state)   co-Ru(bpy)$_3^{2+}$) gel

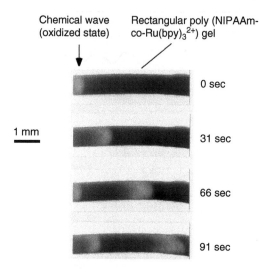

FIGURE 9.14 Propagation of chemical wave in rectangular poly(NIPAAm-co-Ru(bpy)$_3$) gel.

gel length. The dark [Ru (II)] and light [Ru (III)] zones represent the shrunken and swollen parts, respectively. The locally swollen and shrunken parts move with the chemical wave, like the peristaltic motions of living worms.

The propagation of the chemical wave makes the free end of the gel move back and forth at a rate corresponding to the wave propagation speed. As a result, the total length of the gel periodically changes. It was demonstrated by mathematical model simulations that the change in overall gel length is equivalent to that in the remainder of gel length divided by the wavelength, because the swelling and the deswelling cancel each other per one period of oscillation under steady oscillating conditions.[37,38]

Control of Chemical Wavelength by Laser Irradiation to Pacemaker Site

It is well known that the period of oscillation is affected by light illumination for the Ru(bpy)$_3^{2+}$-catalyzed BZ reaction. The excited state of the (Ru(bpy)$_3^{2+*}$) catalyst causes a new reaction process: production of an activator [reaction (R1)] or production of an inhibitor [reaction (R2)], which depends on solute composition.[48]

R1: $Ru(bpy)_3^{2+*} + Ru(bpy)_3^{2+} + BrO_3^- + 3H^+ \rightarrow HBrO_2 + 2Ru(bpy)_3^{3+} + H_2O$

R2: $Ru(bpy)_3^{2+*} + BrMA + H^+ \rightarrow Br^- + Ru(bpy)_3^{3+} + \text{other products}$

Therefore, we can (1) intentionally make a pacemaker with a desired period (or wavelength) by local illumination of a laser beam on the gel or (2) change the period (or wavelength) by local illumination of the pacemaker by a beam that already exists in the gel.

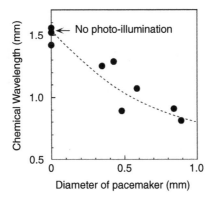

FIGURE 9.15 Relation between diameter of pacemaker and wavelengths of chemical waves.

In a rectangular gel, the corner often becomes a pacemaker from which chemical waves start to propagate. Therefore, the self-oscillating behaviors of the gel can be controlled by irradiating laser light locally to the pacemaker site of the gel. Figure 9.15 shows the effect of laser irradiation on the pacemaker under the condition that photoillumination produces an activator. The size of pacemaker was altered by changing the diameter of an irradiated region on the gel through a pinhole on the light path. The wavelengths of traveling waves in the gel decreased as the size of pacemaker increased. The results were in good agreement with a theoretical model simulation.[49] This result means that we can control the macroscopic swelling–deswelling behavior of a gel by local perturbation, i.e., a small signal can be amplified to produce macroscopic change

Self-Oscillation of Polymer Chains with Rhythmical Soluble–Insoluble Changes

In a self-oscillating gel, redox changes of $Ru(bpy)_3$ catalysts are converted to conformational changes of polymer chains by polymerization. The conformational changes are amplified to macroscopic swelling–deswelling changes of polymer networks by crosslinking. Further, when the gel size is larger than chemical wavelength, the chemical wave propagates in the gel by coupling with diffusion. The peristaltic motion of the gel is created and a hierarchical synchronization process exists in the self-oscillating gel.

It is interesting to clarify the polymerization effect of a catalyst on the oscillating behavior of the BZ reaction, as well as the effects of crosslinking polymer chains on the synchronization of each polymer's oscillation. For this purpose, linear poly(NIPAAm-co-Ru(bpy)$_3$) was synthesized and self-oscillating behavior of polymer chain was investigated through the analysis of transmittance changes of the polymer solution.[50] Gel particles of submicrometer size were prepared. By comparing the oscillating behaviors between them, the effects of polymerization and crosslinking were revealed.

Figure 9.16 shows the oscillation profiles of transmittance for a polymer solution that consisted of linear poly(NIPAAm-co-Ru(bpy)$_3$), MA, NaBrO$_3$ and HNO$_3$ at

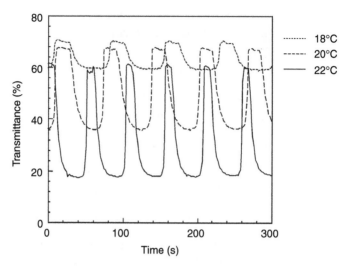

FIGURE 9.16 Oscillating profiles of optical transmittance for poly(NIPAAm-co-Ru(bpy)₃) solution at constant temperatures.

constant temperatures. Synchronized with the periodical changes between Ru (II) and Ru (III) states of the Ru(bpy)₃ site, the polymer became hydrophobic and hydrophilic and exhibited cyclic soluble–insoluble changes. These periodic changes of polymer chains can be easily observed as cyclic transparent and opaque changes for a polymer solution with color changes due to redox oscillation of the catalyst.

Dependence of the oscillation period on initial substrate concentration has been investigated for three systems; (1) a conventional BZ solution using a nonpolymerized catalyst, (2) a polymer solution using a polymerized catalyst (NIPAAm), and (3) a suspension of submicron-sized gel beads, i.e., a crosslinked polymer network of polymerized catalyst. Compared with the period noted under the same substrate concentrations, the period increased in the following order: (1) < (2) < (3).

The reasons for the increases in period can be considered as follows. In the poly(NIPAAm-co-Ru(bpy)₃) case, the charge site is fixed on the polymer chain. Due to the fixation, the increase in electrostatic repulsion between the charge sites may be suppressed. As a result, the change to the oxidation state is restrained. This leads to longer duration of reduced state and elongation of oscillation period. In the case of the crosslinked polymer network (gel beads), polymer chains are constrained to behave cooperatively and diffusion limitation of the substrate from the outer solution into the gel phase will take place. This will result in decreasing effective concentration inside the gel phase and elongation of the oscillation period. Details of the mechanisms are still under investigation.

CILIARY MOTION ACTUATOR USING SELF-OSCILLATING GEL

One of the promising fields of microelectromechanical systems (MEMS) is microactuator arrays or distributed actuator systems. The actuators that have very simple actuation motions such as moving up and down are arranged in an array form. If

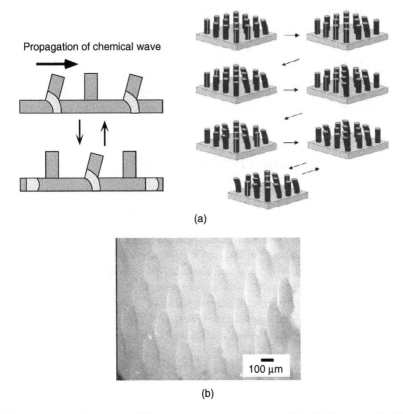

Propagation of chemical wave

(a)

100 μm

(b)

FIGURE 9.17 (a) Concept of ciliary motion actuator using self-oscillating gel. (b) Micro-projection structure array on gel surface fabricated by x-ray lithography technique.

their motions are random, no work can be performed, but by controlling the motions to operate in a certain order, they can generate work as a single system.

One of the typical examples of this kind of actuation array is a ciliary motion microactuator array. Although various actuation principles were proposed, all the early works were based on the concept that the motions of actuators were controlled by external signals. If a self-oscillating gel plate with microprojection structure array on top is used, it is expected that a chemical wave propagates and creates dynamic rhythmic motion of the microprojection structure array (Figure 9.17a). This is the structure of proposed new ciliary motion array that exhibits spontaneous dynamic propagating oscillation.

A gel plate with a microprojection array was fabricated by molding techniques.[51,52] First, the moving mask deep-X-ray lithography technique was utilized to fabricate a poly(methylmethacrylate) (PMMA) plate with a truncated conical shape microstructure array. This step was followed by the evaporation of an Au seed layer and subsequent electroplating of nickel to form the metal mold structure, after which a poly(dimethylsiloxane) (PDMS) mold structure was duplicated from the Ni metal mold structure and utilized for gel molding. The formation of gel was carried out by the vacuum injection molding technique. A structure 300 μm high with a bottom diameter of 100 μm was successfully fabricated by the proposed process (Figure 9.17b). The propagation of the chemical reaction wave and dynamic rhythmic motion of the microprojection array were confirmed by chemical wave observation and displacement measurements.[51,52] The feasibility of the new concept of a ciliary motion actuator made of self-oscillating polymer gel was successfully confirmed. The actuator may serve as a microconveyer to transport micro- or nanoparticles on the surface.

CONCLUDING REMARKS

Several cyclic hydrogel systems have been constructed by utilizing conventional stimuli-responsive gels and designing novel biomimetic gels with self-oscillating functions. The gel system included a cyclic reaction network and it periodically generated mechanical energy from the chemical energy of the BZ reaction — similar to a metabolic reaction. These gel systems may be useful for a number of important applications such as pulse generators, chemical pacemakers, self-walking (automobile) actuators, micropumps with autonomous beating or peristaltic motions, devices for signal transmission utilizing propagation of chemical waves, and oscillatory drug release devices synchronized with cell cycles or human biorhythms. Further studies of the mechanisms of oscillating behaviors and their practical applications are expected.

REFERENCES

1. Okano, T., Ed., *Biorelated Polymers and Gels: Controlled Release and Applications in Biomedical Engineering*, Academic Press, Boston, 1998.
2. Yui, N., Ed., *Supramolecular Design for Biological Applications*, CRC Press, Boca Raton, 2002.
3. Rabai, G. and Beck, M.T., Exotic kinetic phenomena and their chemical explanation in the iodate–sulfite–thiosulfate system, *J. Phys. Chem.*, 92, 2804, 1988.
4. Rabai, G. and Beck, M.T., High-amplitude hydrogen ion concentration oscillation in the iodate–thiosulfate–sulfite system under closed conditions, *J. Phys. Chem.*, 92, 4831, 1988.
5. Lotka, A.J., Undamped oscillations derived from the law of mass action, *J. Am. Chem. Soc.*, 42, 1595, 1920.
6. Yoshida, R. et al., Self-oscillating swelling and deswelling of polymer gels, *Macromol. Rapid Commun.*, 16, 305, 1995.
7. Yoshida, R., Yamaguchi, T., and Ichijo, H., Novel oscillating swelling–deswelling dynamic behaviour for pH-sensitive polymer gels, *Mater. Sci. Eng. C*, 4, 107, 1996.
8. Rabai, G., Kustin, K., and Epstein, I.R., A systematically designed pH oscillator: the hydrogen peroxide–sulfite–ferrocyanide reaction in a continuous-flow-stirred tank reactor, *J. Am. Chem. Soc.*, 111, 3870, 1989.
9. Mori, Y. and Hanazaki, I., Bifurcation structure of the chemical oscillation in the $Fe(CN)_6^{4-}$–H_2O_2–H_2SO_4 system, *J. Phys. Chem.*, 97, 7375, 1993.
10. Crook, C.J. et al., Chemically induced oscillations in a pH-responsive hydrogel, *Phys. Chem. Chem. Phys.*, 4, 1367, 2002.

11. Giannos, S.A., Dinh, S.H., and Berner, B., Temporally controlled drug delivery systems: coupling of pH oscillators with membrane diffusion, *J. Pharm. Sci.*, 84, 539, 1995.

12. Giannos, S.A. and Dinh, S.M., pH oscillation of a drug for temporal delivery, in *Intelligent Materials for Controlled Release*, Dinh, S.M., DeNuzzio, D., and Comfort, A.R., Eds., American Chemical Society, Washington, D.C., 1999, chap. 7.

13. Misra, G.P. and Siegel, R.A., Multipulse drug permeation across a membrane driven by a chemical pH-oscillator, *J. Controlled Release*, 79, 293, 2002.

14. Misra, G.P. and Siegel, R.A., Ionizable drugs and pH oscillators: buffering effects, *J. Pharm. Sci.*, 91, 2003, 2002.

15. Rabai, G. and Hanazaki, I., pH oscillations in bromate–sulfite–marble semibatch and flow systems, *J. Phys. Chem.*, 100, 10615, 1996.

16. Siegel, R.A. and Pitt, C.G., A strategy for oscillatory drug release: general scheme and simplified theory, *J. Controlled Release*, 33, 173, 1995.

17. Baker, J.P. and Siegel, R.A., Hysteresis in the glucose permeability versus pH characteristic for a responsive hydrogel membrane, *Macromol. Rapid Commun.*, 17, 409, 1996.

18. Zou, X. and Siegel, R.A., Modeling of oscillatory dynamics of a simple enzyme-diffusion system with hysteresis: the case of lumped permeabilities, *J. Chem. Phys.*, 110, 2267, 1999.

19. Leroux, J.H. and Siegel, R.A., Autonomous gel/enzyme oscillator fueled by glucose: preliminary evidence for oscillations, *CHAOS*, 9, 267, 1999.

20. Li, B. and Siegel, R.A., Global analysis of a model pulsing drug delivery oscillator based on chemomechanical feedback with hysteresis, *CHAOS*, 10, 682, 2000.

21. Misra, G.P. and Siegel, R.A., New mode of drug delivery: long term autonomous rhythmic hormone release across a hydrogel membrane, *J. Controlled Release*, 81, 1, 2002.

22. Dhanarajan, A.P., Misra, G.P., and Siegel, R.A., Autonomous chemomechanical oscillation in a hydrogel/enzyme system driven by glucose, *J. Phys. Chem. A*, 106, 8835, 2002.

23. Zaikin, A.N. and Zhabotinsky, A.M., Concentration wave propagation in two-dimensional liquid-phase self-oscillating system, *Nature*, 225, 535, 1970.

24. Field, R.J. and Burger, M., Eds., *Oscillations and Traveling Waves in Chemical Systems*, John Wiley & Sons, New York, 1985.

25. Epstein, I.R. and Pojman, J.A., *An Introduction to Nonlinear Chemical Dynamics: Oscillations, Waves, Patterns, and Chaos*, Oxford University Press, New York, 1998.

26. Field, R.J., Körös, E., and Noyes, R.M., Oscillations in chemical systems. II. Through analysis of temporal oscillations in the bromate-cerium-malonic acid system, *J. Am. Chem. Soc.*, 94, 8649, 1972.

27. Field, R.J. and Noyes, R.M., Oscillations in chemical systems. IV. Limit cycle behavior in a model of a real chemical reaction, *J. Chem. Phys.*, 60, 1877, 1974.

28. Chance, B. et al., Eds., *Biological and Biochemical Oscillators*, Academic Press, New York, 1973.

29. Gray, R.A. et al., Mechanisms of cardiac fibrillation, *Science*, 270, 1222, 1995.

30. Winfree, A.T. and Strogatz, S.H., Organizing centres for three-dimensional chemical waves, *Nature*, 311, 611, 1984.

31. Kondo, S. and Asai, R., A reaction-diffusion wave on the skin of the marine angelfish *Pomacanthus*, *Nature*, 376, 765, 1995.

32. Castets, V. et al., Experimental evidence of a sustained standing Turing-type non-equilibrium chemical pattern, *Phys. Rev. Lett.*, 64, 2953, 1990.

33. Kuhnert, L., Agladze, K.I., and Krinsky, V.I., Image processing using light-sensitive chemical waves, *Nature*, 337, 244, 1989.

34. Yoshida, R. et al., Self-oscillating gel, *J. Am. Chem. Soc.*, 118, 5134, 1996.

35. Yoshida, R. et al., Self-oscillating gels, *Adv. Mater.*, 9, 175, 1997.

36. Yoshida, R. and Yamaguchi, T., Self-oscillation of polymer gels coupled with non-linear chemical reaction, in *Biorelated Polymers and Gels: Controlled Release and Applications in Biomedical Engineering*, Okano, T., Ed., Academic Press, Boston, 1998, chap. 3.

37. Yoshida, R., Kokufuta, E., and Yamaguchi, T., Beating polymer gels coupled with a nonlinear chemcial reaction, *CHAOS*, 9, 260, 1999.

38. Yoshida, R., Yamaguchi, T., and Kokufuta, E., Molecular design of self-oscillating polymer gels and their dynamic swelling–deswelling behaviors, *J. Intel. Matl. Syst. Struct.*, 10, 451, 1999.

39. Yoshida, R. et al., Aspects of the Belousov–Zhabotinsky reaction in polymer gels, *J. Phys. Chem. A*, 103, 8573, 1999.

40. Yoshida, R. et al., In-phase synchronization of chemical and mechanical oscillations in self-oscillating gels, *J. Phys. Chem. A*, 104, 7549, 2000.

41. Yoshida, R. et al., Traveling chemical waves for measuring solute diffusivity in thermosensitive poly(N-isopropylacrylamide) gel, *J. Phys. Chem. A*, 105, 3667, 2001.

42. Yoshida, R. et al., Design of novel biomimetic polymer gels with self-oscillating function, *Sci. Tech. Adv. Mater.*, 3, 95, 2002.

43. Yoshida, R., Takei, K., and Yamaguchi, T., Self-beating motion of gels and modulation of oscillation rhythm synchronized with organic acid, *Macromolecules*, 36, 1759, 2003.

44. Yamaguchi, T. et al., Gel systems for the Belousov–Zhabotinsky reaction, *J. Phys. Chem.*, 95, 5831, 1991.

45. Kokufuta, E., Zhang, Y.Q., and Tanaka, T., Biochemo-mechanical function of urease-loaded gels, *J. Biomater. Sci. Polym. Edn.*, 6, 35, 1994.

46. Hirokawa, Y. and Tanaka, T., Volume phase transition in a nonionic gel, *J. Chem. Phys.*, 81, 6379, 1984.

47. Yoshida, R. et al., Comb-type grafted hydrogels with rapid de-swelling response to temperature changes, *Nature*, 374, 240, 1995.

48. Amemiya, T., Ohmori, T., and Yamaguchi, T., An Oregonator-class model for photo-induced behavior in the $Ru(bpy)_3^{2+}$-catalyzed Belousov–Zhabotinsky reaction, *J. Phys. Chem.*, 104, 336, 2000.

49. Mahara, H. et al., "Ring-shaped model" of the pacemaker in oscillatory reaction-diffusion systems, *J. Phys. Soc. Jpn.*, 69, 3552, 2000.

50. Yoshida, R. et al., Self-oscillation of polymer chains with rhythmical soluble–insoluble changes, *J. Am. Chem. Soc.*, 124, 8095, 2002.

51. Tabata, O. et al., Ciliary motion actuator using self-oscillating gel, *Sensors Actuators A*, 95, 234, 2002.

52. Tabata, O. et al., Chemo-mechanical actuator using self-oscillating gel for artificial cilia, *Proc. Int. Conf. MEMS 2003*, pp. 12–15.

10 Cooperative Binding in Surfactant–Polymer Association: A Brief Overview

Rupali Gangopadhyay, Jian Ping Gong, and Yoshihito Osada

CONTENTS

INTRODUCTION

Surfactants are defined as molecules having long hydrophobic tails and strongly hydrophilic head groups. These molecules have a number of interesting and important properties like aggregating into micelles and binding with different organic systems.[1-20] Among these combinations, much attention has been paid to the surfactant–polymer association and different aspects of such combinations have been widely studied. The excellent application potentials of such systems in mimicking biological systems and fabricating fast responsive devices and artificial muscles have been explored. In fact, the surfactant–polymer assembly is considered one of the

0-8493-1487-9/04/$0.00+$1.50

most popular responsive systems. Obviously the thermodynamic and kinetic behaviors of surfactant binding to linear and crosslinked polymers have raised a great deal of scientific interest.

The stoichiometric binding of surfactants with ionic linear polymers or networks is characterized by two processes.[19,20] One is the electrostatic interaction between the surfactant and polymer to form salt-like bridging and the other is the hydrophobic interaction between bound surfactants. The former is an initiation process and the latter is designated as a cooperative or propagation process. In the cases of nonionic polymers, however, the electrostatic attraction does not exist. The side-by-side hydrophobic interaction among the alkyl chains of the surfactant molecules gives rise to a micellar-like structure within the polymer system that signifies the binding of associated surfactant micelles with the polymer systems rather than the separated surfactant molecules.

Cooperative binding is characterized by a sudden occurrence and completion of binding in a very narrow range of equilibrium surfactant concentration (similar to the formation of micelles above critical micelle concentration [CMC]); this behavior is confirmed by the appearance of a sigmoidal-shaped curve of binding isotherm vs. free surfactant concentration. Binding isotherm is defined as the molar ratio of bound surfactant to polymer (β) in the equilibrium surfactant concentration under constant temperature. This chapter will discuss the theoretical and experimental aspects of surfactant binding with linear and crosslinked polymers separately. A few applications of the system will also be discussed.

Considerable research has been performed on surfactant–linear polymer cooperative binding processes involving both ionic and nonionic linear polymers. The nonionic hydrophilic polymers explored in this respect are poly(vinyl pyrrolidone) (PVP),[2,3] poly(ethylene oxide) (PEO),[4,5] and poly(ethylene glycol) (PEG).[6] Polyelectrolytes like poly(methacrylic acid) (PMA),[7,8] poly(styrene sulfonic acid) (PSS), poly(acrylic acid) (PAA), and CMC[9,10] were also studied. A wide range of surfactants bearing both positive and negative charges, namely sodium dodecyl sulfate (SDS, anionic), alkyl trimethyl ammonium bromides (C_nTABs, cationic) were also studied.

Combinations of surfactants with crosslinked polymers and polymer gels are less explored but have given rise to a number of intelligent soft devices. Binding of crosslinked gels of poly(2-acrylamido-2-propane sulfonic acid) (PAMPS), polyacrylic acid (PAA), poly(methacrylic acid) (PMA), and other polyelectrolyte gels with cationic surfactants like alkyl pyridinium chloride with different alkyl chain lengths have been studied in this respect.[19,20] Different aspects of binding of surfactants with some biomolecules and biopolymers have also been studied and important results were obtained. However, in order to exploit the full application potential of such systems, it is very important to understand the details of their binding properties. The kinetics and thermodynamics of surfactant–polymer associations will be discussed in brief in this chapter. Different results obtained from surfactant binding with linear and crosslinked polymeric systems, nonionic polymers, and polyelectrolytes will be addressed separately and discussed in detail.

SURFACTANT–POLYMER ASSOCIATION: EXPERIMENTAL RESULTS

NONIONIC POLYMERS AND POLYELECTROLYTES

Investigations of the interactions of polymers and surfactants in aqueous solution are highly important from the fundamental standpoint of understanding the structures and dynamics of such systems. These interactions resemble phenomena in biological assemblies and have few practical applications; one involves enhanced oil recovery. The interactions of nonionic polymers such as PEO, PVP, and others with SDS has been studied to reveal fundamental characteristics of the system.

When a detergent is added to a water solution of a polymer, two competing phenomena take place: self-aggregation of surfactant molecules to form micelles and interaction of individual surfactant molecules with the monomer units of the polymer chain. As a result, the association between the surfactant and the polymer starts abruptly above a certain detergent concentration (x_1) lower than the critical micelle concentration (CMC) of the surfactant and saturates abruptly above another detergent concentration (x_2) higher than the CMC. The x_1 value is attributed to a process analogous to micelle formation; x_2 corresponds to complete coverage of the polymer by linear adsorption of detergent molecules along its chain; and $x_1 - x_2$ measures the amount of detergent bound to the polymer. Within this region, clusters of SDS molecules cooperatively associate with the polymers.

The nature of the association and relative positions of SDS and nonionic hydrophilic polymers (PEO and PVP) have been monitored using ^{13}C nuclear magnetic resonance (NMR) and fluorescence spectroscopy as the tools.[2] Results showed that the polymer–surfactant interaction is a weak one and some type of mixed micelle is formed by such interaction in which the polar head groups of SDS are bound with the polymer chains while the nonpolar hydrocarbon core is almost retained. Therefore, a polymer–SDS interface where the polymer molecules interact with polar head groups of SDS must occur; in other words, the polar outer phase of the SDS micelle is modified by the presence of the hydrophilic polymer in a fashion schematized in Figure 10.1.

If the association between an ionic polymer (i.e., a polyelectrolyte) and an oppositely charged surfactant is considered, the situation becomes a bit different. If the polymer is a strong electrolyte, an intense association with an oppositely charged

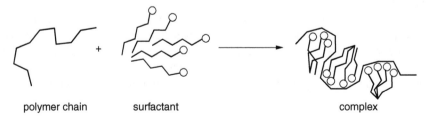

polymer chain   surfactant   complex

FIGURE 10.1 Binding of surfactant molecules with polymer chain.

surfactant takes place because of Coulombic attraction; however, the studies of such compounds were carried out well below the CMC of the surfactant in order to avoid precipitation at higher surfactant concentrations.

Dubin et al.[11] studied the association of poly(dimethyldiallyl ammonium chloride) (PDMDAAC), a strong cationic polyelectrolyte, with Triton-X (a nonionic surfactant) and SDS (an ionic surfactant) by using quasi-elastic light scattering (QELS) data. In the solution of the polycation and oppositely charged surfactant, supramolecular aggregates with hydrodynamic diameters ranging from 30 to 70 nm were confirmed at high ionic strength. The aggregate size was found to be further increased with increases in polymer concentration and hydrodynamic diameters up to 70 nm at polymer concentrations of 1.5 g/l were observed. At very large polymer concentration, these aggregates were in equilibrium with the polymer-rich liquid (coacervate) phase similar to liquid droplets 1 to 75 μm in diameter.

Hyaluronan (Hy) is a linear polysaccharide consisting of alternating units of glucoronic acid and N-acetylglucosamine. It is a polyelectrolyte found in the extracellular matrices of mammals and plays an important role in both mechanical and transport properties. The interaction of Hy and its sodium salt with alkyltrimethyl ammonium bromide (ATMAB) was explored from different aspects[12] by using versatile techniques, namely phase separation, conductivity, self-diffusion, and others. Results demonstrate that binding of the surfactant to Hy takes place for surfactants with more than 10 carbon atoms in their alkyl chains. Because of the low charge density of the Hy surfactant, its binding is weaker than those of other carboxylate-bearing polyelectrolytes.

The interactions between PMA, a weak polyelectrolyte, and cationic surfactants (C_nTABs) was investigated at higher pH (~8) levels by Chu et al.[7,8] Surfactant induced cooperative binding and resulting coiling of PMA chains at higher pH were detected from fluorescence spectroscopic data. The straightened PMA chain at pH 8 was refolded on the addition of C_nTAB and hydrophobic aggregates were formed. This, however, required the surfactant concentration to exceed a certain concentration (*clinical aggregation concentration* or CAC) 1.4 to 1.7 orders magnitude lower than the CMC of the surfactant.

There is a significant effect of chain length and PMA concentration on CAC that is very significant for revealing the nature of the association and the mechanisms of structural transitions in PMA. It was suggested that a PMA–C_nTAB aggregation is a large structure consisting of one coiled polymer chain with 100 surfactant molecules.

A binding isotherm of poly(vinyl sulfate) (PVS), an anionic polymer, and 1-decylpyridinium bromide (DePBr) has been potentiometrically studied at different temperatures.[13] Ising's nearest-neighbor interaction theory[14] was applied and PVS was viewed as a one-dimensional array of binding sites where surfactants were bound stoichiometrically with mutual interaction so that following equilibrium was set up:

$$\text{Polymer} + \text{Surfactant} \xrightleftharpoons{K} \text{Complex}$$

A partition function for such a system is explicitly expressed and yields a lot of important relations, one of which is especially useful:

$$\left[d\beta/d\ln C_s\right]_{0.5} = \sqrt{u/4}$$

Following the Zim–Bragg theory[15] for helix-coil transition of biopolymers, the following expression for cooperative binding[16] can be evolved:

$$K_0 = \left[uC_s(0.5)\right]^{-1}, \; K = \left[C_s(0.5)\right]^{-1}$$

where $C_s(0.5)$ is an equilibrium surfactant concentration corresponding to half binding ($\beta = 0.5$), u is a cooperative parameter or equilibrium constant for an aggregation process among bound surfactants, K_0 is a binding constant for a process of transferring a surfactant ion from aqueous solution to the isolated binding site on the polyelectrolyte, and K is the overall stability constant.

Upon the addition of surfactant to a solution of a nonionic polymer and/or polyelectrolyte, hydrophobic aggregates are formed as result of a cooperative interaction among surfactant molecules. This is analogous to the formation of surfactant micelles and takes place within a narrow range of surfactant concentration. This phenomenon affects different physical properties of the system and is highly dependent on the natures of the polymer and the surfactant.

CROSSLINKED POLYMERS AND GELS

The effect of surfactant binding in a polymeric gel system is as widely explored as linear polymers. Much attention has been paid to the binding aspects of polyelectrolyte-based gel systems; nonionic gels have not been explored as widely.

Tanaka et al.[17] studied swelling equilibrium of N-isopropylacrylamide (NIPA) gel as a function of temperature in aqueous solutions of surfactant and developed the volume phase transition theory for surfactants. They also studied the effects of anionic SDS, cationic dodecyltrimethyl ammonium chloride (DTAC), and nonionic nonaoxyethylene dodecyl ether (NODE) surfactants on the swelling equilibrium and phase transition temperature of NIPA. It was clearly established in pure water that the gel shows a discontinuous volume phase transition at 33.6°C with a volume change of eight times, while in presence of ionic surfactants, the transition temperature and extent of swelling vary remarkably.

The nonionic surfactant has little effect on the volume phase transition of the NIPA gel. The observed effects of ionic surfactants on NIPA gels can be readily understood by assuming that the gel is ionized upon binding of the surfactant molecules to the polymer network. It was concluded that both SDS and DTAC bind to the polymer network within the gel phase through hydrophobic interaction and subsequently convert the neutral gel to a polyelectrolyte gel. The experimental results can be explained qualitatively in terms of the classical Flory–Huggins theory[18] with required modifications for the free energy of associations of surfactant molecules or with the network.

Since a polyelectrolyte gel has deep electrostatic potential valleys along the polymer chains and wells at crosslinked points, it attracts oppositely charged surfactants and forms complexes.[21] Surfactant binding to solvated and crosslinked polyelectrolytes with charges on side chains and backbones has been extensively studied using various kinds of oppositely charged surfactants. Three kinds of surfactant binding were proposed: cooperative and stoichiometric, noncooperative and stoichiometric, and cooperative and nonstoichiometric.[22] Modes of these categories are predominantly determined by the structural and chemical characteristics of the polyelectrolyte, namely its chemical structure, hydrophobicity, charge density, and other factors. Okuzaki et al.[19] carried out a detailed and regular survey of the different aspects of binding of surfactant molecules (C_nPyCl, cationic) to a crosslinked PAMPS gel (anionic).

The effects of different parameters such as chain length of surfactant (n = 4, 8, 10, 12, 16, 18), degree of crosslinking, and activities of counterions were addressed both experimentally and theoretically and important conclusions were drawn. To study these factors, a swollen gel was immersed in a C_nPyCl solution for several days to reach equilibrium. A sudden increase of binding at a critical surfactant concentration indicates the cooperative nature of binding through hydrophobic packing of n-alkyl groups. Association with a surfactant causes the gel to lose its electrostatic energy along with formation of a supramolecular structure in the surfactant-bound gel, resulting in contraction of its volume. Both the binding constant (K) and cooperativity parameter (u) were found to be increased on increasing alkyl chain length, indicating that the binding is cooperative in nature and is dominated by hydrophobic interaction. Thus, increasing the chain length of the surfactant shifts the threshold surfactant concentration for binding toward the lower side and increases the sharpness of the sigmoidal binding curve (Figure 10.2).

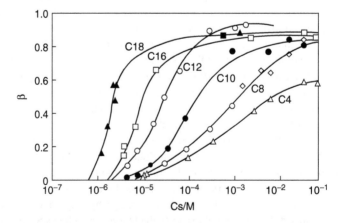

FIGURE 10.2 Binding isotherms of surfactant molecules with PAMPS gel at 25°C: (Δ) C_4PyCl, (◊) C_8PyCl, (•) $C_{10}PyCl$, (o) C12PyCl, (□)$C_{16}PyCl$, (s) $C_{18}PyCl$. Equilibration time = 30 days. (From Okuzaki, H. and Osada, Y., *Macromolecules*, 27, 503, 1994. With permission.)

A comparative study of binding isotherms of linear PAMPS (L-PAMPS) and gels at different temperatures was done using $C_{12}PyCl$ (Figure 10.3). Initiation of binding started at a surfactant concentration as low as 10^{-5} mol L^{-1}, at least one order of magnitude lower than that of a linear polyelectrolyte, indicating favored initiation processes in gels.[20] Binding isotherms of L-PAMPS (Figure 10.3a) showed a very sharp increase in β in a very narrow range that leveled off at β = 0.8. The presence of such a critical surfactant concentration clearly established the cooperative nature of binding. For the PAMPS gel (Figure 10.3b), binding of the surfactant started at around 10^{-6} and continued up to 10^{-3} showing a sigmoidal dependence of β on surfactant concentration.

On the other hand, the cooperativity parameter (u) of a gel system ($u = \sim1$) was more than two orders of magnitude lower than that of the L-PAMPS ($u = 630$), indicating that the propagation process was significantly suppressed and the cooperativity was practically prohibited. Increasing temperatures in both systems resulted in shifting of the curves to lower surfactant concentrations, which indicated favored binding. A highly ordered surfactant gel aggregate was detected from small angle x-ray diffraction patterns and the binding constant was found to increase with the degree of crosslinking.[23] Simulation results revealed that deep electrostatic potential wells existed at every crosslinking point in this system with electrostatic fields as high as 10^8 V/m.[21]

The high electrostatic field potential of the gel resulted in increased local contraction of the surfactant in the network due to Donnan equilibrium and shifted toward the enhanced binding at the given surfactant concentration. Thus, the surfactant is present in three types of equilibria: the equilibrium dispersed in the solution, the one concentrated in the network, and the one bound with the network. As a result, the binding constant increases with the increase in crosslinking density. The large osmotic pressure of the charged network is balanced with the elasticity of the system and is expressed by the reduced cooperativity. An increase in ionic strength of the medium by introduction of a salt has a positive effect on the cooperativity of the system as shown by the increase of u and the steepness of the curves.[21]

This effect is attributed to suppression of the repulsive force between adjacent surfactant molecules in the network. On the other hand, the threshold surfactant concentration is shifted to higher, which accounts for the hampered initiation process by electrostatic shielding of oppositely charged ions of the surfactant and gel.[22]

The effect of the volume collapse of the gel (in presence of a surfactant) on the kinetics of the surfactant uptake was explored. The volume collapse enhanced the velocity of surfactant uptake despite the decreased free space for diffusion of surfactant.[24] This observation agrees with the idea that the kinetics of a surfactant uptake is dominated by electrostatic interactions between oppositely charged moieties. On the other hand, the kinetics of surfactant uptake is shown to be distinctly dependent on the co-ions of the surfactant and counterions of the charged network.[25]

Molecular and supramolecular structures of complexes formed by polyelectrolyte–surfactant association were further studied using a different polymeric system. A sodium salt of poly(styrene sulfonate) and its copolymer with polystyrene were subjected to binding with C_nPyCl (n = 12, 16); the structures of the complexes and the mechanisms of complexation were highlighted accordingly.[26–28] Results of all

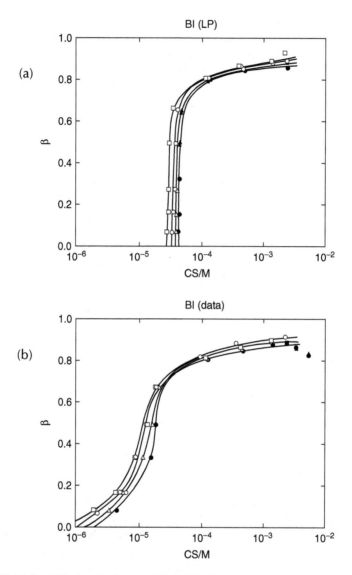

FIGURE 10.3 (a) Binding isotherms of $C_{12}PyCl$ with L-PAMPS under various temperatures: (●) 5°C, (Δ)15°C, (o)25°C, (□) 35°C. Polymer concentration = 3×10^{-3} M. (b) Binding isotherms of $C_{12}PyCl$ with PAMPS gel under various temperatures: (●) 5°C, (Δ)15°C, (o)25°C, (□) 35°C. Degree of crosslinking = 4.5%; degree of swelling (q) = 50. (From Okuzaki, H. and Osada, Y., *Macromolecules*, 28, 4554, 1995. With permission.)

these experiments carried out on crosslinked polymer systems indicated that hydrophobic interactions of alkyl chains play an important role in effective complexation of surfactants. The positively charged surfactants underwent complexation with anionic sites through salt formation; alkyl chains led to lateral hydrophobic interactions to produce micelle-like structures of surfactants within the gels.

The original, stoichiometric binding profile of a surfactant with a polymer gel can be studied if the surfactant itself is not able to undergo hydrophobic interaction. Isogai et al. studied the binding of tetraphenylphosphonium chloride (TPPC) with PAMPS because this surfactant, due to the bulky hydrophobic groups it contains, cannot undergo cooperative binding interaction.[27] When PAMPS gel is immersed in TPPC solution, it shrinks in volume over time. Dilute TPPC solutions result in a gradual and continuous contraction of the gel while concentrated solutions bring about a collapse of the network to 4% of its initial volume. The curve of the binding isotherm was found to be almost similar to that obtained for C_nPyCl although the critical surfactant concentration required for binding shifted to higher by almost two orders of magnitude. In the presence of salt, the threshold surfactant concentration further shifted to a higher one although u increased to some extent. Therefore, initiation process in this case was dominated by electrostatic interaction and formation of a one-to-one stoichiometric complex, but the overall binding process was noncooperative. The abrupt volume change was attributed to intramolecular aggregation of gel-bound TPPC molecules to form aggregates in a very special manner (Figure 10.4).

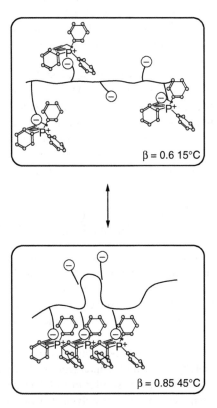

FIGURE 10.4 Reversible aggregate formation in response to change in temperature. (From Isogai, N., Gong, J.P., and Osada, Y., *Macromolecules*, 29, 6805, 1996. With permission.)

This very unusual association and special kind of cooperativity can successfully explain the observed volume contraction and thermosensitivity of the gel. It can be inferred that interaction between nearest-neighbor surfactant molecules is important but not necessary for cooperative binding; geometric structures leading appropriate stacking of the binding molecules can also play an important role. Both types of binding are reversible in nature and on transferring the surfactant bound gel to water, the expansion in volume is observed.

The third category of binding (cooperative and nonstoichiometric) was studied by using a group of amphiphilic polymers like x,y-ionene bromide (IB) (x = 6, 12; y = 4, 6, 12) polymers and acrylate copolymers, with long alkyl side groups and bulky hydrophobic groups exhibiting lower critical solution temperatures (LCSTs). Binding of positively charged 6,12-IB polymer with SDS and acrylate copolymers NIPA-co-AMPS and poly-(12,acryloydodecanoic acid-co-acrylic acid) with C_nPyCl was monitored experimentally.[28,29] In both cases two-step surfactant binding mechanisms were established and soluble complexes were detected. The linear polymers and corresponding gels were studied and identical behaviors were observed. On the addition of surfactant to the respective polymer solutions, insoluble complexes were found to precipitate out from the medium, suggesting the formation of one-to-one stoichiometric complexes. As the surfactant:polymer ratio exceeded 1.0, the precipitate started dissolving and disappeared at a mixing ratio between 1.3 and 1.5.

A remarkable contraction in volume of gel systems was observed initially; it was followed by reswelling, corresponding to the behaviors of linear polymers. As the binding isotherm curve was studied, a two-step surfactant binding phenomenon was established in both systems (Figure 10.5). After the completion of the formation of a one-to-one complex, a second binding took place with the excess surfactant in solution. Since the stoichiometric complex had no electrical charge, the second binding presumably occurred through the hydrophobic interaction of the surfactant and the one-to-one complex. Binding of excess amounts of surfactant produced a negatively charged complex and led to its solubilization.

THEORETICAL MODELING OF SURFACTANT–POLYMER ASSOCIATION

Some theoretical models have been proposed for polymer–surfactant interactions, all based on the structure of the micelle-like clusters bound to the polymers. Gilanyi and Wolfram[30] suggested a simple model with a fixed aggregation number for the free and polymer-bound micelles and a fixed degree of counterion binding; a relation between activity of the surfactant and the total surfactant that could be fitted very well to experimental data was derived.

The model was further modified by Nagarajan[31] who considered variation of the aggregation number, thereby allowing the interactions of uncharged polymers with both ionic and nonionic surfactants. A similar model was suggested by Rukenstein et al.[32] An approach often used in cases of polyelectrolyte–surfactant interaction is to treat the binding of the surfactant as site binding to polymers. Cooperativity of binding is taken into account by an additional cooperativity factor. The well-known

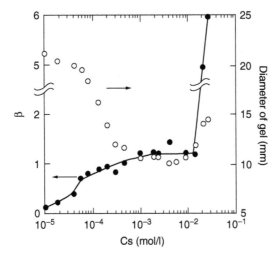

FIGURE 10.5 Binding isotherm of $C_{12}PyCl$ with poly(NIPA-co-AMPS) gel (•) and change in diameter of gel (o). Copolymer contains 10 mol% AMPS unit. Equilibration time = 3 weeks at 25°C. (From Yu, S.Y. et al., *Macromolecules*, 29, 8022, 1996. With permission.)

Zimm and Bragg model,[15] originally proposed for helix-coil transition in biopolymers, can be applied to the array of occupied and unoccupied sites. This treatment is applied to experimentally obtained binding isotherms and provides the values of the intrinsic binding constant K and the cooperativity parameter u, which may be convenient for comparisons of the bindings of different polyelectrolytes and surfactants. Information can also be derived about the aggregation numbers of the clusters adsorbed to the polyelectrolyte and about the number of monomer units in the unoccupied regions of the polyelectrolyte, but the adequacy of these numbers for polyelectrolyte–surfactant interactions remains to be proved.

Theoretical work done on crosslinked polymers is also very limited as compared to the work on linear polymers. Khokhlov et al.[33] proposed a theory of weakly charged polyelectrolyte networks immersed in the solution of an oppositely charged surfactant; swelling and collapse of the network were well described but the electrostatic interaction between the network and the surfactant was not considered

Results obtained by Isogai et al.[27] to experimentally reveal the effect of crosslinking on surfactant binding to linear and network polymer systems has already been discussed. Gong et al. theoretically ascribed the role and effect of the crosslinkage on surfactant binding.[34] The contribution of the hydrophobic interaction has been treated using the nearest-neighbor interaction model originally employed for polyelectrolyte titration by Marcus.[35] General formulas for the binding of a surfactant with a linear polyelectrolyte and with a charged network have been derived. The derived equation showed that the low cooperativity observed for the charged network is due to the high osmotic pressure created by the mobile counterions that tend to expand in competition with the conformational shrinkage on binding. The calculated results showed a fair agreement with the experimental data.

The results obtained from theoretical analyses of linear and crosslinked polymers are discussed separately. In the following sections, superscripts p and g denote binding with a linear polymer and a crosslinked gel, respectively. Rigorous calculations are avoided in some places and only the significant considerations and inferences are presented.

THEORY OF BINDING WITH A LINEAR POLYELECTROLYTE

As noted earlier, the association of surfactant with an oppositely charged polyelectrolyte is characterized by an electrostatic attraction (initiation) followed by a hydrophobic interaction (cooperative binding). During such combination, the CMC of a surfactant is lowered by two to three orders of magnitude. The electrostatic interaction between a solubilized linear polyelectrolyte with negative charges and positively charged surfactants capable of forming micellar-like complexes was taken into account by Gong and Osada.[34] The free energy of the system (F) can be written as a sum of three terms:

$$F = F_{int} + F_{mobile} + F_{comp} \qquad (10.1)$$

where F_{int} is the free energy of the volume interactions of monomer links, F_{mobile} is the free energy of motion of microions in solution, and F_{comp} represents the free energy of surfactants bound with polyions. According to the Flory–Huggins theory:[18]

$$F_{int} = RT \frac{V}{v_c} \left[\frac{\phi}{m} \ln(1-\phi) + (1-\phi)\ln(1-\phi) + \chi\phi(1-\phi) \right] \qquad (10.2)$$

where V is the volume of solution, ϕ is the volume fraction of the polymer, χ is the Flory–Huggins parameter, M is the polymer chain length, v_c is the molar volume of solvent or monomer, assuming they have the same specific volume, and R and T are the gas constant and absolute temperature, respectively.

Since the free energy of the microions largely attributes to the translational entropy of mobile ions in the solution, the molar numbers of counterions of surfactant and polymer are M and N, respectively. F_{mobile} can be obtained as:

$$F_{mobile} = RT \left[(M-N\beta)\ln\frac{(M-N\beta)v_c}{V} + M\ln\frac{Mv_c}{V} + N\ln\frac{Nv_c}{V} \right] \qquad (10.3)$$

N and M are denoted as the total molar numbers of monomeric units of polymers and surfactants, respectively. β is the degree of binding that is the ratio of the molar number of bound surfactants to N, and $C_s^p = (M - N\beta)/V$ represents the equilibrated molar concentration of surfactant in the polymer solution.

If the nearest-neighbor interaction between surfactant molecules is taken into account, the binding of surfactant should occur in a continuous sequence and not in a random distribution along the polymer chain. Theoretical consideration of the nearest-neighbor interaction for the titration curve of a linear polymer chain was given by Marcus[35] and Lifson[36] using the Ising model.[14] When the polymer chains have $N\beta$ already bound groups and $N(1 - \beta)$ unbound groups at a surfactant concentration C_s^p, the total free energy of such an assembly is associated with N_{aa}, the number of pairs of nearest-neighbor surfactant–surfactant binding. Using Marcus' theory:[34]

$$F_{comp} = N_A N\beta\left(\Delta F_e + \Delta F_h\right) - RT \ln \sum g\left[N\beta, N(1-\beta), N_{aa}\right] \exp\left(\frac{N_{ab}\Delta F_h}{2kT}\right) \quad (10.4)$$

and

$$\frac{\partial F_{comp}}{\partial \beta} = N_A N\left(\Delta F_e + \Delta F_h\right) +$$

$$RTN \ln \frac{\left.\right)4\beta(1-\beta)\left[\exp\left(-\Delta F_h/kT\right)-1\right]+1+2\beta-1}{\left.\right)4\beta(1-\beta)\left[\exp\left(-\Delta F_h/kT\right)-1\right]+1+1-2\beta} \quad (10.5)$$

where N_A is Avogadro's number, $N_{ab} = 2(N\beta - N_{aa})$ is the number of nearest-neighbor pairs of bound and unbound groups, $g[N\beta, N(1 - \beta), N_{ab}]$ is the number of ways of binding for a given β and N_{ab}. ΔF_e denotes the free energy change due to the electrostatic binding, which equals the electrostatic potential energy on the surface of the macroion, and ΔF_h represents free energy change through the hydrophobic interaction. For simplification, it is supposed that ΔF_e does not change with respect to the progress of binding; ΔF_h depends on the chemical structure of the surfactant, particularly on the sizes of alkyl chains.

The equilibrium value of β can be determined by minimization of the total free energy of the system $\partial F/\partial \beta = 0$. Thus, we have:

$$\ln C_s^p v_c = \left(\Delta F_e + \Delta F_h\right)/kT - 1 +$$

$$\ln \frac{\left.\right)4\beta(1-\beta)\left[\exp\left(-\Delta F_h/kT\right)-1\right]+1+2\beta-1}{\left.\right)4\beta(1-\beta)\left[\exp\left(-\Delta F_h/kT\right)-1\right]+1+1-2\beta} \quad (10.6)$$

The second term of the above equation is a transition function that becomes steeper with an increase in the value of ΔF_h.

Equation (10.6) indicates that the binding isotherm of the surfactant onto the linear polyelectrolyte consists of two terms: the first characterizes the transition concentration (initiation process) and the second characterizes the steepness of the transition (cooperative process). The initiation process of the binding is determined by the electrostatic interaction and by the hydrophobic interaction, while the cooperative process of the binding is determined only by the hydrophobic interaction obtained from the slope of the binding curve at $\beta = 0.5$.

Lowering of the critical transition concentration (CTC) of the surfactant by two or three orders of magnitude can also be interpreted. Equation (10.6) indicates that two factors contribute to the lowering of CTC. One is the enhanced electrostatic interaction between surfactant ions and macroions. Since the electrostatic potential valley of a polymer chain is much deeper than that of a corresponding monomer ion, the polyelectrolyte is able to effectively bind the surfactant molecules and favors aggregation through hydrophobic interaction. The other factor is a decreased entropy loss of counterions. The formation of aggregates by surfactant molecules does not lead to a loss of translational entropy of the polymer, although the surfactant aggregation would result in a significant loss in the translational entropy of counterions without polyelectrolytes.

BINDING WITH CROSSLINKED POLYELECTROLYTE

In the case of a crosslinked polyelectrolyte immersed in an oppositely charged surfactant solution, the free energy of the system F is the sum of the free energy of the outer solution F_s and the free energy of the polymer network F_g:

$$F = F_s + F_g \tag{10.7}$$

F_g can be expressed as follows:

$$F_g = F_{int} + F_{mobile} + F_{comp} + F_{el} \tag{10.8}$$

where F_{int} is the free energy of the volume interactions of monomer links, F_{comp} represents the free energy of surfactants bound with polyions, F_{mobile} is the free energy of motion of microions in the network, and F_{el} is the elastic free energy of the network. If S_i^+, S_i^-, and P_i^+ are denoted as the molar numbers of surfactant ions, their counterions, and network counterions in the outer solution ($i = s$) and in the network ($i = g$), we have:

$$S_s^+ + P_s^+ = S_s^- \tag{10.9}$$

$$S_g^+ + P_g^+ = S_g^- + N(1 - \beta) \tag{10.10}$$

from the neutrality condition. From the ion number conservation condition:

$$M = S_s^+ + S_g^+ + N\beta \tag{10.11}$$

$$M = S_s^- + S_g^- \tag{10.12}$$

$$N = P_s^- + P_g^-$$ (10.13)

If $\alpha = S_g^+/N$, $\gamma = S_g^-/N$, then $S_s^+ = M - N(\alpha + \beta)$, $S_s^- = M - N\gamma$, $P_g^+ = N[1 + \gamma - (\alpha + \beta)]$, and $P_s^+ = N[(\alpha + \beta) - \gamma]$.

Since the free energy of the outer solution is equal to that of the translational motions of microions in outer solution, we have:

$$F_s = RT \left\{ [M - N(\alpha + \beta)] \ln \frac{[M - N(\alpha + \beta)]v_c}{V - V_g} + (M - N\gamma) \ln \frac{(M - N\gamma)v_c}{V - V_g} + \right.$$

$$\left. N(\alpha + \beta - \gamma) \ln \frac{N(\alpha + \beta - \gamma)v_c}{V - V_g} \right\}$$ (10.14)

where V_g is the equilibrated volume of network in the surfactant solution. It is considered that no micelle formation occurs in the outer solution.

The free energy of the volume interaction of monomer links F_{int} is obtained from Equation (10.2) by putting $m \to \infty$ and substituting the volume of network V_g for the volume of solution V:

$$F_{int} = RT \frac{V_g}{v_c} \left[(1 - \phi) \ln(1 - \phi) + \chi \phi (1 - \phi) \right]$$ (10.15)

where the volume fraction of polymer $\phi = V_0/V_g$ and $V_0 = Nv_c$ is the volume of the polymer network in dry state. The free energy due to the mobile ions in the network is:

$$F_{mobile} = RT \left\{ N\alpha \ln \left(N\alpha v_c / V_g \right) + N\gamma \ln \left(N\gamma v_c / V_g \right) + \right.$$

$$\left. N(1 + \gamma - \alpha - \beta) \ln \left[N(1 + \gamma - \alpha - \beta) v_c / V_g \right] \right\}$$ (10.16)

The elastic free energy for the deformation of the network F_{el}[18] is expressed as:

$$F_{el} = \frac{3}{2} RT v_e \left[(\phi_0/\phi)^{2/3} - 1 - \ln(\phi_0/\phi)^{1/3} \right]$$ (10.17)

where ϕ_0 is the volume fraction of the network at the reference state. The free energy of the surfactant binding with the polymer network F_{comp} should be the same as in Equation (10.4). By minimizing the total free energy of the system $\partial F / \partial \beta = 0$, we get the equilibrium value of β:

$$\ln C_s^g v_c = \left(\Delta F_e + \Delta F_h\right)/kT - 1 + \ln \frac{\left.\right)4\beta(1-\beta)\left[\exp(-\Delta F_h/kT)-1\right]+1+2\beta-1}{\left.\right)4\beta(1-\beta)\left[\exp(-\Delta F_h/kT)-1\right]+1+1-2\beta}$$

$$+ \ln \frac{(\alpha+\beta-\gamma)V_g}{\left[1-(\alpha+\beta-\gamma)\right]\left(V-V_g\right)} \qquad (10.18)$$

where

$$C_s^g = \frac{M - N(\alpha+\beta)}{V - V_g}$$

is the molar concentration of the surfactant in the outer solution and α and γ can be determined from the condition of $\partial F/\partial \alpha = 0$ and $\partial F/\partial \beta = 0$, which give rise to:

$$\alpha(\alpha+\beta-\gamma) = C_s^g\left(V-V_g\right)1+\gamma-\alpha-\beta/N \qquad (10.19)$$

$$\left[C_s^g\left(V-V_g\right)/N+\alpha+\beta-\gamma\right](\alpha+\beta-\gamma) = \gamma\left[1+\gamma-\alpha-\beta\right]\left[\left(V-V_g\right)/V_g\right]^2 \quad (10.20)$$

The equilibrium value of the network volume fraction ϕ can be determined by $\partial F/\partial \phi = 0$:

$$\ln(1-\phi) + \chi\phi^2 + \frac{\phi v_e}{N}\left[\left(\frac{\phi_0}{\phi}\right)^{2/3} - \frac{1}{2}\right] + \phi(\beta-2\gamma) +$$

$$2v_c\left[C_s^g + \frac{N(\alpha+\beta-\gamma)}{V-V_g}\right] = 0 \qquad (10.21)$$

By combining Equation (10.18) through Equation (10.21), the binding isotherms of the surfactant with the polymer network can be obtained.

Comparing Equation (10.18) with Equation (10.6) used for the linear polymer, it can be seen easily that the crosslinking effect is indicated in the last term in Equation (10.18), which can be rewritten as the ratio of polymer counterion concentration distribution in the solution $[P_s^+]$ and within the network $[P_g^+]$:

$$\ln\frac{(\alpha+\beta-\gamma)V_g}{(1+\gamma-\alpha-\beta)(V-V_g)} = \ln\frac{[P_s^+]}{[P_g^+]} \qquad (10.22)$$

and by combining Equation (10.18) and Equation (10.19), we have:

$$C_s^g / C_g^g = \left[P_s^+ \right] / \left[P_g^+ \right] \qquad (10.23)$$

where $C_g^g = N\alpha/V_g$ is the equilibrium-free surfactant concentration in the network.

Thus, the presence of the crosslinkage introduces an extra ionic osmotic pressure difference inside and outside the network. When β is small, $[P_s^+] \ll [P_g^+]$ and the network tends to swell, which is balanced by the elastic force. This swelling ionic osmotic pressure enhances the initial binding process but suppresses the surfactant aggregation compared with aggregations of the linear polyelectrolyte.

As pointed out by Kwak et al.,[9] cooperative binding is sensitively influenced by the chemical structure and flexibility of a polymer chain, and the cooperativity parameter becomes very low when the polymer chain lacks flexibility. If we regard the polymer network as a crosslinked three-dimensional polymer chain in water, the presence of the locally concentrated counterions that originate the swelling osmotic pressure makes the network expand in competition with the conformational shrinkage on binding and thus strongly reduces cooperativity.

It was previously reported that the cooperativity parameter of the binding for the polymer network can be increased by adding a neutral salt in sacrifice of the initiation process.[19] This can be well understood from the present theory. The salt strongly shields the electrostatic repulsions between macroions, thus lowering the electrostatic potential energy ΔF_e. This leads to a shift of the isotherm curve toward a higher equilibrium concentration. On the other hand, a high ionic strength suppresses the network expansion since the addition of salt makes P_s^+/P_g^+ insensitive to β and enhances the cooperative binding, as can easily be predicted from Equation (10.18). By differentiation of the equations for binding in linear and network polymers, i.e., Equation (10.6) and Equation (10.18) at $\beta = 0.5$, the corresponding values of K_0 and u can be calculated. In network systems, the value of u was calculated to be very near to unity that indicates almost absence of cooperative binding in spite of strong hydrophobic interaction.

COMPARISON OF THEORETICAL AND EXPERIMENTAL RESULTS

The described theoretical approach was compared with the experimental data for the binding of dodecylpyridinium chloride ($C_{12}PyCl$) with linear and crosslinked PAMPS.[20] The theoretical curve fit quite well with the observed data when β was less than 0.7 while a deviation was observed when β exceeded 0.7 (Figure 10.6). This may be associated with the drastic conformational change of the polymer chain from the extended random coil to the globules that should have occurred at a certain β value. The conformational change would have largely decreased the surface potential energy ΔF_e and altered the binding equilibrium to produce decreased binding of the surfactant.

Data for the initiation constant K_0 and the cooperativity parameter u for the network with varying degrees of swelling (q) were also compared.[34] The calculated values of u agreed fairly well with those of the observed data, while the K_0 showed a discrepancy between the calculated and the observed data when q became higher. Data for the linear polymer was shown for a comparison. A series of experiments on binding of a single gel ($q = 50$) with surfactants having variable alkyl chain lengths produced a divergence of observed and calculated data as β exceeded 0.7 (Figure 10.7).

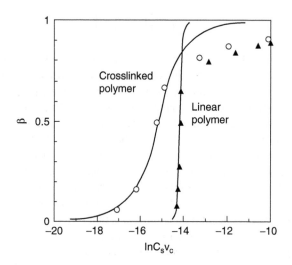

FIGURE 10.6 Binding isotherm of $C_{12}PyCl$ with linear and crosslinked PAMPS. Solid lines are theoretical results using $N = 3 \times 10^{-5}$; $V_0 = 6 \times 10^{-6}$ L; $V = 0.01$ L; $v_c = 0.018$ L/M; $\Delta F_h/kT = -6.2$; $q = 50$. Open circles (crosslinked polymer) and triangles (linear polymer) are experimental results from Okuzaki and Osada.[20] (From Gong, J.P. and Osada, Y., *J. Phys. Chem.*, 99, 10974, 1995. With permission.)

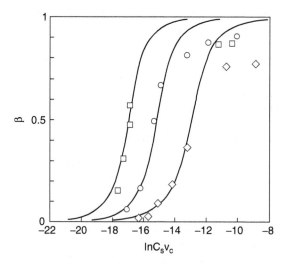

FIGURE 10.7 Binding isotherms of surfactants with different alkyl chain lengths to a network of $q = 50$. Solid lines are calculated using $\Delta F_h/kT = -8.0, -6.2$, and -4.0 (left to right). Other parameters are the same as in Figure 10.6 [($\Diamond$) $C_{10}PyCl$, (o) $C_{12}PyCl$, ($\Box$) $C_{18}PyCl$]. (From Gong, J.P. and Osada, Y., *J. Phys. Chem.*, 99, 10975, 1995. With permission.)

Unlike the linear polymer solution, the electrostatic potential on the polymer network cannot be analytically described by the rod-like model.[37,38] The charged network introduces potential valleys and deep potential wells at every crosslinking point. Therefore, the binding of the surfactant to the network presumably starts at the crosslinking points and later proceeds to the chain. Because the the electrostatic potential distribution along the polymer chain could be a complicating factor, we supposed that the ΔF_e of the network was approximately equal to that of the linear polymer at a corresponding polymer concentration. To simplify the numerical calculation, we assumed that $\alpha \approx \gamma \approx 0$, meaning that all the surfactant molecules penetrated into the network and are bound with the macroions and the equilibrium between the free surfactant ions and the bound surfactant in the network domain was not considered.

This is true only when the surfactant has a very strong hydrophobic interaction and the polymer network has a high crosslinking density. Discrepancies were observed in the system with a lower crosslinking degree (i.e., larger q). A numerical calculation of the general situation in which the equilibrium of surfactants inside the network is considered should be performed for the polymer network having a high degree of swelling. Nevertheless, the calculated isotherms showed fairly good agreement with the experimental data and this confirms the essential feature of the theory. Comparative studies of the cooperative binding of surfactants with linear and crosslinked polymers have been published elsewhere.[39,40]

The experimental results regarding the uptake of surfactant by the polyelectyrolyte gel and the effects of different parameters such as crosslinking degree, ionic strength, counterions, and co-ions were discussed earlier. Narita et al. also described such results.[25,41] It was suggested that the kinetics of surfactant uptake can be well expressed in terms of two processes: diffusion and binding. For the sake of convenience, binding was assumed to be very rapid as compared to diffusion so that a local equilibrium always existed between bound and free surfactants. Diffusion was considered as a one-dimensional process and the diffusion constant (D) was assumed to be constant. Volume changes and ionic properties of the surfactant were ignored. The mathematical modeling cited elsewhere by Gong et al.[40] may explain the fact that the velocity of surfactant uptake was enhanced on binding of the surfactant. However, the effects of the counterion and electrostatic interaction were taken into account in another publication.[25]

CHEMOMECHANICAL SYSTEMS DESIGNED FROM SURFACTANT–POLYMER COMPLEXATION

From the results discussed, it is obvious that surfactant binding in polyelectrolyte gels results in remarkable shrinkage of the gels. Therefore, selective surfactant binding to a particular surface of gel can result in selective shrinking and bending of the gel to a particular direction. Because polyelectrolytes are electroactive in nature and surfactant binding is reversible, it is possible to make a gel stretch and bend selectively and reversibly. These phenomena have been exploited to fabricate gel-based moving objects, namely gel pendulums and gel loopers.[42]

In contrast to motors and hydrodynamic pumps, the movements of polymer gels are produced by the chemical free energies of the polymer networks. Electrical or thermal energy is used to drive the direction and control the state of equilibrium. Thus, a chemomechanical gel driven by an outside stimulus can exhibit a gentle and flexible action; its movement is more like that observed in muscle than in metallic mechanical systems.

Osada et al.[42] developed a novel inchworm-like device that moves by repeatedly curling and straightening itself based on the reversible and cooperative complexations of surfactant molecules on a polymer gel under electric field. The device is a pioneering approach toward man-made soft devices. It consists simply of a strip of PAMPS gel suspended from a plastic ratchet bar and immersed in a dilute solution of $C_{12}PyCl$ and sodium sulfate. When 20 V of direct current (DC) were applied through a pair of long carbon plate electrodes placed at upper and lower positions of the ratchet bar and polarity was altered at 2-sec intervals, the gel moved forward in water, like a looper, by repeated bending and stretching. Figure 10.8a shows time profiles of the "walking" actions of a gel looper at a constant velocity of 25 cm min^{-1} in water at 20 V DC. The electric field drives and controls the direction of

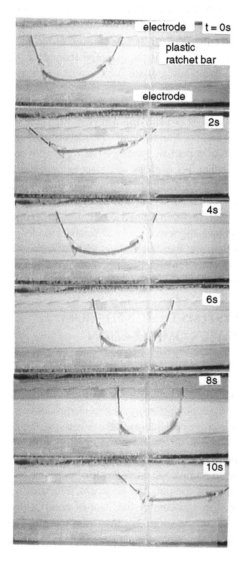

FIGURE 10.8(a) Time profile of the gel looper showing stretching and bending of a $C_{12}PyCl$-bound PAMPS gel under an electric field. Degree of crosslinking = 5 mol%; degree of swelling (q) = 45. (From Osada, Y., Okuzaki, H., and Hori, H., *Nature*, 355, 242, 1992. With permission.)

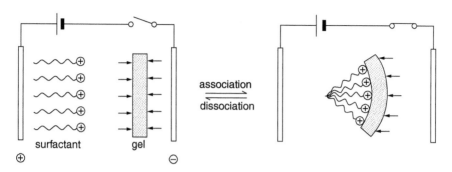

FIGURE 10.8(b) Mechanism of movement of PAMPS gel. Left: Gel is free from electric field. Right: Gel is under voltage with the anode facing the right side.

surfactant–gel equilibrium to give anisotropic complexation. When the DC voltage is turned on, the positively charged surfactant molecules move toward the cathode by electrophoresis and form a complex with the negatively charged gel, preferentially on the side of the strip facing the anode. This causes anisotropic contraction of the gel by bending it toward the anode. When the polarity of the field is reversed, the surfactant molecules absorbed on the gel are released and travel electrophoretically toward the anode. New surfactant molecules complex preferentially to the opposite side and straighten the gel. Thus, the gel strip can be made to bend and stretch repeatedly and the looper moves forward along the bar (Figure 10.8b). By using a longer strip of gel and fixing five pairs of parallel-plate platinum electrodes at specified gaps, an eel-like motion was observed (Figure 10.9). The moving object (designated a *geel*) was able to move 15 cm min^{-1} under a voltage 10 V.[43–45] All these soft devices are discussed in an excellent recent review.[46] The stream of work continues and new findings continue to appear.

CONCLUSIONS

It is evident that the surfactant–polymer associations in linear polymers, networks, and gels has been an area of interest to polymer scientists and physical chemists for a long time. Such systems are dominated by the cooperative binding interactions revealed by experimental results. While the fundamental aspects of linear polymer systems and polyelectrolyte gels have been widely explored, many aspects of non-ionic crosslinked systems warrant further investigation.

Surfactant binding in gels has proven highly promising for applications in soft devices because of the gentle and flexible actions that resemble muscle movements. The surfactant–gel association approaches a perfect "artificial muscle" that appears highly promising for miniaturized applications.

Much work remains to be done on fabricating actuators from these soft gels for robots and other machines that are expected to be more efficient. The molecular machine that is capable of biomimetic mobility through use of a gel will open a new world of gentle, smooth, and noiseless movement. Applications may eventually

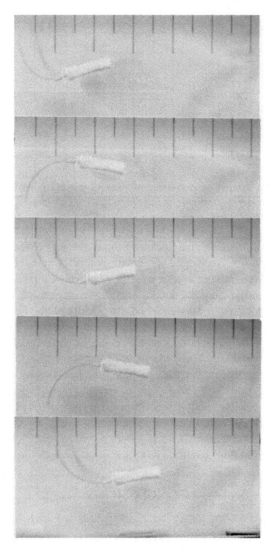

FIGURE 10.9 Time profiles of electro-driven chemomechanical swinging of PAMPS gel in the presence of C_nPyCl (0.01 M) and Na_2SO_4 (0.03 M) under 10 V alternating current every 2 sec. (From Gong, J.P. and Osada, Y., in *Polymer Sensors and Actuators*, Osada, Y. and DeRossi, D.E., Eds., Springer-Verlag, New York, 1999, p. 285. With permission.)

include devices that can be inserted into muscles and emulate nervous systems. It can be concluded that the surfactant–polymer association has established itself as a highly promising field of research and development that will ultimately lead to a group of effective and intelligent materials and devices.

ACKNOWLEDGMENT

RG sincerely acknowledges the Japanese Society for the Promotion of Science for providing a postdoctoral fellowship.

REFERENCES

1. K. Shinoda et al., *Colloidal Surfactants,* Academic Press, New York, 1963.
2. N.J. Turro, B.H. Baretz, and P.L. Kuo, *Macromolecules*, 17, 1321, 1984.
3. G.C. Kresheck and W.A. Hargraves, *Colloid Interface Sci.*, 83, 1, 1981.
4. B. Cabane, *J. Phys. Chem.*, 81, 1639, 1977.
5. R. Zana, P. Lianos, and J. Lang, *J. Phys. Chem.*, 89, 41, 1985.
6. F. Tokiwa and K. Tsujii, *Bull. Chem. Soc. Jpn.*, 46, 2684, 1973.
7. D.-Y. Chu and J.K. Thomas, *Macromolecules*, 17, 2142, 1984.
8. D.-Y. Chu and J.K. Thomas, *J. Am. Chem. Soc.*, 108, 6270, 1986.
9. K. Hayakawa, J.P. Santeree, and J.C.T. Kwak, *Macromolecules*, 16, 1642, 1983.
10. K. Hayakawa and J.C.T. Kwak, *J. Phys. Chem.*, 86, 3866, 1982.
11. P.L. Dubin and D.D. Davis, *Macromolecules*, 17, 1294, 1984.
12. K. Thalberg and B. Lindman, *J. Phys. Chem.*, 93, 1478, 1989.
13. K. Shirahama and M. Tashiro, *Bull. Chem. Soc., Jpn.*, 57, 377, 1984.
14. E. Ising, *Physik*, 31, 253, 1925.
15. B.H. Zimm and J.K. Bragg, *J. Chem. Phys.*, 31, 526, 1959.
16. I. Satake and J.T. Yang, *Biopolymers*, 15, 2263, 1976.
17. E. Kokufuta, Y.-Q. Zhang, T. Tanaka, and A. Mamada, *Macromolecules*, 26, 1053, 1993.
18. P.J. Flory, *Principles of Polymer Chemistry*, Cornell University Press, Ithaca, NY, 1953.
19. H. Okuzaki and Y. Osada, *Macromolecules*, 27, 502, 1994.
20. H. Okuzaki and Y. Osada, *Macromolecules*, 28, 4554, 1995.
21. J.P. Gong and Y. Osada, *Chem. Lett.*, 6, 449, 1995.
22. N. Isogai, T. Narita, L. Chen, M. Hirata, J.P. Gong, and Y. Osada, *Coll. Surf. A Physicochem. Eng. Aspects*, 147, 189, 1999.
23. H. Okuzaki and Y. Osada, *Macromolecules*, 28, 380, 1995.
24. T. Narita, J.P. Gong, and Y. Osada, *Macromol. Rapid. Commun.*, 18, 853, 1997.
25. T. Narita, N. Hirota, J.P. Gong, and Y. Osada, *J. Phys. Chem. B*, 103, 6262, 1999.
26. B. Kim, M. Ishizawa, J.P. Gong, and Y. Osada, *J. Polym. Sci. A Polym. Chem.*, 37, 635, 1999.
27. N. Isogai, J.P. Gong, and Y. Osada, *Macromolecules*, 29, 6803, 1996.
28. S.Y. Yu, M. Hirata, L. Chen, S. Matsumoto, M. Matsukata, J.P. Gong, and Y. Osada, *Macromolecules*, 29, 8021, 1996.
29. L. Chen, S. Yu, Y. Kagami, J.P. Gong, and Y. Osada, *Macromolecules*, 31, 787, 1998.
30. T. Gilanyi and G. Wolfram, *Coll. Surfaces*, 3, 181, 1981.
31. R. Nagarajan, *Coll. Surfaces*, 13, 1, 1985.
32. E. Rukenstein, G. Huber, and H. Hoffmann, *Langmuir*, 3, 382, 1987.
33. A.R. Khokhlov, E.Y. Kramarenko, E.E. Makhaeva, and S.G. Starodubtzev, *Macromol. Chem. Theo. Simul.*, 1, 105, 1992.
34. J.P. Gong and Y. Osada, *J. Phys. Chem.*, 99, 10973, 1995.

35. R.A. Marcus, *J. Phys. Chem.*, 58, 621, 1954.

36. S. Lifson, *J. Chem. Phys.*, 26, 727, 1957.

37. S. Lifson and A. Katchalsky, *J. Polym. Sci.*, 13, 43, 1954.

38. J.P. Gong, T. Nitta, and Y. Osada, *J. Phys. Chem.*, 98, 9583, 1994.

39. T. Narita, J.P. Gong, and Y. Osada, *J. Phys. Chem. B*, 102, 4566, 1998.

40. J.P. Gong, T. Mizutani, and Y. Osada, *Polym. Adv. Tech.*, 7, 797, 1996.

41. T. Narita, J.P. Gong, and Y. Osada, *Wiley Polymer Networks Group Rev. Ser.*, 1, 477, 1998.

42. Y. Osada, H. Okuzaki, and H. Hori, *Nature*, 355, 242, 1992.

43. H. Okuzaki, Y. Eguchi, and Y. Osada, *Chem. Mater. Commun.*, 6, 1651, 1994.

44. Y. Ueoka, J.P. Gong, and Y. Osada, *J. Intel. Syst. Struct.*, 8, 465, 1997.

45. H. Okuzaki and Y. Osada, *Electrochim. Acta*, 40, 2229, 1995.

46. D. Kaneko, J.P. Gong, and Y. Osada, *J. Mater. Chem.*, 12, 2169, 2002.

11 Rate-Limiting Steps in Volume Change Kinetics of Fast Responsive Microporous Gels

Norihiro Kato and Stevin H. Gehrke

CONTENTS

INTRODUCTION

Keen attention has been focused on solvent-swollen gels that alter their structures and properties in response to external stimuli. Such polymer gels have also been termed *smart*, *intelligent*, and *stimuli-responsive*. The swelling degree (swollen volume) is the property of these gels that typically changes most drastically in response to various kinds of chemical and physical stimuli. Other properties like permeability can also be altered as the result of a volume change. Some property changes can also occur at constant volume (e.g., opaque-to-transparent transition). A wide variety of environmental stimuli including temperature, pH, solvent composition, ionic strength, light, electric field, magnetic field, and specific chemical triggers like glucose have been shown to trigger such changes in many types of gels.[1-11] These stimuli can trigger discontinuous changes (thermodynamically identified as phase transitions) or gradual changes that occur over a finite range of stimulus levels. These changes are typically reversible, although hysteresis may occur. These properties have attracted much attention for their potential for use in a wide variety of devices and applications including sensors, drug delivery carriers, tissue engineering, recyclable absorbents, artificial muscles, separation systems, and bioreactors.[11-20]

For most applications of responsive gels, ability to control the response rate is one of the most important factors for technological and commercial success. Analyses of the swelling or shrinking kinetics of gels are essential to the design of most gel applications. Since kinetics may well determine which applications can move from the laboratory to the marketplace, it is necessary to identify the relationships between swelling or shrinking kinetics and the relevant rate-limiting steps. In this chapter, the rate-limiting steps for gel swelling or shrinking are examined, with particular emphasis on maximizing response rates in microporous gels.

EVALUATION OF KEY GEL PROPERTIES

The key properties of hydrogels for most applications include degree of swelling, swelling kinetics, and permeability. Relatively poor mechanical properties can limit their utility or require bonding to stronger substrates. Transparency can be key for some applications such as light sensors or contact lenses. For medical and pharmaceutical applications, *in vivo* properties such as biocompatibility and biodegradability are also important for successful development of applications.[21-23]

The equilibrium swelling degree (ratio of wet mass or volume to dry mass or volume) is the most important property of a hydrogel because it directly affects most of the other properties of the material including kinetics, permeability, and modulus.[24-27] The swelling of a hydrogel at equilibrium with water is determined primarily by the hydrophilic/hydrophobic balance of the base polymer, the concentrations of counterions associated with any ionized groups in the network, and the concentrations of crosslinking junctions.

The microstructure of a gel can also influence the swelling degree of a gel, but this has not been widely studied. Theories for gel swelling thermodynamics assume homogeneous distribution of network chains in the solvent, which works for most conventional (nonporous) gels. The water content of microporous (gels with distinct pores of size on the order of a micron) and macroporous gels (gels with distinct pores about the size of a millimeter) often are strongly influenced by the synthesis conditions in a manner not correlated by the thermodynamic theories developed for nonporous gels.

The widely variable and adjustable permeability of hydrogels is the primary property that makes them useful in drug delivery and separation applications. Since the solute mobility of a gel is hindered by the polymer network, increasing the swelling degree dilutes the network and normally leads to an increased permeability to solutes. Conversely, a decrease of the swelling degree leads to a decrease in permeability. These trends are typically seen in cases where the polymer is inert to the solutes and the microstructure varies affinely with the macroscopic volume change.[26] However, the microstructure of a gel may not maintain geometric similarity with the macroscopic gel as it swells and shrinks. Furthermore, a polymer network often interacts with solutes via hydrogen bonding, electrostatics, and hydrophobic interaction. Thus, a direct relationship between gel swelling degree and permeability to solutes may not always exist.

Permeability (P) has been defined as the product of a thermodynamic property, the partition coefficient (K), and a transport property, the diffusion coefficient (D). The partition coefficient is defined as the ratio of the concentration of the solute inside the gel to that in the solution outside the gel at equilibrium. A value of $K < 1$ means that the solute is excluded from the gel network to some extent (with complete exclusion at $K = 0$), while $K > 1$ indicates that the solute favorably interacts with the gel phase. To understand permeability requires understanding of how the gel network alters the transport and thermodynamic properties of a system.[26]

The release rates of drugs from swelling-controlled delivery devices may be controlled by solvent absorption and the swelling rates. There are many important examples of drug delivery induced by permeability that increases upon solvent uptake. In these cases, the rate of solvent sorption has a major impact on the release rate. This is true both for gels swelling from a dry state and for triggered releases from stimuli-responsive gels whose solvent absorption capacities are controlled by the environmental triggers such as pH, temperature, solvent composition, and electric field.

The mechanical performance of gels is also strongly affected by the swelling degree and the rate by which this changes in a triggered release system. The shear modulus G depends directly upon the water content of the gel. The dependence typically scales with the polymer volume fraction to the 1/3 power, but the relationship between modulus and water content depends upon the specific situation at hand.[27] The relationships between water content and other mechanical properties like tensile strength and elongation at break are less defined. In general, however, mechanical properties decline as a polymer network is diluted upon swelling.

The remainder of this chapter is focused on the swelling kinetics of gels, with particular emphasis on identifying the rate-limiting steps behind environmentally triggered swelling and shrinking and concepts for maximizing the response rates to achieve "flash" response characteristics.

RATE-LIMITING STEPS FOR NONPOROUS GEL SYSTEMS

The swelling rate of a gel immersed in a solvent is affected by a number of variables, and swelling may occur in a series of steps. In most cases, the rate of network motion is the rate-limiting step, but for responsive gels the rate of stimulus change can become rate-limiting. In the case that a single step is rate-limiting, gel swelling kinetics can be predicted with an appropriate model for that step alone, even if that process is not the sorption process. For example, poly(acrylic acid) gels swell and

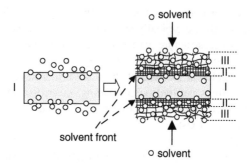

FIGURE 11.1 Gel swelling in solvents from glassy to rubbery gels. I: Glassy core at dry state. II: Transition from glassy to rubbery state. III: Mutual diffusion of polymer network and solvent.

shrink in response to pH changes because they contain carboxylic acid groups whose ionization state varies with pH.

When the pH of the solution is increased from below the pK_a of the gel's acidic groups to a higher pH, it changes from a nonionic form to an ionized form. The gel then absorbs the solution to dilute the cations associated with the negatively charged network. Under some conditions, the swelling rate can be controlled by the rate of pH changes inside gels.[2,28,29]

Accordingly, ion exchange kinetic models can be used to predict the rates of swelling and shrinking for these gels.[2,28] However, the rate of network-solvent diffusion generally is much slower than that of stimuli in nonporous gels.[2,11,30] In contrast, for stimuli-responsive microporous gels, the swelling and shrinking kinetics for the gels are strongly affected by the rates of application of the driving stimuli. For example, the rate of heat transfer often limits the swelling or shrinking rate for the fast responsive gels.[18,31,32] This topic is the focus of the following sections.

Several kinetic parameters are associated with volume change kinetics of gels, including the solvent sorption rate, rate of approach to the equilibrium swelling degree, rate of moving solvent and solute fronts (if present), and transport mechanism of the solvent.[21,22,33–35] Figure 11.1 illustrates the swelling process in an initially glassy gel. The solvent sorption rate, in terms of mass uptake per unit time, usually increases with swelling degree. However, the rate of approach to equilibrium is not directly correlated with the equilibrium swelling degree. In rubbery gels, the swelling can usually be correlated with a diffusion coefficient, as detailed below.

In cases where gel swelling is controlled simply by diffusion, the swelling can be correlated by the diffusion coefficient of the network in the solvent. If glassy gels are contacted with a swelling solvent, a moving solvent front often develops and advances toward the center of the gel. The visually observed solvent front is an area of steep refractive index gradient, and often indicates the boundary between a glassy central core and swollen, plasticized (i.e., rubbery) regions. Since solute diffusivity can be orders of magnitude different in the two regions, this phenomenon can provide the basis for swelling-controlled release systems.[33–46]

The transport mechanism may indicate the degree of deviation from a simple diffusion-controlled swelling process. Such deviations can arise from polymer relaxation processes, boundary layer resistances, anisotropic dimensional changes (such as those that occur upon disappearance of the glassy core), shifts in rate-limiting steps during the swelling process, chemical reactions (such as hydrolysis), and so on.[21,22,33–47] A single general model for treating kinetic data in such complex cases does not exist due to the diversity and complexity of the phenomena. However, a simple empirical model is widely used to identify deviation from simple diffusion-controlled processes, and provides the definition of the transport exponent n. This model fits the first 60% of the absorption or desorption data to the following equation:

$$\frac{M_t}{M_\infty} = kt^n \qquad (11.1)$$

where M_t is the mass absorbed or desorbed at time t, M_∞ is the mass absorbed or desorbed at equilibrium, k is an empirical rate constant, and n is called the transport exponent.[33,47] The value of n indicates rate-controlling steps. In the case of a flat sheet, a value of $n = 0.5$ means that the rate-controlling step is a diffusive process. Exponents between 0.5 and 1.0 are defined as anomalous and indicate non-Fickian transport. A value of $n = 1.0$ is particularly interesting; it indicates a constant swelling rate. Values of $n < 0.5$ and $n > 1.0$ are sometimes observed and can arise from a variety of processes, most of which are difficult to model more quantitatively.

The sorption and desorption of solvents by rubbery polymer gels often occurs by a simple diffusion-controlled process (transport exponent of 0.5 in planar geometry). This usually describes the swelling of responsive gels, as they normally undergo volume changes between two different rubbery states. In such cases, swelling and shrinking kinetics of gels can often be modeled with a single parameter. This parameter is the diffusion coefficient (D), as obtained from the solution of Fick's law of diffusion. Solutions to the Fickian sorption problems for a wide variety of geometries and boundary conditions are given by Crank.[48] For planar geometry, the solvent sorption as a function of time can be calculated from the following equation (for flat sheets with aspect ratios greater than 10):

$$\frac{M_t}{M_\infty} = 1 - \sum_{n=0}^{\infty} \left[\frac{8}{(2n+1)^2 \pi^2} \right] \exp\left[-(2n+1)^2 \pi^2 \frac{Dt}{L^2} \right] \qquad (11.2)$$

where L is the thickness of the gel sheet. If this calculation is applied to a volume-fixed frame of reference (laboratory coordinates), this equation is strictly applicable only to nonswelling systems. In such cases, the diffusion coefficient is given as the polymer–solvent mutual diffusion coefficient (D_v) in a volume-fixed reference frame.[11,48,49]

For an expanding or contracting sheet, the mathematics are the same as for the volume-fixed system except that the length L should be the initial half-thickness and the diffusion coefficient becomes that in the polymer-fixed reference frame (D_p).[48] D_p can be converted to a value in lab coordinates, but in swelling studies it is most useful simply as an empirical parameter.

Tanaka et al. used a different approach to the problem of swelling rubbery gels, starting with the equations of motion instead of Fick's law to define a diffusion coefficient.[50,51] The diffusion coefficient defined in this way is the ratio of the longitudinal bulk modulus of the network to the frictional coefficient between the network and the fluid. This diffusion coefficient is called a collective diffusion coefficient of the network (D_c). The concept of collective diffusion successfully describes the swelling kinetics and the dynamics of density fluctuations of gels as observed by dynamic light scattering spectroscopy. Tanaka and Fillmore solved the equations of motion for a gel swelling in a solvent under nonequilibrium conditions; these equations are often described as the products of the *TF theory*.

$$\frac{L_t}{L_\infty} = 1 - \sum_{n=0}^{\infty} \left[\frac{8}{(2n+1)^2 \pi^2} \right] \exp \left[-(2n+1)^2 \pi^2 \frac{Dt}{L^2} \right] \tag{11.3}$$

Although derived differently, Fick's law and TF theory yield the same functions and correlate different dimensional parameters. The parameter correlated by Fick's law is the normalized approach to the equilibrium mass or volume (M_t/M_∞), while TF theory correlates the normalized approach to the equilibrium of the linear dimension (L_t/L_∞). Fick's law and TF theory are equivalent only in the limit of no volume change, but their D values differ by less than a factor of two in most cases. In practice, both equations have been used to fit the data of a large range of experiments equally well and either can be used to correlate data, although theoretical interpretation of the resulting values is complex.[11]

The swelling and shrinking diffusion coefficients obtained from these analyses are generally on the order of 10^{-7} cm^2/s, a value characteristic of polymers dissolved in solvents, but much lower than the diffusion coefficients of solvents in swollen gels. To demonstrate that the diffusion coefficients of gels were limited by diffusion of the networks through the solvent rather than the diffusion of solvent into the gel, Gehrke and Cussler determined the diffusion coefficient of deuterium oxide (D_2O) inside swollen hydrogels.[2] Poly(acrylamide-co-sodium methacrylate) gels equilibrated in pH 4.0 HCl or pH 9.2 NaOH solution were transferred into limited volumes of solutions of 10 wt% D_2O in water at the same pH levels, and the change in solution density was measured as a function of time. The diffusion coefficients obtained for the D_2O were 2.3×10^{-5} cm^2/s into the ionized pH 9.2 gel and 2.4×10^{-5} cm^2/s into the nonionized pH 4.0 gel. Since the self-diffusion coefficient of D_2O is 2.6×10^{-5} cm^2/s, the diffusion coefficient inside the gels was reduced as expected due to the presence of the polymer in the gel.[2,33,52,53] This result means that solvent molecules can diffuse into or out of a polymer network much faster than the gel swells or shrinks.

The significance of this analysis is that the diffusion coefficient of a polymer network in water is on the order of 10^{-7} cm^2/s and is relatively insensitive to the type of polymer network. This means that diffusion-limited networks of macroscopic size swell or shrink rather slowly. The only way to circumvent this fact is to make the sample dimensions smaller, since the equilibration time scales with the square of the dimension: $t \sim L^2$. However, making a sample smaller to increase response rate is not always feasible. The route to bypass this problem is to develop systems in which convection rather than diffusion is the dominant mass transfer mechanism. This can be achieved in microporous gels, which are the subjects of the remaining sections of the chapter.

FAST RESPONSIVE MATERIALS

PREPARATION OF MICROPOROUS MATERIALS

To overcome diffusion-limited kinetics in macroscopic gel samples, porous structures can be generated. Network diffusion then occurs over the scale of the microstructure rather than in macroscopic dimensions as long as the microstructure allows the fluid to be absorbed or desorbed by convection through the pores. Thus, construction of a sufficiently porous structure can be an effective route to overcoming diffusion limitations and creating fast responsive materials.

Many methods have been used to make various microporous materials. These methods include *in situ* generation of gas bubbles, leaching of embedded soluble particles, copolymerization in one phase of a bicontinuous emulsion, solvent-induced polymer aggregation, and induced phase separation of polymer solutions.

Commercially, porous foams are usually made by the gas generation technique involving dispersion of a gaseous phase throughout a fluid polymer phase (e.g., by a gas-generating reaction) and the solidification of the resultant state. In these macroporous materials, pore size is generally on the order of 100 to 200 μm or larger.[54] Another technique is to disperse solid particles in a polymer melt or in a polymer solution. After solidification of the polymer, the solid particles are leached away by dissolution of the particles in a good solvent or by some other chemical treatment, thus leaving voids that function as pores.

One example of such a process is the preparation of porous polypropylene sheets using calcium carbonate filler. The pore size and porosity can be controlled by the volume fraction and the size of filler particles. A similar technique was used by Mikos et al. to prepare microporous poly(lactic-co-glycolic acid) foams with porosity values as high as 95% and pore size around 200 μm.[55] Materials prepared by such methods are generally macroporous, with pores too big to retain much solvent by capillarity under an applied load. The techniques also tend to create closed-cell pore architectures that are not as effective at allowing solvent sorption or desorption by convection as inherently open-celled architectures.

A microporous polystyrene foam can be produced in water–oil microemulsions. Such foams can have high porosities (greater than 90%) and micron-scale pore sizes, typically in the range of 1 to 30 μm. The technique's generality is limited by the ability to find a suitable solvent and nonsolvent for the comonomers and an emulsifying agent that will form a bicontinuous emulsion.[56–58]

Microporous, poly(vinyl alcohol) (PVA) gels have been prepared by subjecting aqueous polymer solutions to repeated freeze and thaw cycles. Ikada et al. reported that PVA microporous gel can be prepared by cooling concentrated PVA solutions below their freezing points; this was followed by slow crystallization of the frozen polymers above their freezing points. X-ray and scanning electron microscopy (SEM) measurements revealed that the gel had a semicrystalline and microporous structure.[59,60]

Microporous gels and membranes also have been produced by phase inversion processes. Phase inversion is a process by which a polymer solution (where the solvent is a continuous phase) inverts into a three-dimensional macromolecular network or gel where the polymer forms a solid, continuous phase. Phase inversion occurs when the polymer becomes insoluble in the solvent upon changing the system conditions. The three types of phase inversion processes are the dry process, the wet process, and the thermally induced phase separation (TIPS) process.[61]

In the TIPS process, the phase inversion is carried out by changing the temperature of a polymer solution to a value at which the solvent becomes a nonsolvent for the polymer.[62,63] If the polymer-solvent system has an upper critical solution temperature (UCST) — that is, the polymer becomes insoluble in the solvent by lowering the temperature — a permanent microstructure can be achieved by vitrifying the polymer phase simply by lowering the temperature either below the glass transition temperature of the polymer or below the freezing point of the solvent. The phase separation in the TIPS process can occur by spinodal decomposition, which readily yields a microporous structure with interconnected pores. This process is relatively easy to control because temperature is a relatively easy variable to monitor and adjust to desired values.

PREPARATION OF MICROPOROUS FAST RESPONSIVE GELS

Responsive gels can be synthesized by any method that can form a polymer network, including crosslinking of monomers, chemical or physical crosslinking of linear polymers, and chemical conversion of one gel type to another. The chemical reactions of monovinyl monomers and divinyl crosslinkers have been the most widely used methods. A number of studies have been carried out on poly(N-isopropylacrylamide) (PNIPA) gel with particular emphasis on its thermosensitive properties.[1,13,17,64,65] This gel is synthesized in solution by a free radical polymerization with a relatively small amount of a crosslinking monomer, typically N,N'-methylenebisacrylamide. In contrast, thermosensitive cellulose ether gels can be made by crosslinking the polymer with divinyl sulfone.[66–70]

Producing responsive gels by crosslinking linear precursor polymers over the copolymerization-crosslinking technique has several advantages: availability of numerous well-characterized linear polymers, possibility of solute loading during gel preparation, and the potential for easier approval from the U.S. Food and Drug Administration (FDA) of gels made from precursor polymers on the Generally Recognized as Safe (GRAS) list. However, swelling or shrinking rates of ordinary nonporous gels in response to applied stimuli are usually slow, irrespective of synthesis method. The slow responses of ordinary homogeneous gels limit their utility in various applications that require rapid responses to environmental triggers. Thus, control of the microstructure of the polymer network for responsive gels to achieve rapid convective sorption and desorption is an indispensable technique to improve their potential in applications where response time is important.

For acceleration of swelling or shrinking rates, efforts have been made to produce gels with the desired microporous structures. The response times of stimuli-responsive gels can be dramatically reduced by decreasing the characteristic diffusion path lengths since time scales with the square of the dimension for a diffusion-limited process. However, reducing the gel dimension may not be desirable or feasible for practical use as noted earlier.

The response rates can be substantially faster for microporous responsive gels possessing 0.01 to 100 μm pores. Hirasa and coworkers reported on microporous poly(vinyl methyl ether) (PVME) gels prepared by γ-irradiation under conditions that induced microscopic phase separation.[9,31,60] Since high energy radiation can split covalent bonds into unpaired radicals that then recombine randomly, a linear polymer possessing a lower critical solution temperature (LCST) can be crosslinked also by nonchemical means such as irradiation to form a temperature-responsive gel.[71] Yoshida et al. prepared comb-type PNIPA gels with PNIPA graft chains that shrank rapidly in response to temperature.[72]

Wu et al. synthesized microporous PNIPA gels by carrying out the crosslinking reaction entirely above the LCST in the presence of another LCST polymer.[73] Huang et al. reported a PVME gel containing ferric oxide powder that was effective in increasing the heat transfer rate within the gel and in the generation of a porous structure within the gel.[74] Some other approaches for the preparation of fast responsive gels include incorporation of surfactants during gel synthesis and incorporation of microparticles such as silica into a PNIPA gel.[75]

Gehrke and colleagues proposed a technique based on modification of the temperature-induced phase separation (TIPS) process to make chemically crosslinked microporous gels.[30,49,76,77] This technique allowed a great degree of control over porosity, pore size, strut size, and type of gel microstructure.[76,78–80] During gel synthesis, three different time and temperature intervals can be controlled to make micropores, as illustrated in Figure 11.2. Each temperature was controlled by immersing the reaction mold into a water bath at the desired temperature. In the first period (t_{BP}, time before phase separation), crosslinking was conducted in a homogeneous state below the LCST to initiate formation of an embryonic network or microgel. In the following period (t_{DP}, time during phase separation), the temperature was increased above the LCST of the polymer solution into the unstable region of the phase diagram, inducing spinodal decomposition. In the optional final period (t_{AP}, time after phase separation), the temperature was decreased below the LCST of the solution where remixing of phases and further crosslinking could occur before the reaction was quenched.

This TIPS method was applied to PNIPA and cellulose ether gels to make them fast responsive.[30,76,77] Figure 11.3 is a scanning electron microscopy (SEM) photograph of microporous hydroxypropyl cellulose (HPC) gel prepared by the TIPS method. It clearly shows this process is effective in creating permanent micropores from structures generated by the phase separation of LCST polymers. By using the TIPS method, a wide variety of gel morphologies, from unconnected to interconnected, can be created by varying these parameters.[78] At higher crosslinker concentrations, the microstructure becomes more rigid, limiting the volume change. However, such materials make excellent superabsorbents from the dry state.[79,80]

Kato and Takahashi proposed another convenient method to prepare microporous thermosensitive gels.[81] The shrinking rate of PNIPA gel and HPC gel in response to temperature can be accelerated dramatically after treatment by freeze-drying and rehydration. A SEM microphotograph shows the microporous structures formed by the freezing process (Figure 11.4). A heterogeneous polymer network remained after

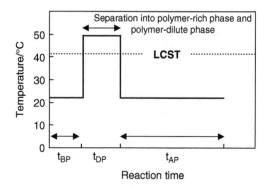

FIGURE 11.2 Modified temperature-induced phase separation (TIPS) method. During t_{BP}, an embryonic network forms, but it is insufficient to stop phase separation. During t_{DP}, phase separation occurs and the crosslinking reaction continues in the polymer-rich regions, forming the pore walls. Then the temperature is dropped below the LCST, where remixing can occur until the reaction is completed during t_{AP}.

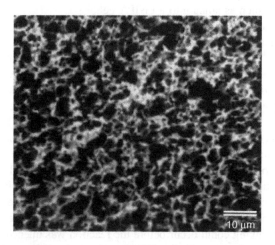

FIGURE 11.3 Representative cross-sectional SEM microphotograph of a microporous HPC gel sample. Interconnected micropores are formed during the TIPS process and range in size from ~0.5 to ~8.0 μm separated by struts ranging from ~0.5 to ~1.0 μm thick. (Adapted with permission from Kabra, B.G. and Gehrke, S.H., in *Superabsorbent Polymers: Science and Technology,* Buchholz, F.L. and Peppas, N.A., Eds., ACS Symposium Series 573, American Chemical Society, Washington, D.C., 1994, p. 76. Copyright 1994 American Chemical Society.)

sublimation of the ice generated by the freezing of the gels. Since the shrinking rate of the gel treated by freeze-thawing was comparable to that of a gel treated by freeze-drying and hydration, the freezing process rather than the drying process is important; ice crystal formation probably promotes aggregation of the polymer chains. The pore size and the shrinking time can be altered with changing the water content within the gel just before freezing.[82] This technique can be applied to most well-known hydrogels as a method for generating micropores.

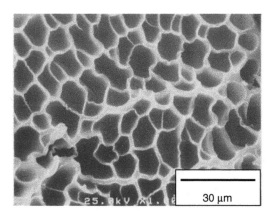

FIGURE 11.4 Representative field-emission scanning electron microscopy (FESEM) view of PNIPA gel crosslinked by 1 mol% N,N'-methylenebisacrylamide, frozen at $-30°C$ within 3 min, and then freeze-dried. The surface of the gel was observed by FESEM. Micropores formed during the freezing process.

A variety of techniques can produce microporous gels. Porosity is a necessary but not sufficient condition for producing fast responsive materials. In general, microporous gels are two-phase systems consisting of a continuous solid phase and numerous pores on the order of a micron in dimension filled with a fluid. If the fluid-filled pores are generally interconnected, the microstructure is termed *open-celled*. If the voids in the structure are largely discrete so that the fluid phase of each pore is separated from all the other pores, then the microstructure is *closed-celled*.

Structures of intermediate connectivity can also be generated. Interconnectivity of micropores is a key to lead to fast volume change of gels; open-celled structures allow the solvent to be expelled or absorbed by convection — a much faster process than diffusion. Also, the characteristic dimension of the network motion for microporous gels is not the macroscopic dimension of the gel, but the thickness of the pore walls or struts that make up the microstructure. In most cases, the strut thickness is on the order of microns. Such micron-scale structures swell and shrink in fractions of a second. In the following section, the rate-limiting steps for the microporous gels will be discussed in detail.

RATE-LIMITING STEPS FOR FAST RESPONSIVE GEL SYSTEMS

In many cases, the volume change kinetics of nonporous rubbery gels can be described by a diffusion coefficient because the rate of stimulus transfer is much faster than the network motion. Kinetic behavior of these gels is determined by the collective diffusion coefficient of polymer chains in solvents, typically on the order of 10^{-7} cm^2/s. Thus a 1-mm thick gel sheet takes several hours to reach a new equilibrium water content in response to a stimulus — too slow for most sensor or "triggered" applications. In contrast, convection through a microporous structure can occur so rapidly that the volume change kinetics of microporous gels may become limited by the rate of stimulus transfer.

Microporous gels, regardless of synthesis method, can swell or shrink in response to a thermal stimulus around 10^3 to 10^4 times faster than conventional homogeneous gels can, as described below. In other words, the rate of volume change of a gel cannot exceed the rate of stimulus transfer. This section will focus on how the microstructure of a gel can affect the volume change kinetics in response to a stimulus. The swelling and shrinking kinetics of stimuli-responsive, microporous gels was carefully studied using thermosensitive HPC gels prepared by the TIPS method. This material will illustrate the concepts of rate-limiting steps in microporous gels.

Microstructure of HPC Gel

The modified TIPS method was described in the previous section (Figure 11.2);[76] the polymer-rich phase forms water-swollen struts while the polymer-dilute phase leads to pores in a microporous gel. The lever rule for phase separation indicates that the ratio of the amount of the polymer-dilute phase to the polymer-rich phase at the phase separation temperature is equal to the ratio of the difference of the polymer-rich concentration and the system's average concentration to the difference of the system's average concentration and the polymer-dilute concentration.

Accordingly, decreasing the initial HPC concentration leads to a greater percentage of the dilute phase and a higher effective porosity. When the reaction time before phase separation (t_{BP}) is greater than the gelation time, the resulting gels are mostly nonporous because too much of the network is formed to allow much phase separation to occur. Increasing t_{BP} allows more crosslinking to occur, locking the polymer chains into a three-dimensional network and restricting the distance a polymer chain can move away from neighboring chains during phase separation. With a reaction time (t_{BP}) less than the gelation time, it is possible to make the microporous gel with interconnected pores. The embryonic network formed during t_{BP} can alter the gel morphology, pore size, strut thickness, and kinetic properties. For the reaction time during phase separation (t_{DP}), sufficient time is needed both to induce phase separation and to allow sufficient crosslinking to occur and preserve the interconnected phase domains.

Microsyneresis during t_{DP} can generate at least two different domains with different polymer concentrations because the crosslinking reaction may not be completed. The reaction temperature after phase separation (t_{AP}) is reduced below the phase separation temperature, which can allow remixing of the phases if they are insufficiently crosslinked. This process may alter the microstructure by altering the extent of crosslinking reaction in the two phases. There is also a complex relationship among synthesis conditions, mechanical properties, and volume changes of the gels, but this review focuses on kinetics.[79,80]

Relative Rates of Heat Transfer and Network Motion

Thermally responsive gels are among the most widely studied responsive systems. Because heat transfer is much faster than any mass transfer steps, it is also the most effective for triggering fast responses in microporous gel systems. The volume change kinetics of thermosensitive gels depends on the various steps: the heat transfer rate as the stimulus change rate, mutual diffusion of water and polymer chains at the struts, and the convective flow of water through the pores. Gehrke and coworkers compared the experimentally measured rates of temperature changes inside gels to the theoretical rates of those from heat transfer by conduction.[30,32]

The theoretical rate of heat transfer by conduction is controlled by a single parameter, the thermal diffusivity (α) of the gel:

$$\alpha = \frac{k}{\rho C_p} \qquad (11.4)$$

where k, ρ, and C_p are thermal conductivity of the gel, density of the gel, and heat capacity of the gel, respectively. The fractional uptake of heat (Q_t/Q_∞), defined as the fraction of total heat lost or gained by the gel, can be analyzed by the following equation:

$$\frac{Q_t}{Q_\infty} = 1 - \sum_{n=0}^{\infty} \left[\frac{8}{(2n+1)^2 \pi^2} \right] \exp\left[-(2n+1)^2 \pi^2 \frac{\alpha t}{L^2} \right] \qquad (11.5)$$

where Q_t and Q_∞ are the heat gained or lost by the gel at time t and at the thermal equilibrium, respectively. This equation is derived analogously to Equation (11.2), with thermal diffusivity replacing the diffusion coefficient D.

The temperature change inside an HPC gel was tracked with thermocouples embedded along the centerline of the sample after immersion of the sample in a water bath at a different temperature. Equation (11.5) was fitted to experimental data to obtain the best fit values of the thermal diffusivity, and found to be approximately 0.001 cm²/s for both nonporous and microporous gels, about the same as that for water (0.0014 cm²/s).[32] This is reasonable because gels are about 90% water. Since the thermal diffusivity values for nonporous and microporous gels are about the same, it is clear that these do not depend upon pore size and porosity, but are probably averages of the values for water and polymer, independent of microstructure. Because thermal diffusivity is three to four orders of magnitude larger than the network diffusion coefficient, the rate-limiting step for a nonporous gel where convection cannot occur is not heat transfer; it is the diffusion of the network in water. In contrast, the swelling and shrinking of microporous gels can occur at rates comparable to Fickian processes, with values of the diffusion coefficients between 10^{-3} and 10^{-7} cm²/s. This broad range of rates is achieved by altering the synthetic parameters of the TIPS method to control pore connectivity, pore size, and porosity (strut thickness can be decreased from between 0.03 to 0.15 and 0.2 to 2.0 μm while preserving interconnection of micropores).

MEASURING RATE OF CONVECTION

In order to directly measure the rate of convection, a technique that decouples the rate of heat transfer from convection was developed to measure the rate of convection

TABLE 11.1
Synthesis and Properties of Microporous HPC Gels with Interconnected Pores

Property	Result
Porosity	0.80
Initial polymer concentration	7.0 wt%
Initial crosslinker concentration	1.3 wt%
Reaction before phase separation	$t_{BP} = 2$ min (22°C)
Reaction during phase separation	$t_{DP} = 5$ min (49°C)
Reaction after phase separation	$t_{AP} = 1433$ min (22°C)
Overall reaction time	24 h
Swelling time and shrinking time	Time to reach 98% of equilibrium
Response time	Time to reach 98% of uptake/square of initial thickness
Heat transfer time	Time taken for thermal equilibrium/square of initial thickness
Thermal diffusivity	$\alpha = 0.0010$ cm²/s

Process	Swelling Ratio at 22–60°C	Swelling or Shrinking Time (s)	Response Time (s/cm²)	Heat Transfer Time (s/cm²)	Convection Time (s/cm²)
Swelling	1.7	30 ± 10	1900 ± 700	400 ± 200	200 ± 100
Shrinking	1.7	20 ± 10	800 ± 400	700 ± 200	—

during swelling. After removing a shrunken gel equilibrated with water at 60°C, the gel was lightly blotted with lint-free tissue paper and allowed to cool in air to room temperature (22°C) for approximately 30 s, which was sufficient to reach thermal equilibrium for a gel sheet of 1.6 mm thick and $\alpha = 10^{-3}$ cm²/s. The gel sheet was immersed in water, also at 22°C. Since no temperature change occurred when the gel was placed into the water, the heat transfer step was eliminated.

The results of this experiment and the comparable temperature-induced swelling and shrinking kinetics are shown in Figure 11.5 and summarized in Table 11.1. In the absence of heat transfer (as described above), the sample absorbed water so quickly that it was essentially at equilibrium in only 2 s. In contrast, the same gel undergoing thermally induced shrinking took more than 10 s to shrink to equilibrium — a rate that matches that predicted for heat transfer with α as measured in the section above covering relative rates of heat transfer and network motion.

Swelling appears to be slightly slower than the heat transfer rate (Table 11.1), but based on similar data for other gels, this may not be statistically significant due to the limited number of points that could be collected for a given trial due to the speed of response.[83] Thus, the data demonstrate that conductive heat transfer is the rate-limiting step and that further optimization of the microstructure to increase the rate would have little value for a fast responsive system. However, further optimization of the microstructure for convection is valuable for the development of superabsorbents designed to rapidly absorb fluid from a dry state.[79,80]

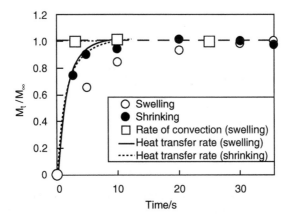

FIGURE 11.5 Weight change kinetics of microporous HPC gel prepared by the TIPS method as described in Table 11.1. This gel has interconnected pores and its mass rapidly changes in response to temperature change. The swelling and shrinking kinetics were determined by a temperature jump between 22 and 60°C. The rates of heat transfer were calculated assuming the thermal diffusivity was $\alpha = 0.0010$ cm²/s.

Another technique for isolating and quantifying the convective process in microporous gels was cooling a rectangular gel sheet in a shrunken state to room temperature and putting one edge of the gel sheet into contact with water at room temperature. Because the water was absorbed through the interconnected pores, the gel sheet expanded gradually from the edge in contact with the water. During this swelling process, the gel sheet was clearly divided into three distinct regions, depending on the degree of swelling: completely swollen, partially swollen, and unswollen.

For microporous gels possessing interconnected pores, the plots of convection front positions indicated by the movement of these regions against the square root of time fell on a straight line, as shown in Figure 11.6. This behavior for unsteady state convection into a random porous medium can be mathematically described by analogy to the process of unsteady state diffusion. Unsteady state convective flow through porous media has been a widely studied problem, and studies of the flow of solvent through porous papers are directly relevant to the problem at hand.[84]

Ruoff et al. succeeded in characterizing this flow through porous papers using the mathematics of diffusion, even though the physical process is not molecular diffusion.[85–89] A parameter analogous to a diffusion coefficient can be extracted from the line in Figure 11.6, but with values up to several orders of magnitude greater than for Fickian diffusion, consistent with Figure 11.5. This analysis also shows that the rate of convection in a microporous gel is inversely proportional to the square of gel thickness, as the mathematical analogy to diffusion suggests. Hence the time required for convection is directly proportional to the square of gel thickness, and the response rates of gels of different thicknesses can be put on the same basis and directly compared by dividing the equilibration time by the characteristic dimension squared.

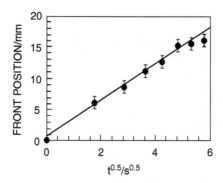

FIGURE 11.6 Isothermal water sorption kinetics of microporous HPC gel shown in Figure 11.3. The moving swelling front advanced with the square root of time, consistent with the theory for wicking of fluid into random porous media.

IDENTIFYING KINETIC LIMITATIONS FOR MICROPOROUS GELS

As mentioned above, the rates of heat transfer, convection, and volume change vary with the square of gel thickness. Thus, the response time of a gel (t_R) can be defined as the time taken to reach 98% fractional uptake divided by the square of the initial thickness of the gel (other bases for a definition of response time could be chosen, but 98% was convenient for these data). Similarly, heat transfer time (t_H) and convection time (t_C) are also defined as the measured time divided by the square of the initial thickness of the gel. This eliminates the effect of gel thickness, allowing direct comparison of samples.

As described earlier, Figure 11.5 shows the time evolution of swelling, shrinking, fractional uptake of heat, and fractional uptake of water due to convection. This microporous gel possesses interconnected pores (porosity 0.80) and can shrink and swell rapidly to its equilibrium mass within 15 to 30 s. The synthesis parameters, response time, heat transfer time, and convection time are summarized in Table 11.1. As indicated in Figure 11.5, convection is much faster than heat transfer and the actual rate of volume change of a microporous gel. These results suggest clearly that convection or heat transfer can limit the swelling and shrinking kinetics of these gels. Unlike convection, the rate of heat transfer is not affected by the gel microstructure; it is only a function of gel thickness, assuming convective heat transfer in the pores is small compared to heat conduction through the sample. Thus the rate of heat transfer remains constant, independent of gel type, unlike the rate of convection that is controlled by the microstructure. Thus, the upper bound on the rate of volume change kinetics is given by the rate of heat transfer, largely independent of gel type.

This is demonstrated in Table 11.1. Convection time (200 s/cm²) is much smaller than heat transfer time (400 to 700 s/cm²), demonstrating that heat transfer plays a major role in determining the volume change kinetics of thermoresponsive microporous gels (although convection can have an influence in gels with microstructures different from those in this example). Since the rate of heat transfer is governed only by gel thickness (assuming a constant thermal diffusivity), the heat

TABLE 11.2
Synthesis and Properties of Microporous PNIPA Gels
with Unconnected Pores

Property	Result
Initial polymer concentration	1.0 M
Initial crosslinker concentration	1.0 mol%
Overall reaction time	24 h
Reaction temperature	22°C
Swelling time and shrinking time	Time to reach 98% of equilibrium
Response time	Time to reach 98% of uptake/square of initial thickness
Heat transfer time	Time taken for thermal equilibrium/square of initial thickness
Thermal diffusivity	$\alpha = 0.0010$ cm²/s

Process	Swelling Ratio at 22–50°C	Swelling or Shrinking Time (s)	Response Time (s/cm²)	Heat Transfer Time (s/cm²)
Swelling	12.5	$(2.9 \pm 0.1) \times 10^4$	$(3.2 \pm 0.1) \times 10^6$	400 ± 200
Shrinking	12.5	40 ± 5	1300 ± 200	600 ± 200

transfer time in the swelling process is always shorter than that in the shrinking process, as observed in Table 11.2. Thus all gels with interconnected pore structures and micron-scale dimensions are expected to display rapid volume changes in response to temperature stimuli, regardless of the specific microstructure. Very small pores will not allow significant convection and very thick walls will respond slowly. The fact that convection can occur so much faster than heat transfer indicates that the kinetics should be reasonably independent of microstructure if the pores remain interconnected throughout the swelling or shrinking processes.

The lower bound of volume change kinetics — that is, the slowest possible rate of volume change kinetics — is obtained when the rate of convection is zero. In cases of nonporous gels or gels with unconnected pores, the convection rate becomes zero and the characteristic lengths of heat transfer and diffusion become equal. The swelling and shrinking kinetics of such thermoresponsive gels are limited by the rate of diffusion of the polymer chains through the solvent (network motion) that is orders of magnitude slower than conductive heat transfer.

However, intermediate cases between the upper bound of heat transfer and the lower bound of network diffusion also exist. This has practical implications in that the kinetics can be adjusted over the entire range between these bounds to match the requirements of a given application. For example, the pores can be small enough that convection occurs more slowly than heat transfer, yet faster than network diffusion.

If the pores are only partially interconnected, convection will occur only through the interconnected channels. In some cases, the degree of interconnectivity may depend upon the swelling state of the gel: the pores may be blocked when shrunken and open when swollen. In such cases, the gel shrinks quickly in the beginning due to convective flow through interconnected pores. The shrinking rate then slows due to blockage of pores upon shrinking that may slow or even stop convection. If the pores become blocked, the characteristic diffusion path length effectively returns to that of a conventional nonporous gel, i.e., the half thickness of a gel sheet or the radius of a gel cylinder or sphere.

Kabra et al. synthesized microporous HPC gels possessing partially interconnected pores and demonstrated this hypothesis experimentally.[76,83] Similar results were obtained with PVME gels made by irradiating the polymer at a rate high enough to crosslink the polymer while heating the solution sufficiently to induce phase separation (another TIPS process).[49,60]

Other techniques have been developed to make fast responsive materials besides those reviewed in the section on preparation of microporous fast responsive gels. However, it is not uncommon for such techniques to create materials that significantly enhance shrinking rates but not swelling rates. This phenomenon has been observed with comb-type polymer networks, materials made by incorporation of silica particles into a PNIPA gel, γ-irradiation of PNIPA solutions, and freeze-drying and hydration for conventional PNIPA gels.[71,72,75]

As an illustration, Kato et al. studied the shrinking and swelling kinetics of a microporous PNIPA gel prepared by freeze-drying and hydration (FD) treatment.[81,82] Synthesis parameters and kinetic data are summarized in Table 11.2. Figure 11.7 clearly indicates that the rate of shrinking (10^{-4} cm^2/s) is much faster than that of swelling (10^{-7} cm^2/s), with swelling occurring at a rate comparable to that of the equivalent nonporous gel.

One of the important properties of the FD-treated PNIPA gel is a high swelling ratio (12.5) that is approximately seven times greater than that of the microporous HPC gel (1.7) cited in Table 11.1. This can be an important variable in applications.[79,80] Because the strut thickness of microporous the PNIPA gel prepared by the FD treatment was 0.1 to 2.0 μm, the network motion of the strut was much faster than the convective flow. When the gel was swollen at 22°C, the microporous gel was slightly translucent while the nonporous gel was transparent. However, this fast-shrinkable gel can expel only a small amount of water under mechanical pressure; the effective porosity is very low and most of its pores are unconnected.

SEM images also suggest that closed cells are generated during the freezing process. The possible explanation is that the pores connect in the beginning of shrinking process followed by the polymer aggregation due to the hydrophobic interaction. The pore water then can be squeezed out through the interconnected channels with a convective flow. Since the rate of heat transfer is much faster than the actual rate of volume decrease, the shrinking kinetics is probably limited by convection through temporarily formed interconnected channels. SEM images also suggest that the micropores disappear after shrinking. This is why the FD-treated gel swelled slowly and behaved like a nonporous gel in the swelling process.

RESPONSES TO CHANGES IN SALT CONCENTRATION

The previous section focused on thermoresponsive gels in which heat transfer was the triggering stimulus. However, gels can be triggered to undergo volume changes

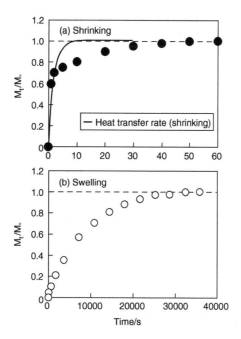

FIGURE 11.7 Weight change kinetics of microporous PNIPA gel prepared by freeze-drying and rehydration as cited in Table 11.2. (a) This gel has unconnected pores and its shrinking is rapid. (b) This gel swells slowly, similar to a nonporous gel. The swelling and shrinking kinetics were determined by temperature-jump between 22 and 60°C. The rates of heat transfer were calculated when the thermal diffusivity was $\alpha = 0.0010$ cm²/s.

upon changes in solution composition and temperature. Other variables in addition to temperature that affect solvent quality include salts and solvents. For example, HPC gels swell and shrink in response to changes in salt, solvent concentration, and temperature.[30] Ionizable gels are also strongly affected by pH.

Since ions and small molecules diffuse at much faster rates ($\sim 10^{-5}$ cm²/s) than polymer networks ($\sim 10^{-7}$ cm²/s), the rate-limiting step for a nonporous gel should be diffusion of the network from one equilibrium conformation to another. If a gel network is uniform down to a submicron scale, significant convection is unlikely to occur and the characteristic dimension for diffusive processes will be that of the entire sample (radius of a sphere or long cylinder; half thickness of a flat sheet). However, in microporous gels with characteristics comparable to the example in Table 11.1, it is possible that the rate of ion transport may be slower than convection, and thus become the rate-limiting step.

When an HPC gel is immersed in a solution of ammonium sulfate after equilibration in pure water, it shrinks due to alteration of hydrogen bonds between the polymer and water and enhancement of hydrophobic interactions between polymer chains.[52,90] The process is reversed upon reimmersion of the gel in water. Experimental data for these kinetic experiments can be fitted by diffusion curves with diffusion coefficients of magnitude 10^{-6} to 10^{-5} cm²/s. These values lie between the rate of convection and the rate of network motion, as noted in earlier sections. In contrast, the diffusion coefficient of ammonium sulfate is estimated from the ionic diffusion coefficients as 1.5×10^{-5} cm^2/s.[29] The diffusion coefficients of solutes inside gels can be estimated with the following relationship:

$$D = D_0 \left(\frac{1 - \phi_p}{1 + \phi_p} \right)^2 \qquad (11.6)$$

where ϕ_p is the polymer volume fraction; D and D_0, respectively, are diffusion coefficients in the gel and in the solution.[2,53,91] The values of ϕ_p for the shrunken state in 1.0 M ammonium sulfate and swollen state in distilled water are 0.26 and 0.11, respectively. Using Equation (11.6), the average diffusion coefficient of ammonium sulfate obtained is 7×10^{-6} cm^2/s. Since the value calculated accords with the experimental value (10^{-6} to 10^{-5} cm^2/s), the rate of salt transport appears to be the rate-limiting step.

When an HPC gel shrinks due to changes in salt concentration, the rate of swelling is observed to be much faster than that of shrinking.[30] This phenomenon can be explained by the effect of the convection on mass transfer. When the salt concentration increases at a given point inside the gel, that part of the gel shrinks, causing a convective flow of the solute from the gel to the outside solution. This convective flow of solution is in the direction opposite to the stimulus and therefore retards the rate of stimulus change. In contrast, convection moves in the same direction as the stimulus in the case of the swelling process. Thus, enhancement of mass transfer results and an increase of the swelling rate is observed.

In summary, the upper bound of volume change kinetics is the rate of ion transport and is a combination of diffusion and convective flow, the latter of which can accelerate or retard the process. The lower bound on the rate remains the network diffusion coefficient, as observed for a nonporous gel. Since the diffusion coefficients of even small ions are much smaller than liquid thermal diffusivities, the difference in these bounds is much smaller than for thermally responsive gels: a range of approximately 50 to 100 times.

RESPONSES TO CHANGES IN SOLVENT COMPOSITION

When a gel is immersed into a solvent with a different composition, its behavior (swelling or shrinking) depends upon whether the new environment is a better or poorer solvent for the polymer. HPC gels swell less in acetone than in water due to less favorable interactions between polymer and solvent.[30] Using microporous HPC gels with interconnected pores, the volume changes of gels were determined by transferring them between water and acetone. The results of this experiment are shown in Figure 11.8. In this case, the volume change of gels can be fitted to the diffusion curves with diffusion coefficients of magnitude 10^{-5} to 10^{-6} cm^2/s.

These values are approximately same as those for salt-induced volume changes and can be interpreted similarly. The relative rates of shrinking and swelling can be interpreted in terms of convective mass transfer. During swelling, convection of the swelling solvent into the gel enhances the swelling stimulus; during shrinking, the

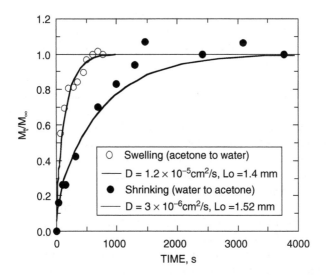

FIGURE 11.8 Normalized mass change kinetics of microporous HPC gel sample shown in Figure 11.3, induced by the indicated solvent changes between acetone and water. The kinetics are dominated by the rate of solvent change within the gel. (Reprinted with permission from Kabra, B.G. and Gehrke, S.H., in *Superabsorbent Polymers: Science and Technology*, Bucholz, F.L. and Peppas, N.A., Eds., ACS Symposium Series 573, American Chemical Society, Washington, D.C., 1994, p. 76. Copyright 1994 American Chemical Society.)

stimulus rate is retarded by the flow of solvent out of the gel. All these observations are consistent with the hypothesis that the rate of solvent transport is the rate-limiting step for the voume change, as noted for salt-induced volume changes.

RESPONSES TO CHANGES IN PH

Polymer chains of pH-sensitive gels usually have ionizable groups, such as carboxylic acid and basic aminoalkyl moieties. When these groups become ionized, a substantial osmotic swelling pressure is generated inside a gel, causing the swelling degree to increase. In general, the rate of actual volume change for nonporous gels is much slower than that of ionization of the polymer network as the rate-limiting step is the network motion rather than the ion exchange kinetics.[2]

The lower bound of volume change kinetics for pH-sensitive gels observed in nonporous gels is set by the rate of network motion. According to previous studies, it is expected that the ion exchange reaction at the ionic site is much faster than the rates of diffusion of ions through the boundary film and the gel.[28,92–94] Thus, the upper bound of volume change kinetics is generally governed by the rate of solute diffusion, similar to a salt-induced process.

DESIRED GEL MICROSTRUCTURE

A variety of protocols have been developed for creating microporous gels. As discussed earlier, interconnected micropores (open-cell structures) are key to the development of fast response swelling and shrinking of gels as they allow convective sorption and desorption of solvent. In contrast, if the pores are discrete so that the fluid phase of each pore is independent of all the other pores (closed-cell structure), convective flow cannot occur and the response kinetics is comparable to nonporous gels.

To a lesser extent, pore size and pore volume fraction also influence convection. The rate of convection and thus the gel response rate can be altered by changing the microstructure. However, above some threshold, the stimulus response becomes rate-limiting and further optimization of the microstructure to enhance convection has no further effect. Convection can have a modest impact on the kinetics in that convective sorption of a stimulus that causes swelling can increase the rate, while sorption of a stimulus that causes shrinking will reduce the rate. These situations can be modeled as moving boundary problems with combined diffusion and convection.

The fastest stimulus is thermal, as the thermal diffusivity in a hydrogel is about 10^{-3} cm^2/s, while diffusion coefficients of even small ions are only about 10^{-5} cm^2/s. Thus, microporosity has the most dramatic effect on temperature-responsive gels. Since the upper bound of the volume change kinetics for thermosensitive microporous gels is the rate of heat transfer, it is worthwhile to identify conditions under which the rate of the network motion in the pore walls becomes faster than the rate of heat transfer through a macroscopic sample under conditions in which convection is not rate-influencing.

The rate of network motion for microporous gels depends upon the network diffusion coefficient and the strut thickness, while the time required for heat transfer is set by the thermal diffusivity of the gel and the macroscopic gel thickness. For both processes, equilibration time scales with the square of the respective characteristic dimension. For the rate of network motion to be faster than the rate of heat transfer, the following equation should be satisfied for a microporous gel with an interconnected structure:

$$\frac{\alpha}{(Gel\ Thickness)^2} \leq \frac{D_p}{(Strut\ Thickness)^2} \qquad (11.7)$$

where D_p is the diffusion coefficient of the polymer network. Using a typical value of diffusion coefficient for rubbery gels ($D_p = 1 \times 10^{-7}$ cm^2/s) and a reasonable value of thermal diffusivity for a water-swollen gel ($\alpha = 1 \times 10^{-3}$ cm^2/s), the following relationship results:

$$\frac{(Strut\ Thickness)}{(Gel\ Thickness)} \leq 0.01 \qquad (11.8)$$

Hence the requirement for the condition under which the rate of network motion becomes faster than the rate of heat transfer is that the gel thickness should be more than 100 times greater than the strut thickness. Comparable relationships can be developed for other stimuli. In addition, the microstructure must have a high level of interconnectivity among the micropores and sufficient porosity to allow convective solvent transport into and out of the gel. In all types of gels, the upper bound on the kinetics is the rate at which the stimulus in question can permeate the gel.

SUMMARY

Microporous gels can be created by a variety of techniques that are fast responsive in comparison to conventional nonporous responsive gels. The response of conventional gels is limited by a network diffusion coefficient that is typically on the order of 10^{-7} cm^2/s. Since the characteristic dimension of nonporous gels is the macroscopic dimension, response times of samples of millimeter dimension can be on the order of hours — too slow for many applications.

Microporous, thermosensitive gels have the fastest response kinetics, over a thousand times greater than chemically similar nonporous gels. Such gels can have struts on the order of a micron in size, and thus can respond to stimuli in fractions of a second. Convection through the pores can occur much more quickly than stimulus transfer. Hence the rate of stimulus transfer can become the upper bound on response rates of microporous fast responsive gels. Since heat transfer occurs with a thermal diffusivity on the order of 10^{-3} cm^2/s while chemical stimuli occur with diffusivities on the order of 10^{-5} cm^2/s, thermally responsive gels can respond over a hundred times faster than microporous gels responding to chemical stimuli. In principle, gels responsive to magnetic or electrical fields could respond even more quickly, at the limit of convective transport, but this has yet to be demonstrated.

REFERENCES

1. Freitas, R.F.S. and Cussler, E.L., Temperature-sensitive gels as extraction solvents, *Chem. Eng. Sci.*, 42, 97, 1987.
2. Gehrke, S.H. and Cussler, E.L., Mass transfer in pH-sensitive hydrogels, *Chem. Eng. Sci.*, 44, 559, 1989.
3. Tanaka, T., Nishio, I., Sun, S., and Ueno-Nishio, S., Collapse of gels in an electric field, *Science*, 218, 467 1982.
4. Tanaka, T., Collapse of gels and the critical endpoint, *Phys. Rev. Lett.*, 40, 820, 1978.
5. Suzuki, A. and Tanaka, T., Phase transition in polymer gels induced by visible light, *Nature*, 346, 345, 1990.
6. Mamada, A., Tanaka, T., Kungwatchakun, D., and Irie, M., Photoinduced phase transition of gels, *Macromolecules*, 23, 1517, 1990.
7. Lee, K.K., Cussler, E.L., Marchetti, M., and McHugh, M.A., Pressure-dependent phase transitions in hydrogels, *Chem. Eng. Sci.*, 45, 766, 1990.
8. Ohmine, I. and Tanaka, T., Salt effects on the phase transition of ionic gels, *J. Chem. Phys.*, 77, 5725, 1982.
9. Huang, X., Ueno, H., Akehata, T., and Hirasa, O., Effects of salt solution on swelling or shrinking behavior of poly(vinylmethylether) gel (PVMEG), *J. Chem. Eng. Jpn.*, 21, 10, 1988.
10. Kato, N., Takizawa, Y., and Takahashi, F., Magnetically driven chemomechanical device with poly(N-isopropylacrylamide) hydrogel containing γ-Fe$_2$O$_3$, *J. Intell. Mater. Syst. Struct.*, 8, 588, 1997.

11. Gehrke, S.H., Synthesis, equilibrium swelling, kinetics, permeability and applications of environmentally responsive gels, *Adv. Polym. Sci.*, 110, 81, 1993.

12. Beltran, S., Hooper, H.H., Blanch, H.W., and Prausnitz, J.M., Swelling equilibria for ionized temperature-sensitive gels in water and in aqueous salt solutions, *J. Chem. Phys.*, 92, 2061, 1990.

13. Bae, Y.H., Okano, T., and Kim, S.W., Temperature dependence of swelling of crosslinked poly(*N*,*N'*-alkyl substituted acrylamides) in water, *J. Polym. Sci., Polym. Phys. Ed.*, 28, 923, 1990.

14. Ilavsky, M., Effect of electrostatic interaction on phase transition in the swollen polymeric network, *Polymer*, 22, 1687, 1981.

15. Osada, Y. and Umezawa, K., Electric responses of chemomechanical systems, *Biomedica*, 2, 75, 1987.

16. Gehrke, S.H., Andrews, G.P., and Cussler, E.L., Chemical aspects of gel extraction, *Chem. Eng. Sci.*, 41, 2153, 1986.

17. Hoffman, A.S., Affrassiabi, A., and Dong, L.C., Thermally reversible hydrogels. II. Delivery and selective removal of substances from aqueous solutions, *J. Controlled Release*, 4, 213, 1986.

18. Gehrke, S.H., Lyu, L.H., and Barnthouse, K., Dewatering fine coal slurries by gel extraction, *Sep. Sci. Technol.*, 33, 1467, 1998.

19. Kato, N., Oishi, A., and Takahashi, F., Enzyme reaction controlled by magnetic heating due to the hysteresis loss of γ-Fe_2O_3 in thermosensitive polymer gels immobilized by β-galactosidase, *Mater. Sci. Eng. C*, 6, 291, 1998.

20. Kato, N., Samejima, S., and Takahashi, F., Isomaltose synthesis in the reversed hydrolysis catalyzed by amyloglucosidase immobilized in the thermosensitive gel, *Mater. Sci. Eng. C*, 17, 155, 2001.

21. Gehrke, S.H. and Lee, P.I., Hydrogels for drug delivery, in *Specialized Drug Delivery Systems: Manufacturing and Production Technology*, Tyle, P., Ed., Marcel Dekker, New York, 1990, p. 333.

22. Gehrke, S.H., Synthesis and properties of hydrogels used for drug delivery, in *Transport Processes in Pharmaceutical Sciences*, Amidon, G.L., Lee, P.I., and Topp, E.M., Eds., Marcel Dekker, New York, 2000, p. 473.

23. Peppas, N.A. and Barr-Howell, B.D., Characterization of the crosslinked structure of hydrogels, in *Hydrogels in Medicine and Pharmacy, Vol. I, Fundamentals*, Peppas, N.A., Ed., CRC Press, Boca Raton, FL, 1987, p. 27.

24. Feil, H., Bae, Y.H., Feijin, J., and Kim, S.W., Molecular separation by thermosensitive hydrogel membranes, *J. Membr. Sci.*, 64, 283, 1991.

25. Bae, Y.H., Okano, T., and Kim, S.W., "On-off" thermocontrol of solute transport. II. Solute release from thermosensitive hydrogels, *Pharmaceutical Res.*, 8, 624, 1991.

26. Gehrke, S.H., Palasis, M., Lund, M., and Fisher, J., Factors determining hydrogel permeability, *Ann. NY Acad. Sci.*, 831, 179, 1997.

27. Oliveira, E.D., Hirsch, S.G., Spontak, R.J., and Gehrke, S.H., Influence of polymer conformation on the shear modulus and morphology of polyallylamine and poly(α,L-lysine) hydrogels, *Macromolecules*, 36, 6189, 2003.

28. Gehrke, S.H., Agrawal, G., and Yang, M.C., Moving ion exchange fronts in polyelectrolyte gels, in *Polyelectrolyte Gels*, Harland, R.S. and Prud'homme, R.K., Eds., ACS Symp. Series 480, American Chemical Society, Washington, D.C., 1992, p. 211.

29. Cussler, E.L., *Diffusion: Mass Transfer in Fluid Systems*, Cambridge University Press, Cambridge, 1984.

30. Kabra, B.G. and Gehrke, S.H., Rate-limiting steps for solvent sorption and desorption by microporous stimuli-sensitive absorbent gels, in *Superabsorbent Polymers: Science and Technology*, Buchholz, F.L. and Peppas, N.A., Eds., ACS Symp. Series 573, American Chemical Society, Washington, D.C., 1994, p. 76.

31. Huang, X., Unno, H., Akehata, T., and Hirasa, O., Analysis of kinetic behavior of temperature-sensitive water-absorbing hydrogels, *J. Chem. Eng. Jpn.*, 20, 123, 1987.

32. Gehrke, S.H., Lyu, L.H., and Yang, M.C., Swelling, shrinking, and solute permeation of temperature-sensitive *N*-isopropylacrylamide gel, *Polym. Prep.*, 30, 482, 1989.

33. Peppas, N.A. and Korsmeyer, R.W., Dynamically swelling hydrogels in controlled release applications, in *Hydrogels in Medicine and Pharmacy, Vol. III, Properties and Applications*, Peppas, N.A., Ed., CRC Press, Boca Raton, FL, 1987, p. 109.

34. Frisch, H.L., Sorption and transport in glassy polymers, *Polym. Eng. Sci.*, 20, 2, 1980.

35. Windle, A.H., Case II sorption, in *Polymer Permeability*, Comyn, J., Ed., Elsevier Applied Science, London, 1985, p. 75.

36. Lee, P.I., Dimensional changes during drug release from a glassy hydrogel matrix, *Polym. Commun.*, 24, 45, 1983.

37. Vrentas, J.S., Jarzebski, C.M., and Duda, J.L., Deborah number for diffusion in polymer–solvent systems, *AIChE J.*, 21, 894, 1975.

38. Davidson, G.W.R., III and Peppas, N.A., Solute and penetrant diffusion in swellable polymers. V. Relaxation-controlled transport in P(HEMA-co-MMA) copolymers, *J. Controlled Release*, 3, 243, 1986.

39. Davidson, G.W.R., III and Peppas, N.A., Solute and penetrant diffusion in swellable polymers. VI. Deborah and swelling interface numbers as indicators of the order of biomolecule release, *J. Controlled Release*, 3, 259, 1986.

40. Thomas, N.L. and Windle, A.H., A theory of case II diffusion, *Polymer*, 23, 529, 1982.

41. Gall, T.P., Lasky, R.C., and Kramer, E.J., Case II diffusion: effect of solvent molecule size, *Polymer*, 31, 1491, 1990.

42. Wu, J.C. and Peppas, N.A., Modeling of penetrant diffusion in glassy polymers with an integral sorption Deborah number, *J. Polym. Sci. Polym. Phys. Ed.*, 31, 1503, 1993.

43. Samus, M.A. and Rossi, G., Methanol absorption in ethylene-vinyl alcohol copolymers: relation between solvent diffusion and changes in glass transition temperature in glassy polymeric materials, *Macromolecules*, 29, 2275, 1996.

44. Kabra, B.G., Gehrke, S.H., Hwang, S.T., and Ritschel, W.A., Modification of the dynamic swelling behavior of PHEMA, *J. Appl. Polym. Sci.*, 42, 2409, 1991.

45. Biren, D., Kabra, B.G., and Gehrke, S.H., Effect of initial sample anisotropy on the solvent sorption kinetics of poly(vinylmethylether) gel, *Polymer*, 33, 554, 1992.

46. Gehrke, S.H., Biren, D., and Hopkins, J.J., Evidence for Fickian water transport in initially glassy poly(2-hydroxyethyl methacrylate), *J. Biomater. Sci. Polym. Ed.*, 6, 375, 1994.

47. Ritger, P.L. and Peppas, N.A., A simple equation for description of solute release. 1. Fickian and non-Fickian release from non-swellable devices in the form of slabs, *J. Controlled Release*, 5, 23, 1987.

48. Crank, J., *Mathematics of Diffusion*, 2nd ed., Oxford University Press, London, 1975.

49. Kabra, B.G., Akhtar, M.K., and Gehrke, S.H., Volume change kinetics of temperature-sensitive poly(vinylmethylether) gel, *Polymer*, 33, 990, 1992.

50. Tanaka, T., Hocker, L.O., and Benedek, G.B., Spectrum of light scattered from a viscoelastic gel, *J. Chem. Phys.*, 59, 5151, 1973.

51. Tanaka, T. and Fillmore, D.J., Kinetics of swelling of gels, *J. Chem. Phys.*, 70, 1214, 1979.

52. Palasis, M. and Gehrke, S.H., Permeability of responsive poly(*N*-isopropylacrylamide) gel to solutes, *J. Controlled Release*, 18, 1, 1992.
53. Crank, J. and Park, G.S., *Diffusion in Polymers*, Academic Press, London, 1968.
54. Aubert, J.H., Isotactic polystyrene phase diagrams and physical gelation, *Macromolecules*, 21, 3468, 1988.
55. Mikos, A.G., Whiteman, A.M., Thorsen, A.J., Stein, J.E., Ingber, D., Vacanti, J.P., and Langer, R., Creep behavior of poly(lactic-co-glycolic acid) foams for liver regeneration, Paper 3f presented at AIChE Annual Meeting, Los Angeles, November 1991.
56. Williams, J.M. and Wrobleski, D.A., Spatial distribution of the phases in water-in-oil emulsions: open and closed microcellular foams from crosslinked polystyrene, *Langmuir*, 4, 656, 1988.
57. Williams, J.M., Toroidal microstructures from water-in-oil emulsions, *Langmuir*, 4, 44, 1988.
58. Hainey, P., Huxham, I.M., Rowatt, B., Sherrington, D.C., and Tetley, L., Synthesis and ultrastructural studies of styrene-divinylbenzene polyhipe polymers, *Macromolecules*, 24, 117, 1991.
59. Hyon, S., Che, W., and Ikada, Y., Preparation of poly(vinyl alcohol) hydrogels by low temperature crystallization of the aqueous poly(vinyl alcohol) solution, *Kobunshi Ronbunshu*, 46, 673, 1989.
60. Suzuki, M. and Hirasa, O., An approach to artificial muscle using polymer gels formed by micro-phase separation, *Adv. Polym. Sci.,* 110, 241, 1993.
61. Kesting, R.E., *Synthetic Polymeric Membranes: A Structural Perspective*, John Wiley & Sons, New York, 1985.
62. Castro, A., Methods for Making Microporous Products, U.S. Patent, 4,247,498, 1981.
63. Young, A.T., Moreno, D.K., and Marsters, R.G., Preparation of multishell ICF target plastic foam cushion materials by thermally induced phase separation processes, *J. Vac. Sci. Technol.*, 20, 1094, 1982.
64. Hirokawa, Y. and Tanaka, T., Volume phase transition in nonionic gels, *J. Chem. Phys.*, 81, 6379, 1984.
65. Hirotsu, S., Hirokawa, Y., and Tanaka, T., Volume-phase transitions of ionized *N*-isopropylacrylamide gels, *J. Chem. Phys.*, 87, 1392, 1987.
66. Davidson, R.L., *Handbook of Water-Soluble Gums and Resins*, McGraw Hill, New York, 1980.
67. Doelker, E., Water-swollen cellulose derivatives in pharmacy, in *Hydrogels in Medicine and Pharmacy,* Vol. II, Peppas, N.A., Ed., CRC Press, Boca Raton, FL, 1987, p. 115.
68. Doelker, E., Swelling behavior of water-soluble cellulose derivatives, in *Absorbent Polymer Technology*, Brannon-Peppas, L. and Harland, R.S., Eds., Elsevier, New York, 1990, p. 125.
69. Harsh, D.C. and Gehrke, S.H., Controlling the swelling characteristics of temperature-sensitive cellulose ether hydrogels, *J. Controlled Release*, 17, 175, 1991.
70. O'Connor, S.M. and Gehrke, S.H., Synthesis and characterization of temperature-sensitive HPMC gel spheres, *J. Appl. Polym. Sci.*, 66, 1279, 1997.
71. Kishi, R., Hirasa, O., and Ichijo, H., Fast-responsive poly(*N*-isopropylacrylamide) hydrogels prepared by γ-ray irradiation, *Polym. Gels Networks*, 5, 145, 1997.
72. Yoshida, R., Katsumi, U., Kaneko, Y., Sakai, K., Kikuchi, A., Sakurai, Y., and Okano, T., Comb-type grafted hydrogels with rapid de-swelling response to temperature changes, *Nature*, 374, 240, 1995.

73. Wu, X.S., Hoffman, A.S., and Yager, P.J., Synthesis and characterization of thermally reversible microporous poly(N-isopropylacrylamide) hydrogels, *J. Polym. Sci. Polym. Chem. Ed.*, 30, 2121, 1992.

74. Huang, X., Unno, H., Akehata, T., and Hirasa, O., Swelling pressure of poly(vinyl methyl ether) gel (PVMEG) in swelling process, *J. Chem. Eng. Jpn.*, 21, 651, 1988.

75. Serizawa, T., Wakita, K., and Akashi, M., Rapid deswelling of porous poly(N-isopropylacrylamide) hydrogels prepared by incorporation of silica particles, *Macromolecules*, 35, 10, 2002.

76. Kabra, B.G., Gehrke, S.H., and Spontak, R.J., Microporous responsive HPC gels. 1. Synthesis and microstructure, *Macromolecules*, 31, 2166, 1998.

77. Kabra, B.G. and Gehrke, S.H., Synthesis of fast response, temperature-sensitive poly(N-isopropylacrylamide) gel, *Polym. Commun.*, 32, 322, 1991.

78. Kabra, B.G. and Gehrke, S.H., Microporous Fast Response Gels and Methods of Use, U.S. Patent 6,030,442, 2000.

79. Kabra, B.G. and Gehrke, S.H., Superabsorbent Foams and Methods for Producing Same, U.S. Patent 5,573,994, 1996.

80. Kabra, B.G. and Gehrke, S.H., Superabsorbent Foams and Methods for Producing Same, U.S. Patent 6,027,795, 2000.

81. Kato, N. and Takahashi, F., Acceleration of deswelling of poly(N-isopropylacrylamide) hydrogel by the treatment of a freeze-dry and hydration process, *Bull. Chem. Soc. Jpn.*, 70, 1289, 1997.

82. Kato, N., Sakai, Y., and Shibata, S., Wide-range control of deswelling time for thermosensitive poly(N-isopropylacrylamide) gel treated by freeze-drying, *Macromolecules*, 36, 961, 2003.

83. Kabra, B.G., Synthesis, Structure and Swelling of Microporous Gels, Ph.D. thesis, University of Cincinnati, Cincinnati, OH, 1993.

84. Pronoy, P.K. and Nguyen, H.V., Mechanism of liquid flow and structure property relations, in *Absorbency*, Pronoy, P.K., Ed., Elsevier, Amsterdam, 1985, p. 29.

85. Ruoff, A.L., Prince, J.C., Giddings, J.C., and Stewart, G.H., The diffusion analogy for solvent flow in paper, *Kolloid Zeitschr.*, 166, 144, 1959.

86. Ruoff, A.L., Stewart, G.H., Shin, H.K., and Giddings, J.C., Diffusion of liquid in unsaturated paper, *Kolloid Zeitschr.*, 173, 14, 1960.

87. Cassidy, H.G., Investigation of paper chromatography, *Anal. Chem.*, 24, 1415, 1952.

88. Fujita, H., On the distribution of liquid ascending in a filter paper, *J. Chem. Phys.*, 56, 625, 1952.

89. Muller, R.H. and Clegg, D.L., Paper chromatography instruments and techniques, *Anal. Chem.*, 23, 396, 1951.

90. Wood, S.E. and Strain, H.E., Flow and distribution of solutions in filter paper, *Anal. Chem.*, 26, 260, 1954.

91. Denton, M.J., The capillary absorption of liquids in paper and other porous materials, *J. Chromatog.*, 18, 615, 1965.

92. Lightfoot, E.J., Kinetic diffusion in polymer gels, *Physica A*, 169, 191, 1990.

93. Rossi, G. and Mazich, K.A., Kinetics of swelling for a cross-linked elastomer or gel in the presence of a good solvent, *Phys. Rev. A*, 44, 4793, 1991.

94. Helfferich, F., Ion-exchange kinetics. V. Ion exchange accompanied by reactions, *J. Phys. Chem.*, 69, 1178, 1965.

Section III

Synthetic Systems

12 Fast Shrinkable Materials

Mitsuhiro Ebara, Akihiko Kikuchi, Kiyotaka Sakai, and Teruo Okano

CONTENTS

INTRODUCTION

Complicated mechanisms of biological activities of peptides and proteins play key roles in many specific physiological and pathological processes in the living body, maintaining homeostasis or producing disease. These interactions and their alterations are of intense general interest in designing therapeutic surrogates.

Biologically active therapeutic peptides have recently been produced through genetic engineering techniques. For these potent drugs, novel and effective administration methods must be developed and improved. Progress in this area has been recently reviewed.[1-3] Since drugs typically act through multidimensional time and space interactions with sites in the body, we must consider adverse physiological side effects that consistently appear independently of targeting sites. This is particularly a concern for drugs with high toxicity or bioactive peptides administered systematically.

Drug delivery systems (DDSs) are technological devices developed to maintain effective drug concentrations in blood over long periods.[4–7] Furthermore, DDSs continuously evolve by incorporating advanced technologies, allowing drugs to act increasingly at targeting sites or making them available when required temporally and locally depending on disease state.

Recent developments of improved polymeric biomaterials have greatly contributed to drug delivery,[1–7] tissue engineering,[8–12] bioseparation technologies,[13–16] and actuators.[17–19] Intelligent materials that change their structures and functions in response to external stimuli have attracted recent attention.[20–22] In fact, temporal control of drug release and surface property control for bioactive molecules and cell interactions have been reported using stimuli-responsive polymers responding to external stimuli including temperature,[3,8–16,20–22] pH,[23–25] chemicals[26–28] and electric fields.[29–31] Stimuli-responsive hydrogels have continued to attract attention due to their varieties of tailored properties including sorption capacities,[32] mechanical properties,[33,34] permeabilities,[35] surface properties,[36] and shape memory properties.[37,38]

This chapter focuses on fast shrinkable hydrogels that respond to external stimuli from the viewpoints of their preparation methods and applications. Special attention has been paid to the effects of hydrogel structural design properties including (1) heterogeneous structure formation, (2) surface skin formation, (3) graft architectural effects, and (4) introduction of newly synthesized functional monomers to stimuli-responsive hydrogels on fast hydrogel shrinking properties.

FAST SHRINKING GELS WITH POROUS OR HETEROGENEOUS BULK STRUCTURES

Rapidly shrinkable hydrogels benefit from converting external stimuli into mechanical or physical property changes that then prompt drug release and smart actuators. However, the kinetics of a given hydrogel's bulk and volume changes is critical to their applications and utility. As gel swelling and shrinking kinetics are typically governed by diffusion-limited polymer network transport in water, the inverse of the rate of gel swelling and shrinking is proportional to the square of the gel dimension.[39]

To increase the responses of gel dynamics, several strategies have been explored. Due to the intrinsic diffusion dependence, reducing gel size is one technique known to achieve rapid kinetics. Other techniques include making a gel heterogeneous by producing a microporous gel structure to increase the contact surface area of polymer and solvent.

Hirasa et al.[40] proposed γ-ray radiation-crosslinked poly(vinylmethylether) (PVME) gels as fast shrinkable hydrogels. PVME gels showed opaque spongy-like structures with a lower critical solution temperature (LCST) of 38°C. Shrinking rates of hydrogels in response to temperature changes were 1000 times faster than the widely studied responsive homogeneous hydrogels (Figure 12.1a). The structures of the PVME gels were determined to be heterogeneous and microporous, quite different from the homogeneous structures of conventionally responsive hydrogels. They also prepared poly(N-isopropylacrylamide) (PIPAAm) gels with microporous structures using the γ-ray irradiated crosslinking method (Figure 12.1b).

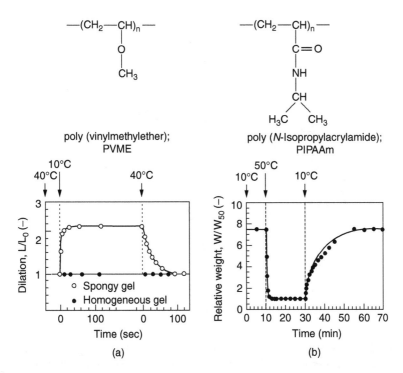

FIGURE 12.1 Reversible volume changes of PVME (a) and PIPAAm gels (b) between two different temperatures across the LCST. L = gel length at time t, L_0 = gel length at initial state, W = gel weight at time t, W_{50} = gel weight at 50°C. Dimension of cubic PIPAAm gel = 1.86 cm per side at 10°C.

The γ-ray irradiation of IPAAm monomer aqueous solutions induced heterogeneous polymerization, resulting in the formation of opaque PIPAAm gels that demonstrated rapid and reversible volume changes with temperature.[41] Kabra and Gehrke[42] designed a microporous PIPAAm gel by increasing solution temperature above the LCST (i.e., 32°C) of PIPAAm during the polymerization reaction in an aqueous milieu. The obtained hydrogels also shrank 3000 times faster than comparable homogeneous PIPAAm gels (Figure 12.2).

Zhang and Zhuo[43] designed a pore structure into PIPAAm gels by using oligo(ethylene glycol) (OEG) with a molecular weight of 400 as a pore-forming agent during the polymerization reaction in water. These gels had significantly larger swelling ratios at 26°C (i.e., below LCST) and exhibited dramatically faster response rates to temperature increases above LCST, releasing 95% of entrapped water in 3 min and over 98% in 8 min. Hoffman et al.[44] designed macroporous structures into PIPAAm hydrogels having large pore volumes. The macroporous gels were synthesized in aqueous solution at 50°C in the presence or absence of another temperature-sensitive polymer, hydroxypropyl cellulose (HPC; LCST, 42°C) as a pore-forming agent. During the polymerization reaction, polymerized PIPAAm

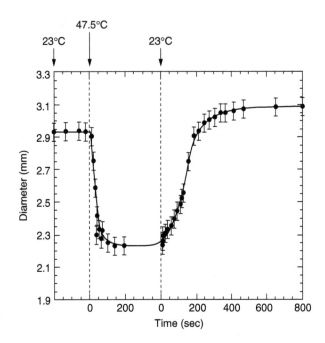

FIGURE 12.2 Swelling/shrinking cycles of phase-separated PIPAAm gel across a volume phase transition temperature of 33°C. The ratio of cylindrical gel length to diameter is 6.9 ± 0.2. (From Kabra, B.G. and Gehrke, S.H., *Polym. Commun.*, 32, 322–323, 1991. With permission.)

chains started to aggregate and the reaction solution became heterogeneous, so that the hydrogel (NV-50) was opaque and showed a heterogeneous structure. Incorporation of temperature-sensitive HPC formed microaggregates dispersed in a monomer solution and polymerized PIPAAm preferentially associated to the surfaces of HPC aggregates. Thus, after removal of HPC, a hydrogel with a macroporous structure (NHV-50) was obtained.

The NHV-50 and NV-50 macroporous gels showed faster deswelling kinetics than conventional N-22 hydrogels upon a temperature increase from room temperature to 50°C (Figure 12.3) because both hydrogels had similar macropore distributions. Permeabilities of both hydrogels to fluorescein isothiocyanate (FITC)–dextran were also similar, while the conventional N-22 PIPAAm gel showed much lower permeability.

Kato and Takahashi[45] accelerated the deswelling ratio of a PIPAAm gel using a freeze-drying and hydration process (Figure 12.4). This treatment resulted in a heterogeneous and porous structure inside the gel by condensing the polymer chains into porous networks. The deswelling rate of the gel prepared by this method was roughly 100 times faster than those of gels not subjected to freeze-drying. These technical methods focusing on reducing gel sizes or introducing micro- or macroporosity for fast responsive gels attempted to accelerate the diffusion processes of polymer networks through increases in their relative surface areas.

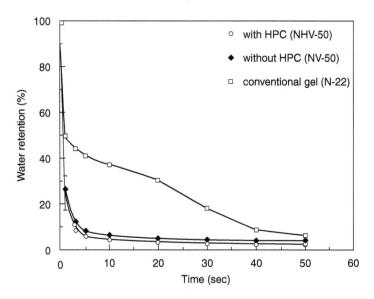

FIGURE 12.3 Deswelling kinetics of macroporous PIPAAm gel prepared in the presence or absence of HPC compared with conventional gel. Gel dimensions = 20 mm diameter, 2 mm thickness. (From Wu, X.S., Hoffman, A.S., and Yager, P., *J. Polym. Sci. A Polym. Chem.*, 30, 2121–2129, 1992. With permission.)

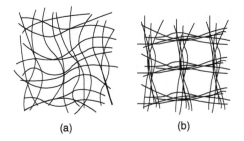

FIGURE 12.4 Polymer networks. (a) Conventional gel. (b) Freeze-dry-treated gel.

FAST ON–OFF GEL SWITCHING MECHANISMS AND APPLICATIONS TO DRUG PERMEATION CONTROL

The next three sections discuss several approaches for achieving fast shrinking hydrogel kinetics. Rapid swelling and deswelling changes of the outermost surface layers used to control rapid on–off regulation of drug permeation in response to stepwise temperature changes of gels will also be discussed.

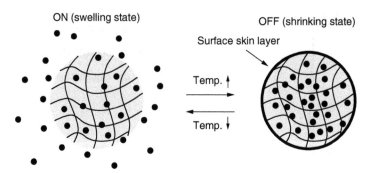

FIGURE 12.5 On–off switching mechanism of drug permeation in response to temperature changes.

Temperature-Responsive Hydrogels

In designing a pulsatile release device, it is desirable to modulate the release rates to release an effective amount of drug during the swollen on state and produce no significant release during the collapsed off state of the gel. Our research group achieved complete and rapid on–off regulation of drug permeation in response to stepwise temperature changes by using temperature-responsive hydrogels comprised of PIPAAm (Figure 12.5).[46–49] A dense gel surface layer (skin layer) was established immediately after a temperature increase above the hydrogel's collapse temperature.[46]

A possible explanation for this skin layer formation is that at a temperature above its collapse point, the outermost gel layer interacts with its environment and then dehydrates quickly, forming a dense surface layer within seconds. The formed skin layer was dense enough to stop or retard the flux of water inside the gel to the outside of the gel.

Gel surface skin layer formation can be controlled by changing the gel polymer chemistry, namely the lengths of alkyl side chains on comonomers used during copolymerization.[47] In Figure 12.6a, remarkable differences are observed in the initial shrinking processes of three types of PIPAAm-derived gels copolymerized with alkyl methacrylate comonomers, butyl methacrylate (BMA), hexyl methacrylate (HMA), and lauryl methacrylate (LMA) after a temperature increase from 20 to 30°C. P(IPAAm-co-HMA) and P(IPAAm-co-LMA) gels, both with longer alkyl side chains, shrunk to 20 to 30% of their original volumes observed at 20°C, while P(IPAAm-co-BMA) gels shrunk up to 80 to 90% in equilibrated conditions. This result indicates that rapid formation of a thin and dense skin layer can be regulated by selecting alkyl side chain lengths. With longer alkyl side chains, denser skin layers were formed, preventing water efflux.

Figure 12.6b shows drug permeation through copolymer gel membranes using two-chamber cells.[48] Two-chamber cells were separated with thermoresponsive copolymer gel membranes, with one side containing indomethacin solution and the other a blank solution. Amounts of drug permeating through the gel membrane were monitored by ultraviolet (UV) absorption. Below the gel transition temperature (20°C), the drug permeated through IPAAm copolymer gel membranes. However,

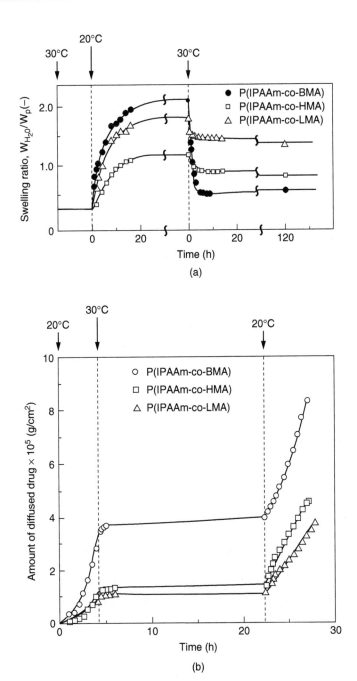

FIGURE 12.6 (a) Swelling/deswelling kinetics of P(IPAAm-co-alkyl methacrylate) gels (alkyl methacrylate = 5 wt%). W_{H_2O} = weight of water, W_P = weight of polymer. (b) diffused amount of indomethacin through P(IPAAm-co-alkyl methacrylate) gels (alkyl methacrylate = 3.7 wt%) in response to stepwise temperature changes between 20 and 30°C. Gel dimensions = 15 mm diameter, 0.5 mm thickness.

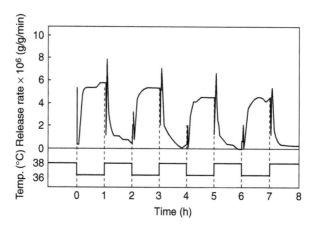

FIGURE 12.7 Release rate of indomethacin from P(IPAAm-co-DMAAm-co-BMA) gel (20 wt% DMAAm, 5 wt% BMA in feed) in response to stepwise temperature changes between 36 and 38°C in PBS. Gel dimensions = 15 mm diameter, 0.5 mm thickness.

just after temperature increases to 30°C (above the transition temperature), the skin layers formed on the gel surfaces immediately blocked further permeation or leakage of drug from the gel interior. By lowering temperature below the gel's transition temperature again, dehydrated shrunken surface layers recovered their equilibrium swelling state, allowing drug permeation. Hydrogels such as P(IPAAm-co-HMA) and P(IPAAm-co-LMA) forming thin and dense surface skin layers exhibited rapid changes in on–off drug release control and maintained constant release rates.

Analogous on–off drug release control over a narrow temperature range near human body temperature (37°C) was also demonstrated.[49] Both hydrophilic *N,N*-dimethylacrylamide (DMAAm) and hydrophobic BMA were incorporated into IPAAm copolymer hydrogels, producing an LCST near 37°C while maintaining high thermosensitivity. Upon temperature increase, the drug release rate increased in a pulsatile fashion, then rapidly decreased to completely stop drug release. The rapid increase in release rate was attributed to squeezing effects of drug molecules resulting from shrinking of the gel surface region. Thus, by using P(IPAAm-co-DMAAm-co-BMA) gels, on–off drug release in response to smaller temperature changes between 36 and 38°C was achieved in phosphate buffered saline (PBS; pH, 7.4) as demonstrated in Figure 12.7. From these results related to gel skin formation processes, it is apparent that the structures of hydrogel skin layers may be controlled by chemical composition and by the molecular structures of the gels.

HYDROGEL RESPONSES TO CHEMICAL CHANGES

Brazel and Peppas[50] reported that pulsatile drug releasing hydrogels created both pH- and temperature-triggered devices for coronary thrombosis-induced heart attack and stroke patients. Thrombolytic and antithrombotic agents such as heparin and streptokinase have minute-order half-lives in circulation and are only required when a blood clot forms and specifically only at the site of the clot. To produce a therapeutic device with responsive hydrogels, they synthesized P(IPAAm-co-methacrylic acid)

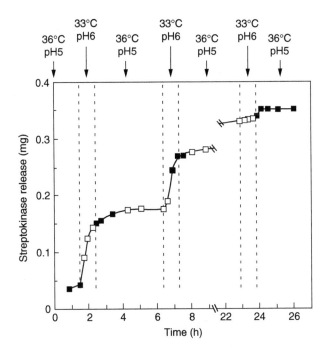

FIGURE 12.8 Streptokinase release from P(IPAAm-co-MAA) gel (IPAAm, 84mol%) upon changes in temperature from 36 to 33°C and pH from 5 to 6 for 1 h, then back to 36°C and pH 5 for a longer interval. Gel dimensions = 14 mm diameter, 0.8 mm thickness in dry state. (From Brazel, C.S. and Peppas, N.A., *J. Control. Rel.*, 39, 57–64, 1996. With permission.)

(MAA) gels and investigated release profiles of biologically active agents as functions of pulsatile pH and temperature (Figure 12.8).

Streptokinase release was seen only when the gels were exposed to low temperature below the LCST and pH value above the pK_a (where K_a is apparent dissociation constant), i.e., gels were swollen due to hydration and electrostatic repulsion between dissociated carboxylate anions. Drug release was observed to immediately decrease and completely stop after simultaneously decreasing pH and increasing temperature. After changes in both pH and temperature, the gel networks began to collapse. Their mesh sizes, representative of the space available for drug diffusion, dropped rapidly from approximately 12.5 to less than 10 nm, making it difficult for streptokinase (approximately 5.5 nm in molecular diameter) to diffuse through the collapsing pores. Heparin release from the gels, however, was not controlled because the mesh sizes of gels were too large to control heparin diffusion (approximately 3 nm in molecular diameter), even in the collapsed gel state.

Another example of on–off drug release control was achieved by using sugar-responsive gels for possible treatment of diabetes mellitus. Pancreatic islets release insulin to lower blood glucose level, and regulate glucose levels ranging from 70 to 110 mg/dl by an autofeedback mechanism in healthy physiological conditions. It is necessary to externally administer exogenous insulin for patients with Type I insulin-dependent diabetes mellitus who cannot control blood glucose levels. However,

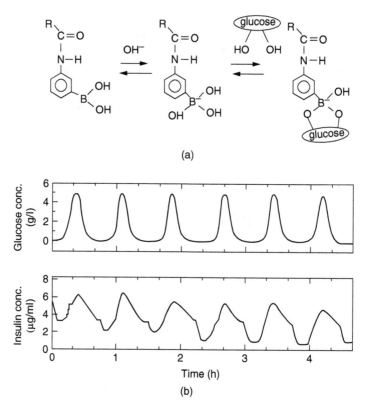

(a)

(b)

FIGURE 12.9 (a) (Alkylamido)phenylboronic acid. (b) Repeated on–off release of FITC-insulin from NB gel at 28°C, pH 9.0, in response to external glucose concentration. Gel dimension =1.0 mm thickness.

overdoses may result in hypoglycemia and coma, which are life-threatening states. Therefore, insulin must be carefully administered to prevent hypoglycemia in these patients.

In order to maintain physiological glucose levels, artificial systems that sense glucose levels and release appropriate amounts of insulin have been investigated.[1,25–28,51] Kataoka et al.[26] designed glucose-responsive NB gels composed of N-isopropylacrylamide derivatized with phenylboronic acid groups as the glucose-sensing moieties. Significantly, phenylboronic acid groups in aqueous solutions are equilibrated between undissociated and dissociated forms as shown in Figure 12.9a. Such equilibrium is shifted in the direction of increasingly charged phenylboronates through complexation with glucose because only charged boronates make stable complexes with cis-diols such as glucose in aqueous conditions.

NB gels have volume transition temperatures that shift with glucose concentrations. Interestingly, NB gels are in collapsed states below 100 mg/dL glucose and in swollen state above 300 mg/dL glucose at 28°C and pH 9. Such glucose concentration ranges correspond to the normal glucose levels in human bodies. Kataoka et al.[26] also performed glucose-responsive insulin release using NB gels. Figure 12.9b shows results of repeated on–off release of insulin from NB gels during repetitive external glucose concentration changes. Rapid release of insulin from the gel at high glucose concentration was effectively shut off by decreasing glucose concentration below the critical value. This on–off regulation of insulin release was achieved through a drastic and rapid change in the gel's solute transport property as a result of formation and disruption of its surface skin layer. Insulin release control was successfully repeated in a synchronized pattern with external glucose concentration changes.

TEMPERATURE-RESPONSIVE MICROCAPSULES AND LIPOSOMES

Okahata et al.[52] prepared large, porous, and ultrathin nylon capsules (diameter, 2.5 mm; membrane thickness 5 μm) with surface-grafted PIPAAm. Grafted PIPAAm molecules were proposed to act as permeation valves in response to temperature changes. Below the LCST of grafted PIPAAm on membrane surfaces (35°C), naphthalene-disulfonate was smoothly released through the porous capsule membrane. Above the LCST, however, the permeability was decreased 12 to 15 times relative to that below LCST because grafted PIPAAm chains dehydrated and covered the porous capsule membranes and closed pores. This thermosensitive permeation was reversibly observed.

Iwata et al.[53] prepared temperature-sensitive poly(vinylidene fluoride) (PVDF) porous membranes with grafted PIPAAm by UV irradiation. Water filtration rates of the PIPAAm-grafted porous membranes increased more than 10-fold above the LCST than the rate below it. The observations, however, were opposite Okahata's.[52] These differences may be explained by hydraulic and diffusional permeability attributed to the surface-grafted polymer density, and/or the sites of PIPAAm modification.

Modification of liposomes with stimuli-responsive polymers was also performed to develop regulated drug release devices responding to such stimuli as pH,[54] light,[55] and temperature.[56] Wu et al.[57,58] synthesized novel PIPAAm-pendant liposomes to conjugate 1-acyl-2-{12-[(7-nitro-2-1,3-benzoxadiazol-4-yl)amino]-dodecanolphos-phatidylethanolamide phospholipids to P(IPAAm-co-N-acryloxysuccinimide) (NAS) copolymers through succinimide active ester groups. These conjugates showed a phase-separated precipitation with increasing temperature. The LCST increased and the temperature range over which the copolymer precipitated also broadened after incorporation of more than 4 mol% of phospholipid. Negative charge remaining on the conjugates may influence LCST behavior.

Kono et al.[59–61] also developed temperature-responsive liposomes to control drug release by using vesicles of egg yolk phosphatidylcholine (EYPC) bearing IPAAm copolymers having long alkyl chains (Figure 12.10a). Temperature-responsive liposomes could regulate the release of drug entrapped in an inner aqueous phase by changing the interaction between polymer and lipid membranes with temperature. Figure 12.10b shows a release profile of carboxyfluorescein (CF) from thermoresponsive liposomes bearing poly(IPAAm-co-octadecyl acrylate (ODA)) in response to repeated temperature changes between 20 and 34°C. Thermoresponsive liposomes showed very fast CF release in response to temperature changes. These results indicate that a rapid increase in hydrophobicity of the copolymer with temperature

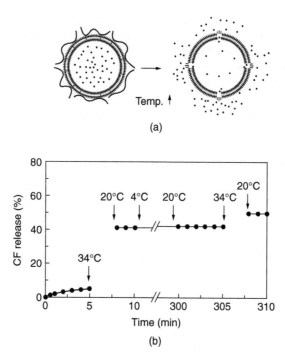

FIGURE 12.10 (a) Liposome-bearing temperature-responsive polymer. (b) Time course of CF release from EYPC liposomes bearing P(IPAAm-co-ODA) prepared by incubation in aqueous solution. Arrows show changes of temperature. Diameter of EYPC liposome is about 100 nm. (From Kono, K. et al., *J. Control. Rel.*, 20, 69–75, 1994. With permission.)

induces disruption of the lipid membrane integrity, forming drug-releasing channels within the lipid membranes. However, the complete drug release was not observed because of the liposomes bearing less amount of the copolymer on these surfaces or the interactions of model drugs and lipid membranes.

In summary, fast on–off PIPAAm switching mechanisms and their applications to drug permeation control are discussed from the viewpoints of rapid shrinking behavior of stimuli-responsive polymers. These polymers demonstrated fast and reversible responses to delicate environmental changes and thus show promise as materials for site-specific drug deliveries triggered by a variety of stimuli.

INTRODUCTION OF GRAFTED POLYMER CHAINS ACCELERATES GEL SHRINKING

COMB-TYPE PIPAAM-GRAFTED HYDROGELS

Tailoring gel architecture at the molecular level greatly influences the swelling and collapse dynamics of a macroscopic gel matrix. Our research group developed novel thermosensitive PIPAAm hydrogels having linear PIPAAm chains grafted onto the gel backbone networks (Figure 12.11a).[20,62,63]

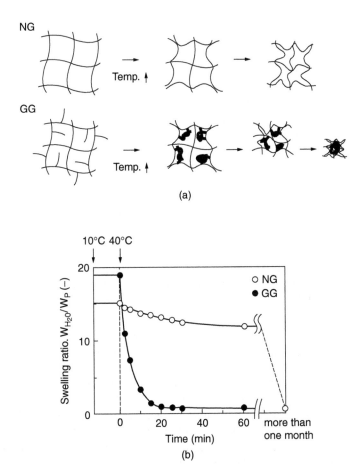

FIGURE 12.11 (a) Structures and shrinking mechanisms of conventional homopolymer gels (NGs) and comb-type grafted PIPAAm gels (GGs) undergoing temperature-induced collapse in aqueous media. (b) Shrinking kinetics for NG and GG in response to temperature changes across the LCST. W_{H_2O} = weight of water, W_P = weight of polymer. Gel dimensions = 15 mm diameter, 2.0 mm thickness.

The comb-type PIPAAm-grafted gels (GGs) had identical chemical composi-tions but different architectures from normal PIPAAm gels (NGs). Both gel types show similar equilibrium swelling ratios with temperature and have the same volume transition temperatures (32°C). It was expected that the GGs would exhibit improved molecular mobility due to the presence of freely mobile grafted chains that showed rapid conformational changes in response to temperature. In fact, GGs and NGs showed different shrinking kinetics with increasing temperature from below to above the transition temperature (Figure 12.11b). Conventional NGs shrank very slowly after temperature increases and required more than a month to reach equilibrium. Because of outside–in thermal conduction, NGs shrank gradually from the surface inward, mediated by diffusion of collapsing polymer networks and the release of entrapped water from the collapsing gel.[46]

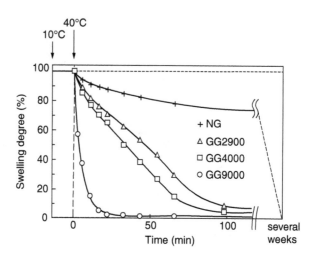

FIGURE 12.12 Time course of shrinking behavior for comb-type grafted gels with various lengths of grafted chains in response to stepwise temperature changes. Gel dimensions = 15 mm diameter, 2.0 mm thickness.

Because a dense, less permeable, and collapsed polymer layer (skin layer) formed at the gel surface before bulk gel collapse was initiated (thermal convection was more rapid than gel mass transfer), gel shrinking stopped after the initial stages via internal hydrostatic pressure. As a result, the gel shrinking rate was limited by the prevention of water permeation from the gel interior through the collapsed polymer skin layer, keeping water within the gel for longer periods.

In contrast, GGs shrank rapidly to equilibrium state at 40°C. In the shrinking process, the gels underwent large and rapid volume changes with marked mechanical buckling. This was a good indication of the much greater aggregation forces operating within PIPAAm graft-type gels. Water was rapidly squeezed from the gel interiors. This fact is supported by the changes in the amount of freezable water within two types of gel matrices determined by a differential scanning calorimeter (DSC). Rapid shrinking was due to the immediate dehydration of single-end free linear polymer chains on the gel networks followed by subsequent hydrophobic interactions between these dehydrated grafted chains that preceded shrinkage of the backbone network and effected rapid expulsion of water from the gel matrix.

Comb-type gels having grafted chains with different molecular weights were synthesized and the effects of graft chain lengths on the dynamic properties of the newly developed comb-type gels were investigated (Figure 12.12).[62] The single-end free, linear grafted chain lengths affected the mobility of the crosslinked main polymer chains. Therefore, the response rate of the gel shrinking process must reflect the influence of graft chain lengths.

In case of the GGs with the longest graft chains [GG9000; molecular weight (MW) of 9000] among the systems examined, the fastest shrinking kinetics were observed in GGs having long graft chains compared to other GGs having shorter chains (MWs of 2900 and 4000 for GG2900 and GG4000, respectively). Attractive forces between dehydrated and aggregated graft chains were more enhanced for grafted gels with longer PIPAAm graft chains.

An increase in the void volume within the gel network resulting from dehydration of grafted PIPAAm chains may also facilitate rapid release of entrapped water to the gel exterior. The collapsed polymer skin layer on the GG9000 gel surface was not observed after a temperature increase. The shrinking rate of GG9000 was faster than that of GG4000 due to the stronger forces operating between the aggregated graft chains and accompanying pressure for expelling bulk water within the gels. In contrast, relative aggregation forces operating between dehydrated grafted chains within GG2900 were significantly weak. The relatively dense shrunken gel surface layers were formed upon temperature increase and entrapped freezable water was released gradually from the interior of GG2900 through the shrunken surface layers. Thus, shrinking rates of gels may be controlled intentionally by changing the grafted PIPAAm chain lengths for applications to drug release mechanisms and actuators. Such intrinsic elastic forces from polymer chains within the network can eliminate current limitations to achieve rapidly acting smart actuators.

POLYETHYLENE OXIDE (PEO)-GRAFTED PIPAAM HYDROGELS

The authors' group developed other comb-type grafted gel architectures using hydrophilic poly(ethylene oxide) (PEO) graft chains instead of linear PIPAAm chains onto PIPAAm networks (Figure 12.13).[63,64] To investigate graft architectural effects of linear PEO graft chains onto PIPAAm gel networks, shrinking and swelling behaviors were investigated for P(IPAAm-g-PEO) gels and random copolymer gels of IPAAm with hydrophilic acrylic acid (AAc) [P(IPAAm-co-AAc)] as control hydrophilic hydrogels.

Equilibrium swelling ratios for P(IPAAm-g-PEO) and P(IPAAm-co-AAc) gels in phosphate buffered saline (PBS; pH, 7.4) are shown in Figure 12.14a and Figure 12.14b. Sensitivities of volume phase transitions for random P(IPAAm-co-AAc) gels were significantly weakened with increasing hydrophilic AAc content, restricting hydrophobic network aggregation. Interestingly, the P(IPAAm-g-PEO) gels showed small magnitudes of LCST shifts while the mole percentages of the hydrophilic PEO moieties in the gels were more than 10 mol%. These results strongly indicate that introduction of hydrophilic moieties as grafted chains maintains the hydrophobic

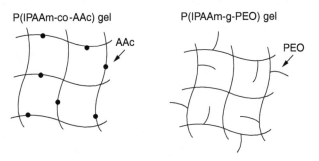

FIGURE 12.13 P(IPAAm-co-AAc) and P(IPAAm-g-PEO) gels.

main network aggregation compared to the random copolymer gels containing hydrophilic moieties.

Chen and Hoffman[23] also reported that graft-type copolymer structures maintain each distinct polymer chain property without interfering with each other. The researchers synthesized graft copolymers comprising side chains of PIPAAm grafted onto poly(acrylic acid) (PAAc) and proved that pendant PIPAAm graft chains have the same phase transition behavior as PIPAAm, independent of the presence of PAAc chains.

Figure 12.14d shows shrinking kinetics for P(IPAAm-g-PEO) gels after temperature jumps from equilibrium states at 10 to 50°C. The normal types of PIPAAm gels (NGs) demonstrated slower shrinking kinetics as noted in the previous section. In contrast, rapid shrinking of P(IPAAm-co-AAc) gels was observed because incorporation of hydrophilic moieties contributed to preventing hydrophobic skin layer formation (Figure 12.14c). The shrinking rate gradually increased with increasing AAc content up to 1.3 wt%. However, shrinking rates of P(IPAAm-co-AAc) gels with AAc contents above 1.3 wt% showed an abrupt decreasing trend. Hydrophobic aggregation forces were significantly weakened due to the break-up of PIPAAm network chains into multiple short segments with hydrophilic chemistry.

In sharp contrast, P(IPAAm-g-PEO) gels maintained large shrinking rates over a wide range of PEO contents. This behavioral difference is attributed to gel architecture. PEO chains were grafted onto the PIPAAm network chains and structurally separated to function independently of the PIPAAm backbone, maintaining hydrophobic aggregation force. The hydrophilic PEO chains formed microphase-separated hydrophilic domains in the dehydrated hydrophobic PIPAAm network due to their hydrated nature and the higher mobility of the freely mobile PIPAAm ends.

These hydrophilic PEG domains act as releasing channels for water molecules within the skin layer, preventing both reduction of the shrinking rate and limitation of water permeation. Above-mentioned results indicate that the balance of hydrophobicity and hydrophilicity and the gel architectural characteristics are important factors for determining gel shrinking kinetics. The method of introducing hydrophilic moieties as graft chains should be designed to maintain the PIPAAm backbone hydrophobic aggregation forces within the gel network.

NOVEL APPROACH FOR FAST SHRINKABLE HYDROGELS USING NEWLY DESIGNED MONOMERS

INCORPORATION OF HYDROPHILIC COMONOMERS

Effects of comonomer properties on temperature-responsive gel shrinking rates were studied for drug release regulation. Gutowska et al.[65] incorporated hydrophilic or hydrophobic components into PIPAAm-derived gels and reported the influence of diffusional barriers (skin layers) on drug release kinetics. Figure 12.15 shows the shrinking kinetics for P(IPAAm-co-BMA) gels and P(IPAAm-co-AAc) gels pre-equilibrated at 1, 15, and 20°C and subsequently immersed in a water bath set at 37°C.

As described in the section covering fast on–off gel switching mechanisms, the sudden temperature changes from below to above the transition temperature led to the formation of dense and less permeable surface skin layers on P(IPAAm-co-BMA)

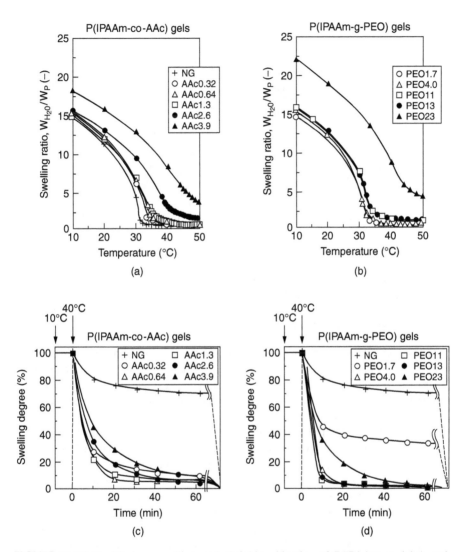

FIGURE 12.14 Equilibrium swelling and shrinking kinetics of P(IPAAm-co-AAc) and P(IPAAm-g-PEO) gels. (a,b) Equilibrium swelling ratios as functions of temperature. W_{H_2O} = weight of water, W_P = weight of polymer. (c,d) Shrinking kinetics. AAcX,X represents feed compositions of AAc wt%. PEOX,X represents feed compositions of PEO wt% at 50 from 10°C. Gel dimensions = 15 mm diameter, 1.0 mm thickness.

gels.[46,66,67] These different gel shrinking kinetics depending on pre-equilibrated temperatures are attributed to the skin layer thickness of the system.

In sharp contrast, the shrinking kinetics of P(IPAAm-co-AAc) gels are very rapid and independent of pre-equilibrium temperatures. Formation of skin-type barriers on PIPAAm gels was suppressed by incorporating hydrophilic comonomers. The authors also reported the same P(IPAAm-co-AAc) gel shrinking behavior as described earlier in the section on grafted polymer chains.[53] However, direct gel

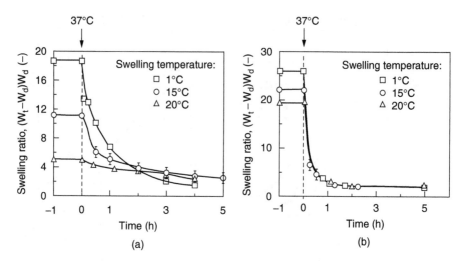

FIGURE 12.15 Shrinking kinetics of (a) P(IPAAm-co-BMA) (BMA = 5 mol%) and (b) P(IPAAm-co-AAc) (Aac = 2 mol%) gels equilibrated at 1, 15, and 20°C and immersed at 37°C at time 0. W_t = weight of gel at time t, W_d = weight of gel at dry state. Gel dimensions = 6 mm diameter, 0.4 mm thickness.

network copolymerization for the hydrophilic (AAc) component incorporation has a limitation related to obtaining fast shrinking kinetics for temperature-responsive hydrogels, restricting the full hydrophobic network aggregations of main PIPAAm networks. More precise molecular designs of gel architectures are necessary to overcome this limitation.

To accelerate gel shrinking without decreasing backbone chain hydrophobic aggregation forces, the introduction of hydrophilic PEO molecules into gels as grafted chains is one promising way as described earlier.[63,64]

Based on these reports, the authors hypothesize that the sensitive temperature response of PIPAAm may arise from reversible associations of critical lengths of repeated isopropylamide groups as seen in PIPAAm homopolymer chains.[68] Random introduction of a large quantities of hydrophilic monomers (e.g., AAc carboxyl groups) into PIPAAm hydrogels without compromising their intrinsic temperature sensitivity has proven difficult.[64,69] To overcome these problems, novel rapid shrinking hydrogels that respond to temperature changes were designed with random-type copolymer architectures by incorporating a newly synthesized monomer, 2-carboxyisopropylacrylamide (CIPAAm) with structural similarities to IPAAm side chains (Figure 12.16, center) along with a carboxylate group.[68]

As shown in Figure 12.17, PIPAAm hydrogels containing as much as 20 mol% CIPAAm exhibited large and sensitive volume phase transitions in response to temperature changes even though carboxylate groups in CIPAAm exist in dissociated states at pH 7.4.[70] These volume phase transition temperatures were nearly identical to those seen for IPAAm homopolymer gels. This is in sharp contrast to P(IPAAm-co-AAc) copolymer gels in which phase transition temperatures increase with AAc contents and eventually disappear at AAc content of 5 mol%.[64,68,69]

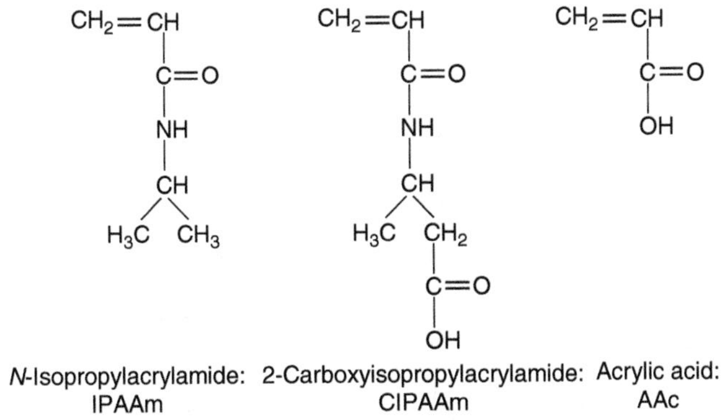

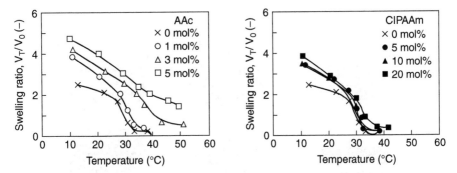

N-Isopropylacrylamide: 2-Carboxyisopropylacrylamide: Acrylic acid:
IPAAm CIPAAm AAc

FIGURE 12.16 Chemical structure of newly synthesized functional monomer, CIPAAm. For comparison, structural formulae of IPAAm and AAc are also shown.

FIGURE 12.17 Equilibrium swelling ratios for P(IPAAm-co-AAc) and P(IPAAm-co-CIPAAm) gels at various compositions as function of temperature in PBS (pH, 7.4). V_T = gel volume at T°C, V_0 = gel volume just after synthesis. Cylindrical gel dimensions = 2 mm length, 0.3 mm diameter.

These results indicate that P(IPAAm-co-CIPAAm) gels maintain their hydrophobic aggregation forces without disruption by ionized carboxyl groups. Because of the apparent differences between the structures of CIPAAm and AAc monomers, differences in respective gel behavior were rationalized to result from the structural analogy of CIPAAm's isopropylamide side groups with those of IPAAm. Therefore, maintenance of isopropylamide side chain alignment within the copolymer chains may facilitate introduction of large amounts of functional groups into IPAAm copolymer gels without losing phase transition behavior. The new monomer, CIPAAm, should prove useful to introduce functional carboxyl groups into temperature-responsive PIPAAm hydrogels while maintaining their intrinsic temperature sensitive behavior.

Figure 12.18a compares the deswelling kinetics of PIPAAm, P(IPAAm-co-CIPAAm), and P(IPAAm-co-AAc) gels exposed to stepwise temperature changes from 10 to 40°C in PBS (pH, 7.4).[71] All hydrogel samples were pre-equilibrated at

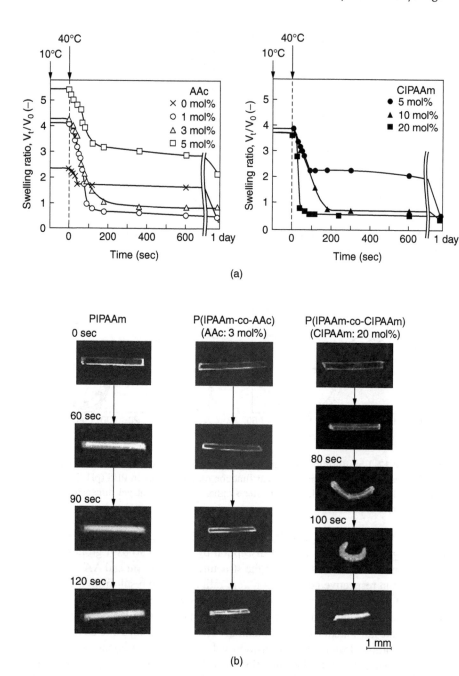

FIGURE 12.18 (a) Shrinking kinetics for P(IPAAm-co-AAc) and P(IPAAm-co-CIPAAm) gels in response to temperature changes from 10 to 40°C. (b) Photographs of shrinking process observed for PIPAAm, P(IPAAm-co-AAc) (AAc, 3 mol%), and P(IPAAm-co-CIPAAm) (CIPAAm, 20 mol%) gels in response to a temperature increase from 10 and 40°C. Cylindrical gel dimensions = 2 mm length, 0.3 mm diameter.

10°C in PBS. Gels then transferred to another water bath equilibrated at 40°C, and gel deswelling kinetics were obtained by recording video images.

The PIPAAm gel changed from transparent to opaque within 60 s after temperature change and stopped deswelling, suggesting skin layer formation.[46] In contrast, introduction of small amounts of AAc to PIPAAm gels induced rapid gel shrinking to a new equilibrium state at 40°C after 100 s for a copolymer gel with 1 mol% AAc and 200 s for gels with 3 mol% AAc. Figure 12.18b (middle column) shows the changes in appearance of the deswelling gel containing 3 mol% AAc at 0, 60, 90, and 120 s that indicate rapid shrinking while maintaining transparency. However, the magnitude of gel deswelling decreased with increasing AAc content in P(IPAAm-co-AAc) gels. In particular, IPAAm copolymer gels containing 5mol% AAc did not dehydrate completely over the examined time range. In contrast, P(IPAAm-co-CIPAAm) gel deswelling rates and collapse magnitudes increased with increasing CIPAAm content.

The volume changes in gels containing 5 mol% of CIPAAm stopped upon skin layer formation observed on their surfaces after 80 s of temperature change. Despite their charged, albeit small, monomer contents, P(IPAAm-co-CIPAAm) gels maintained strong hydrophobic aggregation forces — an effect distinct from those of analogous P(IPAAm-co-AAc) gels and attributed to the unique CIPAAm structure.

From the photographs showing the shrinking of gels containing 20 mol% of CIPAAm (Figure 12.18b, right column), initially transparent gels turned opaque within 80 s upon heating from 10 to 40°C, probably due to skin layer formation at the gel surface. However, gel deswelling was not stopped, regardless of the skin layer formation, due to sufficient hydrophilic carboxylate content that allowed water movement. More specifically, the density of the collapsed polymer layers in 20 mol% CIPAAm-containing gels must have been lower than those of pure PIPAAm gels to permit squeezing water efflux and avoid hydrostatic pressure increases. Additionally, chain aggregation forces between polymer chains producing collapse were maintained compared with those of P(IPAAm-co-AAc) gels. This was evidenced by mechanical buckling of the shrinking gels that occurred between 80 and 100 s (Figure 12.18b, right column). Water within the collapsing gels readily permeated out through the CIPAAm copolymer gel skin layer.

These results emphasize the importance of the balance of two factors for producing rapid shrinking of IPAAm copolymer gels: (1) maintenance of effective hydrophobic aggregation forces between collapsing polymer chains and (2) fabrication of water-permeable networks to readily release water through the collapsing gel skin layer. When the chain aggregation force is too strong and the resulting gel skin layer density becomes very high, water inside the gel cannot permeate and the deswelling change is halted by hydrostatic pressure as seen in PIPAAm gels. Conversely, as aggregation forces were weakened by the introduction of hydrophilic comonomer moieties, deswelling rates slowed and collapse magnitudes became small as seen in P(IPAAm-co-AAc) gels.

Deswelling rates and magnitudes in PIPAAm copolymer gels are readily controlled using CIPAAm because the collapsed skin layer density is altered by changing CIPAAm content. In addition to accelerating gel shrinking, the CIPAAm carboxyl groups introduced into PIPAAm gel have a potential utility for immobilizing further moieties including bioactive peptides and proteins to control cell proliferation and differentiation by temperature changes. These issues are currently under investigation by the authors.

CONCLUSIONS

This chapter focused on the effects of hydrogel architectures to accelerate gel shrinking rates in response to external stimuli. Swelling and deswelling changes in conventional hydrogels are driven by the collective and cooperative network diffusion of polymer networks in a bulk water phase. Such chain and network movement and response to changing environment are dependent upon the relative constraints of the network due to crosslinking and mobility, relative rates of thermal conduction versus polymer mass transfer, and subsequently entrapped water.

These effects all depend on relative diffusion times and scaling effects of gel network size versus surface area. Due to size dependency, the utility of manipulating the swelling and deswelling kinetics of conventional hydrogels for practical applications is limited. To overcome these constraints, novel strategies focusing on different hydrogel architectures were proposed. More rapid network deswelling changes were achieved by introducing freely mobile graft chains into gel backbones to increase the overall polymer network mobility.

The comb-type gel system has the advantage that the deswelling kinetics are independent of matrix size and surface area. Moreover, a newly designed functional hydrophilic comonomer matching the physical chemistry of the stimuli-sensitive polymer matrix was incorporated to accelerate gel shrinking kinetics in response to temperature increase. The incorporation of hydrophilic moieties into PIPAAm gel networks is generally believed to lead not only to acceleration of gel shrinking rates, but also to decreases in hydrophobic aggregation forces between polymer network chains.

CIPAAm, a new comonomer, has been used to show how chemistry matching can overcome water efflux problems during collapse by introducing a large number of hydrophilic carboxylate groups into PIPAAm gels while maintaining intrinsic temperature-sensitive gel behavior. These new approaches can overcome the constraint inherent in bulk gel shrinking rates by collective diffusion mechanisms and are potentially advantageous for applications in the biomedical, separation, biotechnology, and other fields.

REFERENCES

1. S.W. Kim, C.M. Pai, K. Makino, L.A. Seminoff, D.L. Holmberg, J.M. Gleeson, D.E. Wilson, and F.J. Mack, Self-regulated glycosylated insulin delivery, in *Advances in Drug Delivery Systems 4*, J.M. Anderson et al., Eds., Elsevier, Amsterdam, 193–201, 1990.
2. A.S. Hoffman, Applications of thermally reversible polymers and hydrogels in therapeutics and diagnostics, in *Advances in Drug Delivery Systems 3*, J.M. Anderson et al., Eds., Elsevier, Amsterdam, 297–305, 1987.

3. T. Okano and R. Yoshida, Intelligent polymeric materials for drug delivery, in *Biomedical Applications of Polymeric Materials*, T. Tsuruta et al., Eds., CRC Press, Boca Raton, FL, 407–428, 1993.

4. R.A. Lipper and W.I. Higuchi, Analysis of theoretical behavior of a proposed zero-order drug delivery system, *J. Pharm. Sci.* 66, 163–164, 1977.

5. T. Okano, M. Miyajima, F. Kodama, G. Imanidis, S. Nishiyama, S.W. Kim, and W.I. Higuchi, Control of concentration-time profiles *in vivo* by zero-order transdermal delivery systems, *J. Control. Rel.* 6, 99–106, 1987.

6. T. Okano, Ed., *Biorelated Polymers and Gels: Controlled Release and Applications in Biomedical Engineering,* Academic Press, Chestnut Hill, MA, 1998.

7. F.D. Theeuwes, D. Swanson, P. Wong, P. Bonsen, V. Place, K. Heimlich, and K.C. Kwan, Elementary osmotic pump for indomethacin, *J. Pharm. Sci.* 72, 253–258, 1983.

8. A. Kikuchi, M. Okuhara, F. Karikusa, Y. Sakurai, and T. Okano, Two-dimensional manipulation of confluently cultured vascular endothelial cells using temperature-responsive poly(*N*-isopropylacrylamide)-grafted surfaces, *J. Biomater. Sci. Polym. Edn.* 9, 1331–1348, 1998.

9. T. Shimizu, M. Yamato, Y. Isoi, T. Akutsu, T. Setomaru, K. Abe, A. Kikuchi, M. Umezu, and T. Okano, Fabrication of pulsatile cardiac tissue grafts using a novel 3-dimensional cell sheet manipulation technique and temperature-responsive cell culture surfaces, *Circ. Res.* 90, e40–e48, 2002.

10. M. Yamato, M. Utsumi, A. Kushida, C. Konno, A. Kikuchi, and T. Okano, Thermo-responsive culture dishes allow the intact harvest of multilayered keratinocyte sheets without dispase by reducing temperature, *Tissue Eng.* 7, 473–480, 2001.

11. M. Hirose, O.H. Kwon, M. Yamato, A. Kikuchi, and T. Okano, Creation of designed shape cell sheets that are noninvasively harvested and moved onto another surface, *Biomacromolecules* 1, 377–381, 2001.

12. M. Harimoto, M. Yamato, M. Hirose, C. Takahashi, Y. Isoi, A. Kikuchi, and T. Okano, Novel approach for achieving double-layered cell sheets co-culture, overlaying endothelial cell sheets onto monolayer hepatocytes utilizing temperature-responsive culture dishes, *J. Biomed. Mater. Res.* 62, 464–470, 2002.

13. T. Yakushiji, K. Sakai, A. Kikuchi, T. Aoyagi, Y. Sakurai, and T. Okano, Effects of cross-linked structure on temperature-responsive hydrophobic interaction of PIPAAm hydrogel modified surfaces with steroids, *Anal. Chem.* 71, 1125–1130, 1999.

14. K. Yoshizako, Y. Akiyama, H. Yamanaka, Y. Shinohara, Y. Hasegawa, E. Carredano, A. Kikuchi, and T. Okano, Regulation of protein binding toward a ligand on chromatographic matrixes by masking and forced-releasing effects using thermoresponsive polymer, *Anal. Chem.* 74, 4160–4166, 2002.

15. H. Kanazawa, K. Yamamoto, Y. Matsushima, N. Takei, A. Kikuchi, Y. Sakurai, and T. Okano, Temperature-responsive chromatography using poly(*N*-isopropylacrylamide)-modified silica, *Anal. Chem.* 68, 100–105, 1996.

16. J. Kobayashi, A. Kikuchi, K. Sakai, and T. Okano, Aqueous chromatography utilizing hydrophobicity-modified anionic temperature-responsive hydrogel for stationary phases, *J. Chromatogr. A* 958, 109–119, 2002.

17. Y. Osada and M. Sato, Conversion of chemical into mechanical energy by contractile polymers performed by polymer complexation, *Polymer* 21, 1057–1061, 1980.

18. Y. Osada, E. Katsumura, and K. Inoue, Photomechanochemical energy conversion in a polyamide containing a stilbene structure in the backbone, *Makromol. Chem. Rapid Commun.* 2, 411–415, 1981.

19. T. Kurauchi, T. Shiga, Y. Hirose, and A. Okada, Deformation behaviors of polymer gels, in *Polymer Gels*, D. DeRossi et al., Eds., Plenum, New York, 237–246, 1991.

20. R. Yoshida, K. Uchida, Y. Kaneko, K. Sakai, A. Kikuchi, Y. Sakurai, and T. Okano, Comb-type grafted hydrogels with rapid deswelling response to temperature changes, *Nature* 374, 240–242, 1995.

21. A. Kikuchi and T. Okano, Intelligent thermoresponsive polymeric stationary phase for aqueous chromatography of biological compounds, *Prog. Polym. Sci.* 27, 1165–1193, 2002.

22. A. Kikuchi and T. Okano, Pulsatile drug release control using hydrogels, *Adv. Drug Delivery Rev.* 54, 53–77, 2002.

23. G. Chen and A.S. Hoffman, Graft copolymers that exhibit temperature-induced phase transitions over a wide range of pH, *Nature* 373, 49–52, 1995.

24. L.C. Dong and A.S. Hoffman, A novel approach for preparation of pH-sensitive hydrogels for enteric delivery, *J. Control. Rel.* 15, 141–152, 1991.

25. J. Heller, A.C. Chang, G. Rodd, and G.M. Grodsky, Release of insulin from pH-sensitive poly(ortho esters), *J. Control. Rel.* 13, 295–302, 1990.

26. K. Kataoka, H. Miyazaki, M. Bunya, T. Okano, and Y. Sakurai, Totally synthetic polymer gels responding to external glucose concentration: their preparation and application to on–off regulation of insulin release *J. Am. Chem. Soc.* 120, 12694–12695, 1998.

27. Y. Ito, M. Casolaro, K. Kono, and Y. Imanishi, An insulin-releasing system that is responsive to glucose, *J. Control. Rel.* 10, 195–203, 1989.

28. K. Ishihara, M. Kobayashi, and I. Shinohara, Control of insulin permeation through a polymer membrane with responsive function of glucose, *Makromol. Chem. Rapid. Commun.* 4, 327–331, 1983.

29. I.C. Kwon, Y.H. Bae, and S.W. Kim, Electrically erodible polymer gel for controlled release of drugs, *Nature* 354, 291–293, 1991.

30. T. Tanaka, I. Nishio, S.T. Sun, and S. Ueno-Nishio, Collapse of gels in an electric field, *Science* 218, 467–469, 1982.

31. K. Sawahata, M. Hara, H. Yasunaga, and Y. Osada, Electrically controlled drug delivery system using polyelectrolyte gels, *J. Control. Rel.* 14, 253–262, 1990.

32. J. Chen, H. Park, and K. Park, Synthesis of superporous hydrogels: hydrogels with fast swelling and superabsorbent properties, *J. Biomed. Mater. Res.* 44, 53–62, 1999.

33. R. Kishi, M. Hara, K. Sawahata, and Y. Osada, Conversion of chemical into mechanical energy by synthetic polymer gels (chemomechanical system), in *Polymer Gels*, D. DeRossi et al., Eds., Plenum, New York, 205–220, 1991.

34. M. Suzuki, Amphoteric polyvinyl alcohol hydrogel and electrohydrodynamic control method for artificial muscles, in *Polymer Gels*, D. DeRossi et al., Eds., Plenum, New York, 221–236, 1991.

35. H. Feil, Y.H. Bae, J. Feijen, and S.W. Kim, Molecular separation by thermosensitive hydrogel membranes, *J. Membrane Sci.* 64, 283–294, 1991.

36. N.P. Desai and J.A. Hubbell, Tissue response to intraperitoneal implants of polyethylene oxide-modified polyethylene terephthalate, *Biomaterials* 13, 505–510, 1992.

37. A. Lendlein, A. Schmidt, and R. Langer, AB-polymer networks based on oligo(ε-caprolactone) segments showing shape-memory properties, *Proc. Natl. Acad. Sci. USA* 98, 842–847, 2001.

38. Y. Osada and A. Matsuda, Shape memory in hydrogels, *Nature* 376, 219, 1995.

39. E. Sato-Matsuo and T. Tanaka, Kinetics of discontinuous phase transition of gels, *J. Chem. Phys.* 89, 1695–1703, 1988.

40. O. Hirasa, S. Ito, A. Yamauchi, S. Fujishige, and H. Ichijo, Thermoresponsive polymer hydrogel, in *Polymer Gels*, D. DeRossi et al., Eds., Plenum, New York, 247–256, 1991.

41. R. Kishi, O. Hirasa, and H. Ichijo, Fast responsive poly(*N*-isopropylacrylamide) hydrogels prepared by γ-ray irradiation, *J. Polym. Sci. A Polym. Chem.* 30, 2121–2129, 1992.

42. B.G. Kabra and S.H. Gehrke, Synthesis of fast response, temperature-sensitive poly(*N*-isopropylacrylamide) gel, *Polym. Commun.* 32, 322–323, 1991.

43. X.-Z. Zhang and R.-X. Zhuo, Preparation of fast responsive, thermally sensitive poly(*N*-isopropylacrylamide) gel, *Euro. Polym. J.* 36, 2301–2303, 2000.

44. X S. Wu, A.S. Hoffman, and P. Yager, Synthesis and characterization of thermally reversible macroporous poly(*N*-isopropylacrylamide) hydrogels, *J. Polym. Sci. A Polym. Chem.* 30, 2121–2129, 1992.

45. N. Kato and F. Takahashi, Acceleration of deswelling of poly(*N*-isopropylacrylamide) hydrogel by the treatment of a freeze-dry and hydration process, *Bull. Chem. Soc. Jpn.* 70, 1289–1295, 1997.

46. T. Okano, Y. H. Bae, H. Jacobs, and S.W. Kim, Thermally on–off switching polymers for drug permeation and release, *J. Control. Rel.* 11, 255–265, 1990.

47. R. Yoshida, K. Sakai, T. Okano, Y. Sakurai, Y. H. Bae, and S.W. Kim, Surface-modulated skin layer of thermal responsive hydrogels as on–off switches. I. Drug release, *J. Biomater. Sci. Polym. Ed.* 3, 155–162, 1991.

48. R. Yoshida, K. Sakai, T. Okano, and Y. Sakurai, Surface-modulated skin layer of thermal responsive hydrogels as on-off switches. II. Drug permeation, *J. Biomater. Sci. Polym. Ed.* 3, 243–252, 1992.

49. R. Yoshida, K. Sakai, T. Okano, and Y. Sakurai, Modulating the phase transition temperature and thermosensitivity in *N*-isopropylacrylamide copolymer gels, *J. Biomater. Sci. Polym. Ed.* 6, 585–598, 1994.

50. C.S. Brazel and N.A. Peppas, Pulsatile local delivery of thrombolytic and antithrombotic agents using poly(*N*-isopropylacrylamide-co-methacrylic acid) hydrogels, *J. Control. Rel.* 39, 57–64, 1996.

51. T.A. Horbett, B.D. Ratner, J. Kost, and M. Singh, A bioresponsive membrane for insulin delivery, in *Recent Advances in Drug Delivery Systems*, J.M. Anderson et al., Eds., Plenum, New York, 209–220, 1984.

52. Y. Okahata, H. Noguchi, and T. Seki, Thermosensitive permeation from a polymer-grafted capsule membrane, *Macromolecules* 19, 493–494, 1986.

53. H. Iwata, M. Oodate, Y. Uyama, H. Amemiya, and Y. Ikada, Preparation of temperature-sensitive membranes by graft polymerization onto a porous membrane, *J. Membr. Sci.* 55, 119–130, 1991.

54. M.B. Yatvin, W. Kreutz, B.A. Horwitz, and M. Shinitzky, pH-Sensitive liposomes: possible clinical implications, *Science* 210, 1253–1255, 1980.

55. C. Pidgeon and C.A. Hunt, Light sensitive liposomes, *Photochem. Photobiol.* 37, 491–494, 1983.

56. M.B. Yatvin, J.N. Weinstein, W.H. Dennis, and R. Blumenthal, Design of liposomes for enhanced local release of drugs by hyperthermia, *Science* 202, 1290–1293, 1978.

57. X.S. Wu, A.S. Hoffman, and P. Yager, Conjugation of phosphatidylethanolamine to poly(*N*-isopropylacrylamide) for potential use in liposomal drug delivery systems, *Polymer* 33, 4659–4662, 1992.

58. X.S. Wu, A.S. Hoffman, and P. Yager, Effect of conjugation of phospholipid to poly(*N*-isopropylacrylamide) on its critical solution temperature, *Makromol. Chem. Rapid Commun.* 14, 309–314, 1993.

59. K. Kono, H. Hayashi, and T. Takagishi, Temperature-sensitive liposomes, bearing poly(*N*-isopropylacrylamide), *J. Control. Rel.* 30, 69–75, 1994.

60. H. Hayashi, K. Kono, and T. Takagishi, Temperature sensitization of liposomes using copolymers of *N*-isopropylacrylamide, *Bioconjugate Chem.* 10, 412–418, 1999.

61. K. Kono, K. Yoshino, and T. Takagishi, Effect of poly(ethylene glycol)-grafts on temperature-sensitivity of thermosensitive polymer-modified liposomes, *J. Control. Rel.* 80, 321–332, 2002.

62. Y. Kaneko, K. Sakai, A. Kikuchi, R. Yoshida, Y. Sakurai, and T. Okano, Influence of freely mobile grafted chain length on dynamic properties of comb-type grafted poly(*N*-isopropylacrylamide) hydrogels, *Macromolecules* 28, 7717–7723, 1995.

63. Y. Kaneko, S. Nakamura, K. Sakai, A. Kikuchi, T. Aoyagi, A. Kikuchi, Y. Sakurai, and T. Okano, Deswelling mechanism for comb-type grafted poly(*N*-isopropylacrylamide) hydrogels with rapid temperature responses, *Polym. Gels Networks* 6, 333–345, 1998.

64. Y. Kaneko, S. Nakamura, K. Sakai, T. Aoyagi, A. Kikuchi, Y. Sakurai, and T. Okano, Rapid deswelling response of poly(*N*-isopropylacrylamide) hydrogels by the formation of water release channels using poly(ethylene oxide) graft chains, *Macromolecules* 31, 6099–6105, 1998.

65. A. Gutowska, Y.H. Bae, J. Feijen, and S.W. Kim, Heparin release from thermosensitive hydrogels *J. Control. Rel.* 22, 95–104, 1992.

66. Y.H. Bae, T. Okano, and S.W. Kim, On–off thermocontrol of solute transport. I. Temperature dependence of swelling of *N*-isopropylacrylamide networks modified with hydrophobic components in water, *Pharm. Res.* 8, 531–537, 1991.

67. Y. Kaneko, R. Yoshida, K. Sakai, Y. Sakurai, and T. Okano, Temperature-responsive shrinking kinetics of poly(*N*-isopropylacrylamide) copolymer gels with hydrophilic and hydrophobic comonomers, *J. Membr. Sci.* 101, 13–22, 1995.

68. T. Aoyagi, M. Ebara, K. Sakai, Y. Sakurai, and T. Okano, Novel bifunctional polymer with reactivity and temperature sensitivity, *J. Biomater. Sci. Polym. Ed.* 11, 101–110, 2000.

69. H. Feil. Y.H. Bae, J. Feijen, and S.W. Kim, Effect of comonomer hydrophilicity and ionization on the lower critical solution temperature of *N*-isopropylacrylamide copolymer, *Macromolecules* 26, 2496–2500, 1993.

70. M. Ebara, T. Aoyagi, K. Sakai, and T. Okano, Introducing reactive carboxyl side chains retains phase transition temperature sensitivity in *N*-isopropylacrylamide copolymer gels, *Macromolecules* 33, 8312–8316, 2000.

71. M. Ebara, T. Aoyagi, K. Sakai, and T. Okano, The incorporation of carboxylate groups into temperature-responsive poly(*N*-isopropylacrylamide)-based hydrogels promotes rapid gel shrinking, *J. Polym. Sci. A Polym. Chem.* 39, 335–342, 2001.

13 Fast Swelling Hydrogel Systems

Richard A. Gemeinhart and Chunqiang Guo

CONTENTS

INTRODUCTION

There are many applications in which a material is needed to swell rapidly in a fluid. Materials that imbibe large volumes of water are very functional in daily use and in specialized applications. Everyday materials such as diapers and sanitary napkins must rapidly contain large volumes of biologic fluids and retain strength without losing fluid to the surrounding areas.[1] These materials are typically made of hydrophilic polymers that can swell in biologic fluids and will not dissolve.

Hydrogels were first described in the last century as networks that contain small fractions of polymers and large fractions of water; hydrogels maintain their shapes while they imbibe fluids or are dried.[2] Figure 13.1 is a representation of the structure of a hydrogel. When a hydrogel is in a dehydrated or deswollen state, its polymer chains are in close proximity with little room for diffusion of molecules. As the material swells, the polymer chains separate to an extent determined by the properties of the solvent in which the hydrogel has been placed. Under certain conditions, the polymer chains will extend to the greatest extent possible and little interaction will take place between the chains. In this state, the swelling pressure on the polymers is counteracted by the crosslinkers in the hydrogel; the mesh size (Figure 13.1) is greatest, and diffusion of small molecules approaches the diffusion coefficient in pure fluid.

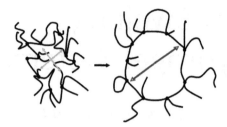

FIGURE 13.1 Swelling of a hydrogel. Left: Hydrogel in a deswollen or dry state. The polymer chains are in close proximity and may interact with each other. As a fluid enters the hydrogel, the polymer chains undergo hydration and other interactions such as hydrophobic or electrostatic interactions. Light gray arrows indicate pressure on the system to swell. Right: When appropriate conditions are met, the hydrogel will reach a state where the polymer chains are fully extended and only the crosslinks prevent the material from dissolution. The mesh size ξ is indicated by the dark arrow.

Medical uses of hydrogels and other materials that swell rapidly in fluids have been the major areas of research in the last several decades. Absorbent sponges made of materials that are similar to diapers have been produced with great success. Embolic agents are currently placed in the blood vessels of patients who would otherwise bleed to death.[3] Embolic agents must swell quickly when placed in blood or they may disperse from the site of administration and become problematic downstream.[4]

The materials cited in these examples may be used in a dehydrated state and swell upon placement in fluid. Other materials can swell rapidly when placed in an appropriate environment that contains a certain pH,[5,6] temperature,[7] electric field,[8–10] light,[11–14] pressure,[15,16] or specific molecule.[17–21] With the advent of nanotechnology, rapidly swelling and shrinking (deswelling) materials have been suggested as actuators in nanodevices.[22–24] These materials require extreme sensitivity and speed for sensing their environments. The need for materials that swell quickly when placed in fluid is quite obvious. Depending upon the type of sensing necessary, problems with speed of sensing, swelling or deswelling, and methods for increasing the speed of transition from deswollen to swollen or the reverse are being vigorously investigated.[25] Diversity of applications for rapidly swelling materials is especially important because materials that are inexpensive to produce in any size and shape would produce benefits for many areas of society, in particular medicine and drug delivery,[26] although applications in other areas are suggested as well.[24]

In this chapter, we discuss methods that have been used to create rapidly swelling hydrogels and crosslinked polymeric systems. Chapter 12 by Ebara et al. discusses materials used in applications in which rapid shrinking (deswelling) is needed. This chapter will focus primarily on applications in which fast swelling is needed and methods for improving the rate at which materials respond to stimuli in the environment. The next section will present materials that swell from a desolvated or dehydrated state, followed by discussion of applications for environmentally sensitive materials that swell rapidly in appropriate environments. By choosing the appropriate techniques, one can create rapid swelling systems that can be used in both aqueous and organic environments.

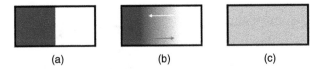

(a)   (b)   (c)

FIGURE 13.2 Movement of fluid into a crosslinked polymer. (a) When a hydrogel (dark) and fluid (clear) are placed in proximity, the fluid diffuses into the hydrogel and the polymer chains begin to relax and diffuse into the fluid. At an intermediate point (b) between the dry (a) and fully swollen (c) states, the system will contain three distinct phases: dry hydrogel, swollen hydrogel with fluid, and fluid. Two interfaces are present: swollen hydrogel–dry hydrogel and swollen hydrogel–fluid.

POLYMER SWELLING

The thermodynamics of polymer swelling has been widely examined and has been well understood for several decades,[27–29] but the kinetics of hydrogel swelling has not been as thoroughly examined. Section II of this text is dedicated to the theoretical considerations of environmentally sensitive polymers and hydrogels. Of particular interest for fast swelling materials is that the uptake of fluid into the network of the polymer occurs while the polymer is relaxing.[30] Diffusion of solvent (typically water) and solutes into the polymer network has been shown to exhibit a Fickian type diffusion, but the diffusion is retarded compared to that expected.

Diffusion has been characterized by Tanaka et al. as related to the bulk modulus K, the shear modulus μ, and the coefficient of friction f between the polymer and solvent [Equation (13.1)].[30–32] Figure 13.2 represents the swelling process of a polymeric network. When dry, the polymer is placed in contact with a fluid, the fluid begins to enter the dry, solid polymer network by diffusion, and the polymer begins to diffuse into the fluid. Over time, the polymer relaxes and reaches equilibrium with the fluid and an interface is formed between the dry and swollen hydrogel. When all the fluid has been absorbed or the hydrogel reaches chemical equilibrium with the fluid, a single interface is again achieved between the hydrogel and the fluid.

Tanaka and Filmore[32] established a theory for swelling of hydrogels that presents a parameter that has been used to describe the kinetics of transport of fluid into swelling materials [Equation (13.2)]. In this relationship the characteristic time for swelling τ is related to the characteristic length of the gel a and the diffusion coefficient D in the network.

$$D = \frac{K + \dfrac{4\mu}{3}}{f} \tag{13.1}$$

$$\tau = \frac{a^2}{D} \tag{13.2}$$

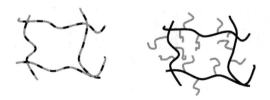

FIGURE 13.3 Alternating and graft copolymers. In the alternating copolymer (left), the two monomers (black and gray) are both in the polymer backbone. In the graft copolymer (right), the polymer backbone has only one monomer (black) and the grafts are repeating units of the copolymer (gray).

This descriptor of swelling is not without some criticism. Additional studies from this laboratory[30,31] and others[33–36] have further developed the kinetics of swelling of polymers in a good solvent. What is most important in these discussions is that the fact that the characteristic length of the polymer is directly related to the swelling time is not in dispute. This suggests that large polymeric networks will respond significantly slower than smaller polymeric networks. For this reason, reducing the size of the polymeric network has been chosen as the primary method of reducing the time for environmental response or for swelling from the dry state.[26] Others have suggested that an alternative to producing smaller systems is introducing a method of rapid mass transport into the polymer networks.

IDEAS FOR RAPID SWELLING

A few methods have been proposed to increase the swelling rate for polymeric networks. Reduction of the size of hydrogels was the first and most utilized method to reduce the swelling time as we stated earlier.[7,30–32] Several investigators have suggested using graft polymers (Figure 13.3) to increase the sensitivity of the polymer network and allow rapid transport in the hydrogels.[37,38] This idea works well for materials that rapidly deswell, but has not been nearly as successful for materials that must swell since the kinetics of diffusion through the hydrogel is limiting.

A comb-type grafted poly(N-isopropylacrylamide) (nIPAAm) hydrogel was synthesized by Okana and coworkers.[39] The comb-type hydrogel had the same chemical composition but a different architecture from normal-type hydrogels and exhibited fast deswelling kinetics responding to changes of temperature. The N-isopropylacrylamide (nIPAAm) monomer chains were grafted to the nIPAAm backbone in the presence of a crosslinker. The backbone and graft chains cooperatively aggregated during dehydration and excluded the entrapped water in 20 min. The swelling kinetics of the grafted hydrogel remained low (800 min) because mass transport into the dehydrated system is predominantly diffusive/relaxive in nature.[37,40] Increasing the porosity of the hydrogels to enlarge the contact area between the hydrogel and the fluid has been achieved by freeze-drying and porogen techniques.[41,42] Microporous materials swell at a much faster rate than the equivalent nonporous materials, but do not swell with sufficient speed for many uses in which diffusion distances are large. This is due to the fact that the porous structure is not intercon-nected in a manner that allows fluid transport to be convective in nature.

SUPERPOROUS HYDROGELS

Superporous hydrogels (SPHs) are a new generation of hydrogels with pore size in the range of 100 μm or larger; the mesh size of a conventional hydrogel is below 100 nm.[43,44] The most remarkable property of superporous hydrogels is their fast swelling ability. The swelling kinetics of SPHs is a few minutes — much faster than that of conventional hydrogels. It usually takes hours to days for conventional hydro-gels to swell to equilibrium when their dimensions are on the order of centimeters. Rapid swelling of SPHs is due to the interconnected pore networks that are formed.[45]

Gas blowing techniques are used to synthesize superporous hydrogels. Control of foaming and polymerization is necessary to form homogeneous open capillary channels in SPHs.[45] The commonly used foaming agents are inorganic carbonates such as Na_2CO_3 and $NaHCO_3$ which have been safely applied in drug delivery systems. Carbon dioxide gas bubbles are generated by the reaction of Na_2CO_3 or $NaHCO_3$ with acid. Other methods may also be utilized as the formation of an SPH is similar to the process of forming Styrofoam.

Factors Affecting Synthesis of Superporous Hydrogel

The major differences in methods of preparing superporous hydrogels and conven-tional hydrogels are the additions of foaming agents and foam stabilizers to the monomer solutions. The pore size of an SPH is largely determined by the amount of gas blowing. It is essential to synchronize the foaming and the polymerization processes to make homogeneous superporous hydrogels. Foam stabilizers are sur-factants that stabilize the gas bubbles produced so that the gas bubbles are sustained for a long period. Many surfactants have been shown to allow gas generated during polymerization to enable interconnected pores.[43]

The formation of pores on the surface of an SPH is also affected by the surface of the polymerization vessel.[45] Polymerization vessels were modified with various silane molecules of varying polarity and ionic content. Hydrophobic surfaces pro-duced porous surface structures while hydrophilic surfaces produced nonporous sur-faces. Gas bubbles have a tendency to close off on the hydrophilic surface of a polymerization vessel. Surprisingly, no great difference was noted for SPHs produced in various polymerization vessels despite obvious surface morphology differences.[45] This can be explained by the interconnection of pores along the axis of gas formation.

The drying process also contributes to the properties of SPHs. When there is no closing or collapse of the pore structure during drying, the swelling kinetics and swelling ratio will be maintained. Methods such as organic solvent drying (e.g., with ethanol or acetone) and freeze drying are better than direct air drying. During air drying, pores in SPHs collapse as water is removed. In contrast, organic solvents have lower surface tension than water, leaving capillary channels intact after evap-oration.[43,46,47] One can maintain the interconnected pore structure under appropriate conditions, even when the SPH has been reduced in size.[47] It was found that by maintaining the interconnectivity of the pores, the swelling kinetics were only marginally reduced, despite a dramatic (up to 83%) reduction in the dry volumes of the hydrogels. This increased the overall volume swelling ratios of the hydrogels without changing the mass swelling ratios, while only increasing the equilibrium swelling time slightly (2 vs. 10 min).

Scanning electron microscopy (SEM) is a typical method to examine the morphology of dried samples of porous hydrogels. Many investigators examine hydrogels under dehydrated conditions and note that they have fine porous structures that are typically artifacts of drying processes such as freeze-drying. Upon placement in fluid, the polymer network hydrates and no longer contains pores.

CryoSEM techniques have shown that superporous hydrogels have extensive open capillary channels interconnected with each other even when hydrated.[48] SPHs swollen in various solutions with varying pH levels exhibit dramatically different pore dimensions as illustrated in Figure 13.4. Open pore structures can be noted in all pH conditions. No fine structures can be seen in these images since the polymer–water network is complete. Upon removal of water by warming the samples (similar to freeze-drying), a lacy structure can be seen in the network areas via cryoSEM (data not shown). This is due to the collapse of the polymer network and is an artifact of the SEM methodology.

SWELLING KINETICS OF SPHS

The swelling kinetics of SPHs is much faster than that of conventional (nonporous, microporous, and macroporous) hydrogels. SPHs swell to equilibrium size in minutes, while it takes hours or days for conventional hydrogels of equal size to swell to equilibrium. This difference of swelling can be interpreted based on the morphology of these two types of hydrogels. Since the mesh sizes of conventional hydrogels are very small (~10 nm) and mostly closed, the swelling process is predominantly determined by water diffusion through the glassy polymer matrix.

SPHs have very large pore sizes (100 μm to 300 μm) and extensive interconnected capillary channels that make their surfaces accessible to water through capillary effects [Equation (13.3)]. In this equation, the rate of fluid uptake $\delta l/\delta t$ is related to the diameter of the capillary d, surface tension of the liquid γ_l, contact angle between hydrogel and fluid θ, and viscosity of the solution η.[49] The pore structures of SPHs are not completely straight,[45] but it has been stated that even under constricted pore conditions, the general form of this equation holds.[50]

Capillary rise is much faster than the diffusion process, and it can be calculated for materials with low contact angles. The typical time for a 1-cm rise of fluid in a narrow capillary (~100 μm) would be on the order of milliseconds.[48] Following capillary rise, diffusion into the polymer network from the pores must then take place. The diffusive part of fluid transport is similar to the process for conventional hydrogels, but much shorter diffusion distances are present because of the relatively small volume of polymer network in the total volume of the hydrogel.

$$\frac{\partial l}{\partial t} = \frac{d\gamma_l \cos\theta}{8\eta l} \qquad (13.3)$$

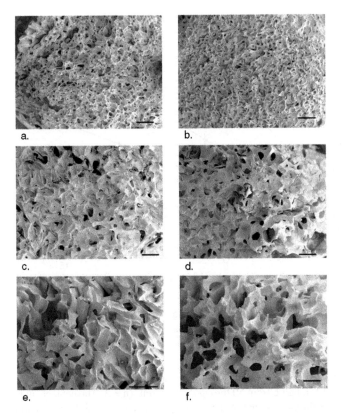

FIGURE 13.4 Scanning electron micrographs of swollen SPHs immersed in buffer solutions of pH 2 (a), 3 (b), 4 (c), 4.5 (d), 5.0 (e), and 7.4 (f) for at least 1 day and examined using cryoSEM. The micrographs were taken at 15× magnification. The scale bar represents 1 mm.

Based on Equation (13.3), the viscosity of the fluid in which a material is swollen has an impact upon the swelling rates of SPHs. For solutions with equivalent ionic contents and ionic strengths and varying viscosities, the swelling rates of SPHs vary dramatically with viscosity (Figure 13.5). The equilibrium swelling times vary from seconds for low viscosity conditions to hours for higher viscosity solutions. The effect of viscosity on the fluid also plays a part in the diffusional process [Equation (13.4)].[31] The frictional component of diffusion in the polymeric network is related to the viscosity of the solutions and inversely related to the square of the mesh size of the network. The cooperative diffusion coefficient is related to the friction coefficient by Equation (13.1). This suggests that the change in viscosity plays a role in both the diffusional and convective transport of the fluid in the porous network, but visual observation attests to the fact that the convective transport of fluid in the hydrogels is significantly slower when viscosity is increased.

$$f \propto \frac{\eta}{\xi^2} \qquad\qquad (13.4)$$

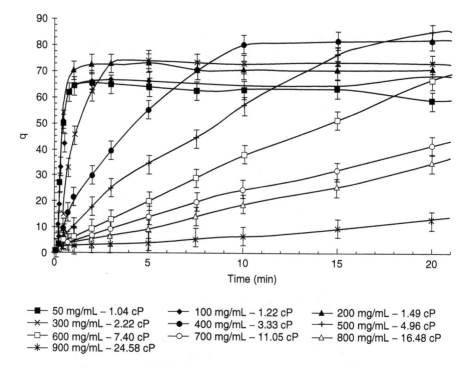

Legend:

- ■ 50 mg/mL – 1.04 cP
- ✕ 300 mg/mL – 2.22 cP
- □ 600 mg/mL – 7.40 cP
- ✳ 900 mg/mL – 24.58 cP
- ◆ 100 mg/mL – 1.22 cP
- ● 400 mg/mL – 3.33 cP
- ○ 700 mg/mL – 11.05 cP
- ▲ 200 mg/mL – 1.49 cP
- ＋ 500 mg/mL – 4.96 cP
- △ 800 mg/mL – 16.48 cP

FIGURE 13.5 Dynamic swelling ratios (q) of superporous hydrogels swollen in sucrose solutions in PBS ranging from 50 through 900 mg/mL (n = 3) The contact angle between the hydrogel and solution was not statistically significant for the different solutions. For each sucrose concentration (mg/mL), the viscosity η (cP) is also presented.

Theoretical analysis and observation were not in perfect agreement in this case. Despite the imperfect fit to capillary rise, the idea that capillary uptake of fluid increases the rate of swelling of SPHs cannot be disputed. Better models that take into account that constricted pore structure may yield a better comparison between theoretical analysis and experimental observation.

ENVIRONMENTALLY SENSITIVE SPHs

Poly(acrylamide-co-acrylic acid) (pAM-AA) SPHs are pH-sensitive and fast swelling.[51] They can swell or collapse with changes of environmental pH due to the presence of carboxyl groups in the polymers. SPHs swollen at a pH of 1.2 and then transferred to a pH of 7.5 swell significantly faster than nonporous hydrogels of similar dimensions. Repeated swelling and deswelling were observed (Figure 13.6). The SPHs swelled at pH 7.5 and then shrank at pH 1.2 in approximately 1 min in either direction; this compared to hours for a similar sized nonporous hydrogel of equivalent composition. CryoSEM studies showed that pore size varied substantially while the SPHs were still hydrated and maintained at various pHs (Figure 13.7). The pore diameter was nearly constant while the pH was raised from 2 to 4, but

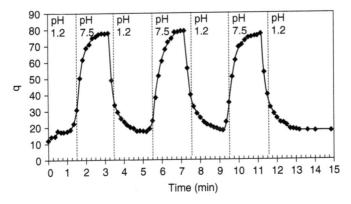

FIGURE 13.6 Swelling of poly(acrylic acid-co-acrylamide) SPH in simulated gastric fluid (SGF; pH, ~1.2) and simulated intestinal fluid (SIF; pH, ~7.5). The SPHs were removed from one solution and inserted in the other solution at the times indicated by the lines ($n = 3$). (From Gemeinhart, R.A. et al., *J. Biomater. Sci. Polym. Ed.*, 11, 1371, 2000. With permission.)

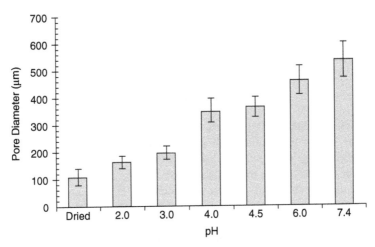

FIGURE 13.7 Pore diameters of swollen poly(acrylic acid-co-acrylamide) SPHs in buffers at different pH levels and equivalent ionic strengths ($n = 3$).

increased dramatically when raised from 4 to 7.4. This was not unexpected since the pK_a of acrylic acid is approximately 4.5.

Poly(n-isopropylacrylamide-co-acrylamide) [p(nIPAAm-AM)] SPHs are temperature-sensitive and have been shown to exhibit rapid swelling characteristics.[44] They showed fast swelling and deswelling kinetics when transferred repeatedly between fluids maintained at 10°C and 65°C. They shrank at 65°C from 36 cm³ to 6.5 cm³ in 72 ± 14 s and swelled to 36 cm³ again when transferred back to 10°C in 78 ± 15 s. The conventional hydrogel did not swell appreciably in 90 s. The lower critical solution temperature (LCST) of the poly(NIPAM-AM) SPHs used in this experiment was determined to be 42°C; this can be controlled by the exact polymer composition as is true with conventional hydrogels.[52] These types of hydrogels have been shown to rapidly respond to their environment in a fashion significantly different from other types of hydrogels. The interconnected pores allow for convective mass transport exterior to the polymer network, thus reduced swelling and deswelling times.

SUMMARY

Many types of hydrogels have been produced in the last half century, but no material has been produced with swelling characteristics similar to the superporous hydrogels developed by Park and coworkers.[43–45,47,51] These materials are capable of rapid swelling from a dehydrated state even when the pore structure is mechanically reduced. Attempts to use other methods of creating porous networks have failed to achieve the rapid swelling possible in SPHs because the porous structures are not present.

Polymer modifications, such as graft copolymers, are insufficient to overcome the slow response due to diffusional limitations as well as polymer relaxation, which is kinetically slow. We have presented basic analyses of hydrogel swelling and some of the methods various investigators have used to increase the swelling and environmental swelling rates for hydrogels. Finally, we presented the concepts of superporous hydrogel production and their use as environmental-sensitive systems.

FUTURE CONSIDERATIONS

Fast swelling hydrogels are being investigated for many biomedical and technology applications. When a material with a large initial and final volume is needed, superporous hydrogels and other hydrogels with large interconnected pores become of particular interest. These materials utilize capillary uptake of fluid that is much more rapid than the diffusion–relaxation phenomena that predominate in nonporous hydrogels. Care must be taken, however, as the mechanical properties of porous hydrogels can be significantly lower than nonporous hydrogels. Methods for improving this quality of porous hydrogels is of particular interest, but must be balanced with ability to swell significantly and rapidly.

Many applications, such as nanoactuators,[22,23,25,53] do not need the large volumes needed for applications such as gastric retention drug delivery devices. The small size allows for sensing even when a porous network is not present. In these applications, the pores would also allow transport of the fluid being analyzed when not desired. For this reason, conventional nonporous hydrogels are optimal, but possible modifications such as graft copolymerization may be desired to increase sensitivity. Care must be taken when determining the type of material desired for a particular application. New ideas, including composite materials, may allow for future materials to be even more sensitive to the external environment, but mass transfer limitations create a need for porous materials when rapid swelling is needed for a large volume of material.

REFERENCES

1. Masuda, F., Trends in the development of superabsorbent polymers for diapers, in *Superabsorbent Polymers*, F.L. Buchholtz and N.A. Peppas, Eds., Chemical Society, Washington, D.C., 1994, pp. 88–98.
2. Wichterle, O. and D. Lim, Hydrophilic gels for biological use, *Nature,* 185, 117, 1960.
3. Matsumaru, Y. et al., Embolic materials for endovascular treatment of cerebral lesions, *J. Biomater. Sci. Polym. Ed.,* 8, 555, 1997.
4. Cummings, J., Microspheres as a drug delivery system in cancer therapy, *Expert Opin. Ther. Patents,* 8, 153, 1998.
5. Park, H. and J.R. Robinson, Mechanisms of mucoadhesion of poly(acrylic acid) hydrogels, *Pharm. Res.,* 4, 457, 1987.
6. Lowman, A.M. et al., Oral delivery of insulin using pH-responsive complexation gels, *J. Pharm. Sci.,* 88, 933, 1999.
7. Tanaka, T., Collapse of gels and critical endpoint, *Phys. Rev. Lett.,* 40, 820, 1978.
8. Frank, S. and P.C. Lauterbur, Voltage-sensitive magnetic gels as magnetic resonance monitoring agents, *Nature,* 363, 334, 1993.
9. Osada, Y., H. Okuzaki, and H. Hori, A polymer gel with electrically driven motility, *Nature,* 355, 242, 1992.
10. Shiga, T. et al., Electric field-associated deformation of polyelectrolyte gel near a phase transition point, *J. Appl. Poly. Sci.,* 46, 635, 1992.
11. Mamada, A. et al., Photoinduced phase transition of gels, *Macromolecules,* 23, 1517, 1990.
12. Suzuki, A., T. Ishii, and Y. Maruyama, Optical switching in polymer gels, *J. Appl. Phys.,* 80, 131, 1996.
13. Suzuki, A. and T. Tanaka, Phase transition in polymer gels induced by visible light, *Nature,* 346, 345, 1990.
14. Andreopoulos, F.M., E.J. Beckman, and A.J. Russell, Light-induced tailoring of PEG-hydrogel properties, *Biomaterials,* 19, 1343, 1998.
15. Zhong, X., Y.X. Wang, and S.C. Wang, Pressure dependence of the volume phase-transition of temperature-sensitive gels, *Chem. Engr. Sci.,* 51, 3235, 1996.
16. Lee, K.K. et al., Pressure-dependent phase transition in hydrogels, *Chem. Eng. Sci.,* 45, 766, 1990.
17. Byrne, M.E., K. Park, and N.A. Peppas, Molecular imprinting within hydrogels, *Adv. Drug Del. Rev.,* 54, 149, 2002.
18. Peppas, N.A. and Y. Huang, Polymers and gels as molecular recognition agents, *Pharm. Res.,* 19, 578, 2002.
19. Watanabe, M. et al., Molecular specific swelling change of hydrogels in accordance with the concentration of guest molecules, *J. Amer. Chem. Soc.,* 120, 5577, 1998.
20. Miyata, T. et al., Preparation of poly(2-glucosyloxyethyl methacrylate) concanavalin: a complex hydrogel and its glucose sensitivity, *Macromol. Chem. Phys.,* 197, 1135, 1996.
21. Miyata, T., N. Asami, and T. Uragami, Preparation of an antigen-sensitive hydrogel using antigen–antibody bindings, *Macromolecules,* 32, 2082, 1999.
22. Van Der Linden, H. et al., Development of stimulus-sensitive hydrogels suitable for actuators and sensors in microanalytical devices, *Sens. Mater.,* 14, 129, 2002.
23. Strong, Z.A., A.W. Wang, and C.F. McConaghy, Hydrogel-actuated capacitive transducer for wireless biosensors, *Biomed. Microdevices,* 4, 97, 2002.
24. Chatterjee, A.N. et al., Mathematical modeling and simulation of dissolvable hydrogels, *J. Aerosp. Eng.,* 16, 55, 2003.

25. Van Der Linden, H.J. et al., Stimulus-sensitive hydrogels and their applications in chemical (micro)analysis, *Analyst,* 128, 325, 2003.

26. Qiu, Y. and K. Park, Environment-sensitive hydrogels for drug delivery, *Adv. Drug Deliv. Rev.,* 53, 321, 2001.

27. Flory, P.J., *Principles in Polymer Chemistry,* Cornell University Press, Ithaca, NY, 1953.

28. Mikos, A.G. and N.A. Peppas, Flory interaction parameter chi for hydrophilic copolymers with water, *Biomaterials,* 10, 95, 1988.

29. Kumagai, H., A. Mizuno, and T. Yano, Analysis of water sorption isotherms of superabsorbent polymers by solution thermodynamics, *Biosci. Biotechnol. Biochem.,* 61, 936, 1997.

30. Li, Y. and T. Tanaka, Kinetics of swelling and shrinking of gels, *J. Chem. Phys.,* 92, 1365, 1990.

31. Tokita, M. and T. Tanaka, Friction coefficient of polymer networks of gels, *J. Chem. Phys.,* 95, 4613, 1991.

32. Tanaka, T. and D.J. Fillmore, Kinetics of swelling gels, *J. Chem. Phys.,* 70, 1214, 1970.

33. Hakiki, A. and J.E. Herz, A study of the kinetics of swelling in cylindrical polystyrene gels: mechanical behavior and final properties after swelling, *J. Chem. Phys.,* 101, 9054, 1994.

34. Tomari, T. and M. Doi, Swelling dynamics of a gel undergoing volume transition, *J. Phys. Soc. Jpn.,* 63, 2093, 1994.

35. Barriere, B. and L. Leibler, Kinetics of solvent absorption and permeation through a highly swellable elastomeric network, *J. Polym. Sci. B Polym. Phys.,* 41, 166, 2003.

36. Peters, A. and S.J. Candau, Kinetics of swelling of spherical and cylindrical gels, *Macromolecules,* 21, 2278, 1988.

37. Annaka, M. et al., Transport properties of comb-type grafted and normal-type n-isopropylacrylamide hydrogel, *Langmuir,* 18, 7377, 2002.

38. Lu, S.J., M.L. Duan, and S.B. Lin, Synthesis of superabsorbent starch graft–poly(potassium acrylate-co-acrylamide) and its properties, *J. Appl. Polym. Sci.,* 88, 1536, 2003.

39. Kaneko, Y. et al., Influence of freely mobile grafted chain length on dynamic properties of comb-type grafted poly(n-isopropylacrylamide) hydrogels, *Macromolecules,* 28, 7717, 1995.

40. Annaka, M. et al., Fluorescence study on the swelling behavior of comb-type grafted poly(n-isopropylacrylamide) hydrogels, *Macromolecules,* 35, 8173, 2002.

41. Serizawa, T. et al., Thermoresponsive properties of porous poly(n-isopropylacrylamide) hydrogels prepared in the presence of nanosized silica particles and subsequent acid treatment, *J. Polym. Sci. Pol. Chem.,* 40, 4228, 2002.

42. Omidian, H. and M.J. Zohuriaan-Mehr, Dsc studies on synthesis of superabsorbent hydrogels, *Polymer,* 43, 269, 2002.

43. Chen, J., H. Park, and K. Park, Synthesis of superporous hydrogels: hydrogels with fast swelling and superabsorbent properties, *J. Biomed. Mater. Res.,* 44, 53, 1999.

44. Chen, J. and K. Park, Superporous hydrogels: fast responsive hydrogel systems, *J. Macromol. Sci Pure Appl. Chem.,* A36, 917, 1999.

45. Gemeinhart, R.A., H. Park, and K. Park, Pore structure of superporous hydrogels, *Polym. Adv. Technol.,* 11, 617, 2000.

46. Dorkoosh, F.A. et al., Preparation and NMR characterization of superporous hydrogels (SPH) and SPH composites, *Polymer,* 41, 8213, 2000.

47. Gemeinhart, R.A., H. Park, and K. Park, Effect of compression on fast swelling of poly(acrylamide-co-acrylic acid) superporous hydrogels, *J. Biomed. Mater. Res.,* 55, 54, 2001.
48. Gemeinhart, R.A., Properties of Superporous Hydrogels for Drug Delivery, Ph.D. thesis, Purdue University, West Lafayette, IN, 1999.
49. Lightfoot, E.N., *Transport Phenomena and Living Systems: Biomedical Aspects of Momentum and Mass Transport,* John Wiley & Sons, New York, 1974.
50. Sharma, R. and D.S. Ross, Kinetics of liquid penetration into periodically constricted capillaries, *J. Chem. Soc. Faraday Trans.,* 87, 619, 1991.
51. Gemeinhart, R.A. et al., pH-sensitivity of fast responsive superporous hydrogels, *J. Biomater. Sci. Polym. Ed.,* 11, 1371, 2000.
52. Kabra, B.G. and S.H. Gehrke, Synthesis of fast response, temperature-sensitive poly(isopropylacrylamide) gel, *Polymer Commun.,* 32, 322, 1991.
53. Selic, E. and W. Borchard, A new apparatus for the characterization of the swelling behavior of micro-gel particles, *Macromol. Chem. Phys.,* 202, 516, 2001.

14 Fast Sliding Motions of Supramolecular Assemblies

Nobuhiko Yui and Tooru Ooya

CONTENTS

INTRODUCTION

Supramolecular chemistry is a highly interdisciplinary field of science that covers chemical, physical, and biological features relating intra- or intermolecular interactions (noncovalent binding). Supramolecular chemistry is still a new area and the study of supramolecular assemblies has progressed as biomimetic and/or bioinspired chemistry such as the design of artificial receptor systems.[1] Recently, molecular motors and machines seen in biological fields have served as models for smart material systems. For example, biological motors are classified as rotary and linear motors; adenosine triphosphate (ATP) synthase is the most aggressive and well studied rotary motor.[2]

Based on these biological molecular machine systems, attempts have been made to create artificial molecular machines and motors in the past decade.[3,4] Clearly, one representative linear motor is a skeletal muscle consisting of a thin filament (actin) and a thick filament (myosin). Actin–myosin sliding action has been extensively studied in the last three decades. Muscle contraction is caused by the sliding of myosin filaments through actin filaments. In terms of synthetic models of the molecular sliding motion, a combination of rings threaded onto the filaments (or rods) displays functional analogy with the myosin–actin complex.

The inclusion complexation between cyclic hosts and lower molecular-weight guests gives us a simple equilibrium equation:

$$[Host] + [Guest] \leftrightarrow [Complex] \tag{14.1}$$

Cyclodextrins, cyclophanes, and calixarenes have been frequently used as host molecules. The driving forces to make the inclusion complexes include hydrophobic interactions, van der Waals interactions, hydrogen bondings and electrostatic interactions. When the guest molecules are linear polymers, some or many cyclic molecules can be threaded onto the linear polymers:

$$m[Host] + [Polymer] \leftrightarrow [(Poly)pseudorotaxane] \tag{14.2}$$

where the polypseudorotaxane is an inclusion complex consisting of cyclic molecules and a linear polymer (Figure 14.1a). Inclusion complexex with bulky blocking groups in which $n-1$ cyclic molecules are threaded (Figure 14.1b) are called [n]-rotaxanes. An [n]-rotaxane consisting of many cyclic molecules is called a polyrotaxane.

These polypseudorotaxanes and [n]-rotaxanes have been recently recognized as *molecular shuttles* or *muscles* because the threading of cyclic molecules (Figure 14.2a) and changing the positions of cyclic molecules in the [n]-rotaxanes (Figure 14.2b) are of special interest in the sliding motion of cyclic molecules due to the noncovalent interactions with linear polymers that may lead to new bases of artificial muscles. This chapter will present an overview of recent progress on the sliding motions of cyclic molecules in both polypseudorotaxanes and [n]-rotaxanes. The dynamics of sliding motion will be summarized from the viewpoints of kinetic theory, stimuli-responsive properties, hydrogel formation, and biorecognition.

THEORETICAL ASPECTS OF SLIDING MOTIONS OF CYCLIC COMPOUNDS ALONG POLYMERIC CHAINS

KINETICS OF POLYPSEUDOPOLYROTAXANE FORMATION
WITH CRYSTALLIZATION

Polypseudorotaxane formation is defined as the inclusion complexation between many cyclic molecules and a linear polymer chain in a certain solvent.[5] Many combinations of cyclic molecules and polymers have been reported.[6] The representative

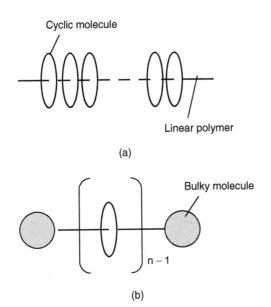

FIGURE 14.1 (a) Polypseudorotaxane; (b) [n]-rotaxane.

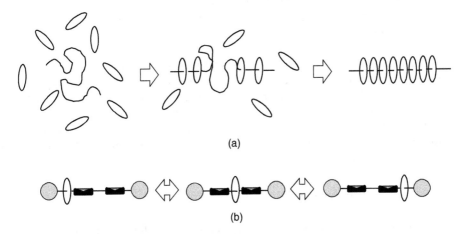

FIGURE 14.2 (a) Threading and sliding processes of cyclic molecules on polypseudorotaxane formation; (b) changing positions of cyclic molecules in [n]-rotaxane.

cyclic molecules are cyclodextrins (CDs) — homochiral cyclic oligosaccharides, most of which are composed of 6, 7, or 8 α-1,4-linked D-glucopyranose units. CDs composed of 6, 7, and 8 glycopyranose units are usually referred to as α-, β- and γ-CDs, respectively.

Polypseudorataxane formation has been extensively studied by Harada et al.,[7,8] Wenz et al.,[9–11] Baglioni et al.,[12–15] and Li et al.[16] Generally, CDs are threaded onto a linear polymer chain in water. Polypseudorotaxanes are often obtained as white

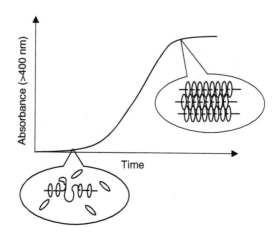

FIGURE 14.3 Relationship between turbidity and time during polypseudorotaxane formation.

crystals after precipitation and filtration from water dispersions. As seen in the Harada's report,[17] this phenomenon includes:

1. Threading of CDs on a linear polymeric chain
2. Sliding of CDs on a polymeric chain
3. Dethreading of CDs from a polymeric chain
4. Precipitation of polypseudorotaxanes due to crystallization (increment in turbidity)

The final process (precipitation) causes an increase in turbidity ($\lambda > 400$ nm) although the other processes are assumed not to increase absorbance (Figure 14.3). The region that does not increase absorbance corresponds to processes 1 through 3 so that the time for this region is defined as *threading time* (t_{th}).[13] Baglioni et al. developed a simple model that attempts to capture the above-mentioned processes[12,14] based on the transition state equation (Eyring theory).[18] They depict polypseudorotaxane formation as a pseudo-first order process:

$$\text{Polymer} + m\text{CD} \leftrightarrow \sigma^* \rightarrow \text{Polypseudorotaxane} \qquad (14.3)$$

where σ^* is the activated complex in polypseudorotaxane formation (rate step) and m is the number of CD molecules that participate in the threading process. From Equation (14.3), the formation of σ^* can be written:

$$\frac{d[\sigma^*]}{dt} = k^*[\sigma^*] = k^* K^{\neq}[Polymer][CD]^m \qquad (14.4)$$

where k^* is the rate constant and $K^{\neq}$ the equilibrium constant. This rate is assumed to be so fast that the polypseudorotaxane is immediately formed after the activation state. Based on the Eyring theory, Equation (14.3) can be written:

$$\frac{d[\sigma^*]}{dt} = \frac{d[Polypseudorotaxane]}{dt} = C[Polymer]_t \tag{14.5}$$

$$C = \frac{k_B T}{h} [CD]^m \exp\left(-\frac{\Delta G^{\neq}}{RT}\right) \tag{14.6}$$

where k_B is the Boltzmann constant (1.38×10^{-23} J/K), T is the absolute temperature (K), h is the Planck constant (6.62×10^{-34} J·s), R is the gas constant (8.31 J·mol^{-1}·K^{-1}), and $\Delta G^{\neq}$ is the Gibbs free energy change of activation (kJ/mol).

Generally, the concentration of CD is in large excess compared to the guest polymer in the preparation of polypseudorotaxane. It is assumed that the CD is not changed after time t. At time t, the concentration of polypseudorotaxane can be written as:

$$[Polypseudorotaxane] = [Polymer]_0 - [Polymer]_t \tag{14.7}$$

where $[Polymer]_0$ and $[Polymer]_t$ are the concentrations of used polymer at times 0 and t, respectively. From this:

$$\frac{d[Polypseudorotaxane]}{dt} = -\frac{d[Polymer]_t}{dt} = C[Polymer]_t \tag{14.8}$$

$$\int_{[Polymer]_0}^{[Polymer]_t} \frac{d[Polymer]}{[Polymer]} = -C \int_0^t dt \tag{14.9}$$

$$\ln\left(\frac{[Polymer]_t}{[Polymer]_0}\right) = -Ct \tag{14.10}$$

taking the $[Polymer]_t < [Polymer]_0$ into account:

$$\ln\left(\frac{[Polymer]_t}{[Polymer]_0}\right) \approx -\left(1 - \frac{[Polymer]_t}{[Polymer]_0}\right) - \frac{1}{2}\left(1 - \frac{[Polymer]_t}{[Polymer]_0}\right)^2 + \ldots\ldots = -Ct \tag{14.11}$$

Therefore,

$$[Polymer]_t = \left(2 - \sqrt{1 + 2Ct}\right)[Polymer]_0 \tag{14.12}$$

After inserting Equation (14.12) into Equation (14.5), the equation can be integrated between 0 and t_{th} when the final concentration of pseudorotaxane is assumed to be the same as $[Polymer]_0$:

$$\int_0^{t_{th}} d[Polypseudorotaxane] = [Polymer]_0 = C[Polymer]_0 \int_0^{t_{th}} \left(2 - \sqrt{1+2Ct}\right)dt \quad (14.13)$$

from which

$$\frac{1}{t_{th}} \approx \frac{3C}{2} = \frac{3k_BT}{2h}[CD]^m \exp\left(-\frac{\Delta G^{\ne}}{RT}\right) \quad (14.14)$$

$$\ln\left(\frac{1}{Tt_{th}}\right) = 24.17 - 2.78m - \frac{\Delta G^{\ne}}{RT} \quad (14.15)$$

Using Equation (14.15) and data of t_{th} values at various temperatures, the value of m and $\Delta G^{\ne}$ can be calculated in order to estimate the threading and sliding processes in various conditions.

KINETICS OF POLYPSEUDOROTAXANE FORMATION WITHOUT CRYSTALLIZATION

When cationic polymers such as protonated poly(iminooligomethylene) and ionenes are used as guest polymers of CDs, polypseudorotaxane formation can be followed in homogeneous condition.[9-11] Since the cationic groups disfavor hydrophobic cavities of CDs,[19] the position of which should be an energetic barrier to sliding on the polymer chain, Wenz et al. proposed a theoretical model in which the real polymer chain is substituted by a one-dimensional periodic potential (Figure 14.4). The inclusion process is controlled by the threading of CDs [Equation (14.16)] sliding along the polymeric chain [Equation (14.17)] and dissociation from the polymeric chain [(Equation (14.18)].[9]

$$-\frac{d[CD]}{dt} = k_f[CD]\frac{2[P]_0}{P_n}(1-Y_1) \quad (14.16)$$

$$-\frac{2[P]_0}{P_n}\frac{dY_i}{dt} = k_{pi}\frac{2[P]_0}{P_n}\{Y_i(1-Y_{i+1}) + Y_i(1-Y_{i-1})\} \quad (14.17)$$

for segment numbers $i = 1$ to $P_n/2$.

$$\frac{d[CD]}{dt} = k_d\frac{2[P]_0}{P_n}Y_1 \quad (14.18)$$

where [CD] is the concentration of free CDs, t is time, $[P]_0$ is the initial concentration of the repeat units of the polymer, P_n is the number average of the degree of

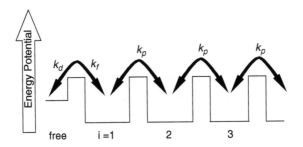

FIGURE 14.4 One-dimensional periodic potential of CD threading process.

polymerization, Y_1 is the relative coverage of the first polymer segment, Y_i is the relative coverage of the ith polymer segment, k_f is the threading rate constant, k_{pi} is the sliding rate constant and k_d is the dissociation rate constant. By using the equations, one can simulate the relative coverage Y vs. time and also determine experimentally the value of Y. This inclusion kinetics is fitted to the function:

$$Y = Y_\infty \left(1 - \exp\left(k_f [P]_0 t\right)\right) \tag{14.19}$$

for a pseudo-first order rate law. The value k_f can be calculated from Equation (14.19) when the time to reach ∞, the rates of threading and dissociation, and $Y_i = Y_\infty$ become equal. Therefore, an equilibrium constant K can be calculated:

$$K = \frac{Y_\infty}{[CD](1 - Y_\infty)} \tag{14.20}$$

Since it can be assumed that $k = k_{pi} = k_d$ and $K = k_f/k$, we can calculate the value of k.

Kinetics of Molecular Shuttles Using [2]- and [3]-Rotaxanes

In 1991, Stoddart et al. first reported a molecular shuttle based on a [2]-rotaxane consisting of a polyether having two hydroquinol "stations" and a bipyridinium ring.[20] In their report, they characterized the shuttling properties using nuclear magnetic resonance (NMR) line shape analysis to estimate exchanging NMR signals associated with the shuttling. This method was based on the method originally reported by Sutherland.[21]

If either of the exchange rates is slow, at least on the NMR time scale, or if the retaining strength on the station is high enough, the signals of some protons attributed to the guest polymer chain should be separated into two chemical shifts. When the exchange rates become much higher, the separated signals coalesce at certain rates. In other words, the material can stay well below the coalescence point. The rate of shuttling at the coalescence point (k_c) is expressed as the following equation:

$$k_c = \frac{\pi(\Delta v)}{2^{1/2}}$$
                                                                            (14.21)

where Δv is the chemical shift difference (Hz) between coalescing signals in the absence of exchange. When the coalescing phenomena are dependent on temperature, temperature at the coalescent point is represented as T_c. By using Eyring equation, the free energy of activation for shuttling ($\Delta G_c^{\neq}$) is given by T_c and k_c:

$$\Delta G^{\neq} = -RT_c \ln\left(\frac{k_c h}{k_B T_c}\right)$$
                                                                            (14.22)

where R, h, and k_B correspond to the gas, Planck, and Bolzmann constants, respectively.

THREADING AND SLIDING OF CYCLODEXTRINS ON POLYPSEUDOROTAXANE FORMATION

"THREADING TIMES" OF CYCLODEXTRINS ONTO VARIOUS GUEST POLYMERS

Cyclodextrins form polypseudorotaxanes with various guest polymers such as alkanes,[22] ethers,[23] amines,[24] polypeptides,[25] esters,[26,27] and siloxanes[28,29] in water. The driving forces of the polypseudorotaxane formation involve hydrophobic interactions[24] and hydrogen bonds between hydroxyl groups on adjacent CDs (Figure 14.5).[30] As mentioned in the section on kinetics of polypseudopolyrotaxanes with crystallization, the threading time t_{th} onto a polymeric chain involves the processes of threading, sliding, and dethreading of CDs (Figure 14.3).

Generally, large amount of CDs are required because the processes are in equilibrium with the solution. The t_{th} values of polypseudorotaxane formation are in the range of 20 to 2400 s, depending on the chemical structures of the guest polymers (Table 14.1). The $\Delta G_c^{\neq}$ values calculated using Equation (14.15) are negative except for α-CD/PPG-PEG-PPG systems.[16] The positive $\Delta G_c^{\neq}$ values indicate that α-CD molecules must overcome the first energy barrier (PPG segments) of threading and sliding processes to form a stable polypseudorotaxane.

The threading time may be modulated by some preparative conditions. Significant increases in t_{th} were observed when temperature increased.[12] Free energy change ($\Delta G^{\neq}$) can be calculated using the Equation (14.15). Both enthalpy ($\Delta H^{\neq}$) and entropy ($\Delta S^{\neq}$) can be calculated by changing temperature using the following equation:

$$\Delta G^{\neq} = \Delta H^{\neq} - T\Delta S^{\neq}$$

Both $\Delta H^{\neq}$ and $\Delta S^{\neq}$ values decrease with increasing temperature, indicating that the sliding process is driven by the enthalpic factor. Concentrations of CDs and polymers are other factors. The higher the concentrations of CDs and guest polymers with fixing CD/polymer ratios, the shorter the t_{th}.[12]

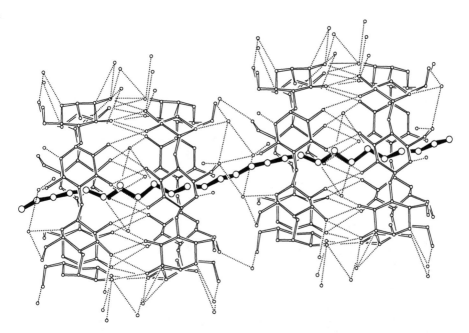

FIGURE 14.5 Crystal structures of inclusion complexes of β-cyclodextrin with poly(trime-thylene oxide). Intermolecular hydrogen bonds are shown as dotted lines. Solvent molecules that form direct hydrogen bonds with β-CDs are shown as open circles with hydrogen bonds. See Reference 30.

The sliding process is apparently favored when the initial concentrations of CDs and polymers become higher. In addition to the effect of temperature and whole concentrations, water structure is also effective for controlling t_{th}. Heavy water (D_2O) forms stronger hydrogen bonding and is a more strongly associating liquid than light water (H_2O). This nature of D_2O produces much stronger hydrophobic interactions and dissolves small nonpolar molecules much better than H_2O.[31]

Nostro et al. reported that the addition of D_2O to H_2O decreased t_{th} of polyp-seudorotaxane formation.[13] Similar effects were observed when sugars such as D-sucrose are added to water.[15] Sugars are known to act as water structure makers and to strength hydrogen bond networks as well as D_2O. Interestingly, the order of decreasing t_{th} is related to an isomer of sugar. Urea is a water structure breaker and weakens hydrophobic effects,[32] which increase over a certain concentration.[15]

Therefore, the sliding process is apparently related to the hydrogen bonding network in water, which depends on the specific sugar isomer and on specific chiral discrimination of CDs. Salts, related to the nature of cations and anions, significantly affected t_{th}. In the case of β-CD/PPG systems, positive ions can interact with donor oxygen atoms of PPG chains and partially displace water of hydration from the PPG chains. The least hydrophilic anions can diffuse from aqueous environment and induce surface charge perturbations that push the PPG chain to thread more easily the hydrophobic cavities of β-CD.

TABLE 14.1

Threading Times and $\Delta G^{\ddagger}$ Values of CDs on Polymeric Chains in Water at 298 K

Guest Polymer		Concentration of Guest Polymer (mg/ml)	Type of Cyclodextrin (Concentration)	Threading Number, m	t_{th} (s)	$\Delta G^{\ddagger}$ (kJ/mol)	Ref.
Type	Molecular Weight						
Poly(ethylene glycol) (PEG)	3350	3.66	α-CD (60.0 mg/ml)	20	200	−53.7	15
Poly(ethylene glycol) (PEG)	8000	6.32	α-CD (85.8 mg/ml)	31	24	−101.5	15
Poly(propylene glycol) bis-2-aminopropyl ether (PPGBA)	2000	0.15	β-CD (9.50 mg/ml)	16	209	−104.4	15
Dimethoxy-poly(ethylene glycol) (DMPG)	2000	3.34	α-CD (47.7 mg/ml)	15	53	−46.0	15
PEG-PPG-PEG triblock copolymer	PEG: 1500 × 2 PPG: 3500	0.95	γ-CD (25.2 mg/ml)	19	60	−101.7	15
PPG-PEG-PPG triblock copolymer	PEG: 1000 PPG: 460 × 2	6.5	α-CD (126 mg/ml)	11[a]	60	8.37[b]	16
PPG-PEG-PPG triblock copolymer	PEG: 1050 PPG: 870 × 2	6.5	α-CD (126 mg/ml)	11[a]	240	11.8[b]	16
PPG-PEG-PPG triblock copolymer	PEG: 525 PPG: 1450 × 2	6.5	α-CD (126 mg/ml)	6[a]	2400	51.9[b]	16

[a] Using number determined by ^{1}H-NMR spectroscopy.
[b] Calculated using Equation (14.15) based on results in each reference.

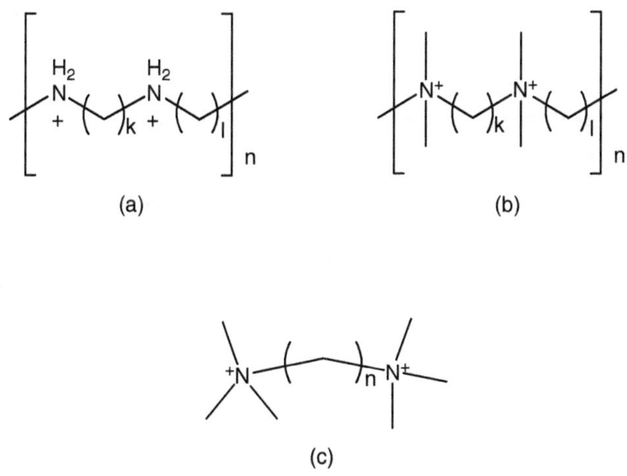

FIGURE 14.6 Various cationic guest polymers for polypseudorotaxane formation with α-CD. (a) Poly(iminooligomethylene)s; (b) inonenes-6,10; and (c) N, N, N, N', N', N'-hexamethyl-1,10-diaminodecane.

SLOW SLIDING OF CYCLODEXTRIN ONTO CATIONIC POLYMERS

When cationic charges and/or methyl groups are located on a guest polymer, they act as barriers for the sliding of cyclodextrins.[9–11] Poly(iminooligomethylene)s (a), inonenes-6,10 (b), and N,N,N,N',N',N'-hexamethyl-1,10-diaminodecane (c) as a monomeric model of (b) were investigated as guest polymers for polypseudorotaxane formation with α-CD (Figure 14.6). From the results of ^{1}H-NMR spectroscopy of an aqueous solution of α-CD and guest cationic polymers, new separate signals arose due to polypseudorotaxane formation.

Signals of internal protons of α-CD (H-3 and H-5) shifted upfield and those of methylene protons of the guest polymers shifted upfield and downfield, respectively. Since the chemical shifts of the new signals did not depend on the concentrations of both components, the threading and sliding steps had to be slow on the NMR time scale. From the peak integration of the shifted peaks, yield of polypseudorotaxane based on α-CD (Y) could be calculated. At a certain time, Y reached maximum values, at which the polypseudorotaxane formation was in an equilibrium state (Y_∞). By using Equation (14.19), the threading rate constant (k_f) could be calculated (Table 14.2).

The Y_∞ value of (a) did not reach 100%, indicating that protonated imonogroups actually act as energy barriers. The lengths of methylene chains in poly(iminooligomethylene)s also affect sliding time: smaller segments of poly(iminooligomethylene)s cannot slide α-CD molecules until both nitrogens in one repeating unit are deprotonated before they can move to the next segment.[9] Trimethylammonium groups in (c) decreased k_f compared with (a) (see Table 14.2). The activation energy of threading determined from temperature dependence of k_f, is 63.4 kJ/mol.[11] This high activation energy is likely due to the steric repulsion between the bulky trimethylammonium group and the cavity size of α-CD. In the similar energy barrier

TABLE 14.2
α-CD Threading Rates and Times to Reach Equilibrium State
of Polypseudorotaxanation and Various Cationic Guest Polymers
in D$_2$O at pD 6.7 and 298 K

Guest Polymers[a]	M_n	Y_∞ (%)[b]	Time to Reach Y_∞ (min)	k_f (10^{-2} s^{-1} M^{-1})[c]	Ref.
Poly (iminooligomethylene)	5,800	48	~180	116[d]	9
N, N, N, N', N', N'-hexamethyl-1,10-diaminodecane	258	98	~50	3.6	11
Inonene-6,10	34,000	55	~1.05 × 10^6 (~2 years)	0.31	11

[a] Chemical structures are shown in Figure 14.6.
[b] The limited value of yield (based on α-CD).
[c] Threading rate constant.
[d] Calculated from data of yield in reference.

mechanism, the k_f of the polymeric form of (c), inonene-6,10 (b), is much smaller than (a). Surprisingly, it took 2 years to reach an equilibrium state of polypseudo-rotaxane formation at room temperature. The number of energy barriers for threading may be important to control threading and sliding speed.

SHUTTLING MOTION OF A CYCLIC COMPOUND ALONG A LINEAR CHAIN IN [2]- AND [3]-ROTAXANES

PRINCIPLE OF SHUTTLING MOTION

One of the characteristic features of rotaxanes is the movement of cyclic molecules (beads) in the interrlocked structure. The first concept of a *molecular shuttle* using [2]-rotaxanes was produced by Stoddart et al.[20] The beads were expected to move back and forth like shuttles between two or more groups (stations) in the rotaxanes. Several research groups have designed [2]- or [3]-rotaxanes aimed at molecular shuttling in solution and kinetically characterized using NMR spectroscopy (Table 14.3).[19–20,33–36]

In order to synthesize rotaxanes for molecular shuttles in high yields, template action between the beads and the station is generally utilized and includes electrostatic pole–dipole attractions, dispersive forces such as π/π stacking, and charge–transfer interactions.[37] Those attractive forces must be eliminated if one wants to shuttle the beads between stations. By using external stimuli such as temperature and solvent exchange, the beads can move along the polymeric chain with solvating. Stoddart et al. designed the first molecular shuttle consisting of a polyether chain that had two hydroquinone rings (molecular station) and a macrocycle with bipyridium units terminated by two triisopropylsilylether groups.[20] In a ^{1}H-NMR spectrum of

TABLE 14.3
Shuttling Properties of [2]- and [3]-Rotaxanes

Components of molecular shuttle		Interaction at the station	Driving force for shuttling	Solvents	k_c (sec⁻¹)	T_c (°C)	$\Delta G^\#$ (kcal/mol)	Ref.
Cyclic molecule	Guest polymer having station							
		π-π stacking, charge transfer interactions	Temperature	Acetone	2360	34	13	20
		Electrostatic pole-dipole attraction	Temperature	DMSO CH$_2$Cl$_2$ Acetone CH$_3$NO$_2$	62~182	-56~150	10~21	34
		Electrostatic pole-dipole attraction	Temperature	DMSO	105	127	20	36
		Hydrogen bonds	Solvents	DMSO CHCl$_3$ [CHCl$_3$+ CH$_3$OH]	5200~62000 [>3 million]	-70~25	11~12 [2.1~2.3]	35
		Repulsive force between an α-CD and a linker	Temperature	DMSO Water	80	130	20	19

the [2]-rotaxane in CD_3COCD_3, chemical shifts attributed to hydroquinone rings of the polymer backbone merged with the baseline at ambient temperature.

On the other hand, the proton was separated into two peaks attributed to the "unoccupied" and "occupied" hydroquinone rings at $-50°C$. The observed two peaks indicate that the site exchange was slower than the NMR time scale and became faster with increasing temperature. The two peaks on the ${}^1H$-NMR spectrum coalesced. In similar manner, shuttling motions of [2]- and [3]-rotaxanes based on a dibenzo[24]-crown-8 macrocycle and a polymer backbone having dialkylammonium ions was observed in various organic solvents (Table 14.3).[36] Electrostatic pole–dipole attractiond and hydrogen bonds between $-CH_2NH_2^+CH_2-$ and ether oxygen of the macrocyle were responsible for the self-assembly. Temperature can also eliminate the noncovalent bonds to show the shuttling motion.

Another principle of molecular shuttle is to control hydrogen bonds at the station and/or repulsive force between a cyclic molecule and a linker. Leigh et al. synthesized peptide-based [2]-rotaxanes, condensing appropriate aromatic diacid chlorides and benzylic diamines with dipeptide derivatives.[35] The dipeptide moiety, Gly–Gly, templates the formation of benzylic amide macrocyles around them. Hydrogen bonding between the macrocycles and peptide linkages is maintained in nonpolar solvents such as $CHCl_3$.

In the polar solvents, the intramolecular hydrogen bonding is switched off, resulting in nonspecific location of macrocycles along the backbone. Molecular shuttling utilizing a combination of hydrogen bonding and donor–acceptor interaction was achieved in both nonpolar and polar solvents.[36] Harada et al. prepared an α-CD-based molecular shuttle containing energetically favored and disfavored portions.[19] Both hydrophobic interaction between an α-CD ring and a station and a repulsive force between an α-CD ring and a linker were utilized for controlling shuttling behavior.

CONTROLLING SHUTTLING RATES

The shuttling rates are usually estimated by k_c using Equation (14.21), and the representative k_c values are summarized in Table 14.3. When the intramolecular interaction between the station and the macrocycles is electrostatic pole–dipole attraction, the order of magnitude of k_c is $10-10^2$ s^{-1}. In these cases, a temperature increase is needed to eliminate the dibenzo[24]-crown-8 macrocycle with 10 to 20 kcal/mol of the free energy of activation for shuttling ($\Delta G_c^{\neq}$).

Since the spacer part of the linear backbone is usually an alkyl chain or aromatic rings, the electrostatic pole–dipole attraction does not exist in organic solvents. Therefore, the only factor to control the shuttling motion should be the electrostatic –pole–dipole attraction. On the other hand, the order of magnitude of k_c is 10^4 s^{1} when the interaction at the station is based on π–π stacking (Table 14.3). The solvation of acetone, a good solvent for the macrocycle, is preferable to the shuttling motion. By changing solvents, the shuttling rate can be controlled in some cases as seen in [2]-rotaxane consisting of a benzylic amide macrocyle with dipeptide derivative (Table 14.3). The solvent-dependent translation isomerism of the peptide-based [2]-rotaxane is characterized by chemical shifts on ${}^1H$-NMR spectra in DMSO-d_6, CDCl$_3$, and CD$_2$Cl$_2$/CD$_3$OD.[35]

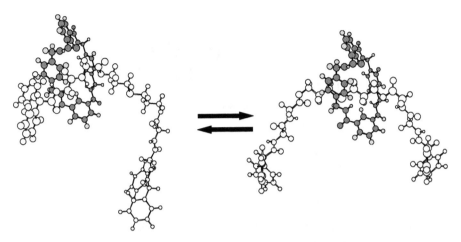

FIGURE 14.7 Sliding image of macrocycle between two peptide stations.

In response to those changes in the polarity of the environment, the macrocyle changes position due to the mechanisms of formation and elimination of hydrogen bonding. The addition of small quantities of CD_3OD to the [2]-rotaxane dissolved in CD_2Cl_2 partially eliminates the intramolecular hydrogen bonding, decreasing $\Delta G_c^{\neq}$ and speeding the sliding of the macrocycle between the two peptide stations (Figure 14.7). For example, in 5% CD_3OD/CD_2Cl_2 at room temperature, $\Delta G_c^{\neq}$ is 2.1 to 2.3 kcal/mol and k_c is 62,000 to more than 3 million s^{-1}.

When [2]-rotaxane consists of α-CD and a dodecamethylene–bipyridinium copolymer (2:1 unit ratio), the shuttling motion can be controllable by either solvent or temperature.[19] The k_c levels at 130 and 30°C in dimethyl sulfoxide (DMSO)-d_6 are 80 and 0.015 s^{-1}, respectively. On the other hand, the site exchange is much slower in D_2O than in DMSO-d_6. Increasing temperature in D_2O did not change the splitting peak attributed to dodecamethylene peaks on a ^{1}H-NMR spectrum, indicating that α-CD ring stays at one of dodecamethylene stations on the NMR time scale.

STIMULI-RESPONSE SLIDING OF CYCLIC COMPOUNDS ALONG A POLYMERIC CHAIN IN ROTAXANES AND POLYROTAXANES

As mentioned earlier, the threading and sliding of cyclic molecules on polypseudo-rotaxane formation processes are dependent on the concentrations of the cyclic molecules. After capping both ends of linear polymeric chains in the polypseudo-rotaxanes, the threading of the cyclic molecules from the medium is impossible. However, the cyclic molecules in the polyrotaxanes can slide if the positions of the cyclic molecules are changeable by attractive or repulsive interactions between the cyclic molecules and the linear polymeric chains in rotaxanes and polyrotaxanes.

Nakashima et al. proposed a light-responsive rotaxane.[38] They synthesized a photoswitchable rotaxane consisting of α-CD, azobenzene, and 2,4-dinitrobenzene

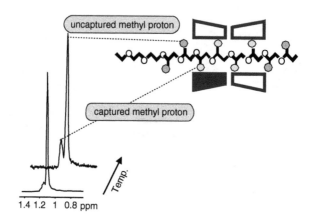

FIGURE 14.8 ^{1}H-NMR peak split attributed to captured and uncaptured PPG segments of triblock copolymer by β-CD.

groups. The photoswitchable function was characterized by ultraviolet–visual (UV–VIS) spectroscopy, circular dichroism, and nuclear Overhauser effect (NOE) differential spectroscopies. Before photoirradiation, a positive-induced ICD band at 360 nm and a negative ICD band at 430 nm assigned to $\pi-\pi*$ and n-$\pi*$ transitions, respectively, were observed in an aqueous solution. The positive ellipticity indicated that the long axis polarized transitions of arene guests parallel to the axis of the α-CD cavity. These results suggest that the azobenzene group is captured by α-CD. After UV irradiation, the positive ICD at 360 nm decreased. The results of NOE spectra after UV irradiation suggest that α-CD exists at methylene spacer parts in the rotaxanes. This photoswitching is reversible.

Controlling hydrophobic interaction between CD cavities and polymeric chains in a polyrotaxane is a prompt way to change the localization of CDs in the polyrotaxane.[39,40] Temperature is a good model of a physical stimulus to control the hydrophobic interaction. Yui et al. synthesized thermoresponsive polyrotaxanes, in which β-CDs were threaded on a triblock copolymer of poly(ethylene glycol) (PEG) and poly(propylene glycol) (PPG) capped with fluorescein-4-isothiocyanate (FITC). β-CDs can form polypseudorotaxanes with PPG but not PEG in aqueous conditions,[41,42] so that PEG segment of the triblock copolymer was considered to be exposed to the aqueous medium.[43] With an increase in temperature of an alkaline solution containing the thermoresponsive polyrotaxanes, a ^{1}H-NMR peak attributed to PG units split and changed the relative peak area. This peak split suggests that two states of PPG segments exist in the NMR time scale: PGs captured and uncaptured by β-CDs (Figure 14.8).

From the relative peak area, the number of β-CDs on the PPG segment was calculated. It was found that 70 to 80% of β-CDs in the polyrotaxanes were localized on the PPG station at 40°C, although β-CDs were dispersed on the triblock copolymer at 20°C (Figure 14.8). The enhanced hydrophobic interaction between the β-CD cavity and the PPG segment at higher temperature should be a dominant driving force to change the localization of β-CDs in the polyrotaxane.

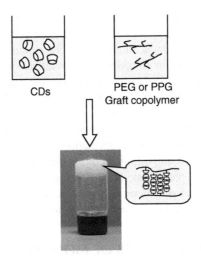

FIGURE 14.9 Hydrogel formation caused by mixing α-CD saturated aqueous solution and aqueous solution of PEG or PPG graft copolymer.

SLIDING OF CYCLIC COMPOUNDS IN HYDROGEL FORMATION

Generally, the polypseudorotaxane formation of cyclodextrins and water-soluble polymers such as PEG leads to precipitation due to crystalline structure of the polypseudorotaxane as mentioned earlier. Even when multiarm PEGs with relatively lower molecular weights (1000 to 7400) are used as guest molecules for CDs, the obtained polypseudorotaxanes are crystalline.[44] This means that most of the PEG chains should be captured by CDs, indicating no ethylene glycol units for hydration.

However, with increases in the molecular weight of PEG and the concentrations of PEG and CDs, the polypseudorotaxane formation leads to a hydrogel.[45] Aqueous solutions of α-CDs and PEG with molecular weights above 2000 form hydrogels rather than crystalline complexes. There are both complexed and uncomplexed α-CDs in the hydrogels — as confirmed by powder x-ray diffraction pattern. The percentage of uncomplexed α-CDs decreased with the increasing molecular weight of PEG. Therefore, the complexed fraction of α-CD–PEG aggregated as well as the crystalline complex of α-CD and PEG with a lower molecular weight and acted as a crosslinking point in the hydrogels.

Polypseudorotaxane formation of CDs and PEG or PPG grafted to polysaccharides resulted in hydrogel formation (Figure 14.9).[46,47] Threading α-CDs onto PEG-grafted dextran produced a crystalline domain and an α-CD–PEG inclusion complex, but the dextran backbone was uncomplexed with α-CDs and easily hydrated. The hydrogels exhibited transition from gel to sol with an incease in temperature. The gel–sol transition was based on the threading and dethreading of α-CDs, and the transition was reversible with hysteresis. The transition temperature was controllable by variation in the concentration and the PEG content in the graft copolymers as well as the stoichiometric ratio between the guest and host molecules.

In a similar manner, supramolecular-structured hydrogels were prepared by mixing PPG-grafted dextrans with β-CDs. These hydrogels also showed a thermoreversible sol–gel transition induced by reversible supramolecular assembly and dissociation. The induction time for gelation was relatively short, and varied depending on the concentrations or feed ratios of the host and guest molecules.

Another type of hydrogel based on polypseudorotaxane formation resulted from a combination of Pluronics (triblock copolymers of PEG–PPG–PEG) and α-CDs.[48] Aqueous solutions containing 13 wt% Pluronics and 9.7 wt% of α-CD turned into viscous gels at 22°C. However, the gel formation was not observed at 4°C. Micelle formation of Pluronic was important in the hydrogel formation. At the elevated temperature (22°C), hydrophobic interaction between the PPG segments of Pluronics facilitated the formation of polymeric networks. At 4°C, the interaction between the PPG segments was weak and the micelle tended to dissociate.[49]

BIOLOGICAL ASPECTS OF MOLECULAR SLIDING IN POLYROTAXANES

The most characteristic structure of polyrotaxanes consisting of α-CDs and PEG is that all the α-CDs are mechanically locked by the PEG chains and each α-CD is expected to slide[12] and rotate along a PEG chain. This dynamic feature may affect intermolecular interactions between CDs and biological components, mimicking a combination of DNA and DNA polymerase. Recently, Yui et al. designed a CD movement-based molecular recognition system using polyrotaxanes.[50] They found that ligand–polyrotaxane conjugates, in which many ligands were covalently bound to α-CDs, recognized those binding proteins in a multivalent manner.[51–53]

They also investigated how α-CDs and ligand mobility in ligand–polyrotaxane conjugates affected multivalent interactions with binding proteins using maltose and concanavalin A (Con A) as the ligand and binding protein, respectively.[50] Three types of maltose–polyrotaxane conjugates were synthesized by a condensation reaction between β-maltosylamine and carboxyethylester-polyrotaxanes[54] in the presence of benzotriazol-1-yl-oxy-tris(dimethylamino) phosphonium hexafluorophosphate (BOP) reagent and 1-hydroxybenzotriazole (HOBt) (Figure 14.10).

The stoichiometric number of an α-CD is generally defined as the number of α-CDs when two ethylene glycol units are included in each α-CD cavity. From the stoichiometric number, the α-CD threading percents are calculated as 22, 38, and 53%, respectively.

The effects of mechanically locked structures in the maltose–polyrotaxane conjugates on multivalent interactions were assessed using a Con A-induced hemagglutination inhibition assay. The maltose-polyrotaxane conjugates inhibited Con A-induced hemmaglutination and the extent became greater with the number of maltose groups in the polyrotaxane. This result was consistent with the multivalent effects in terms of increasing the number of saccharide groups conjugated with polymeric backbones. However, the extent of the inhibition varied with the threading percents of α-CDs in the conjugates. The polyrotaxanes with α-CD threading of 38% exhibited much greater inhibitory effects than any other conjugates examined and the

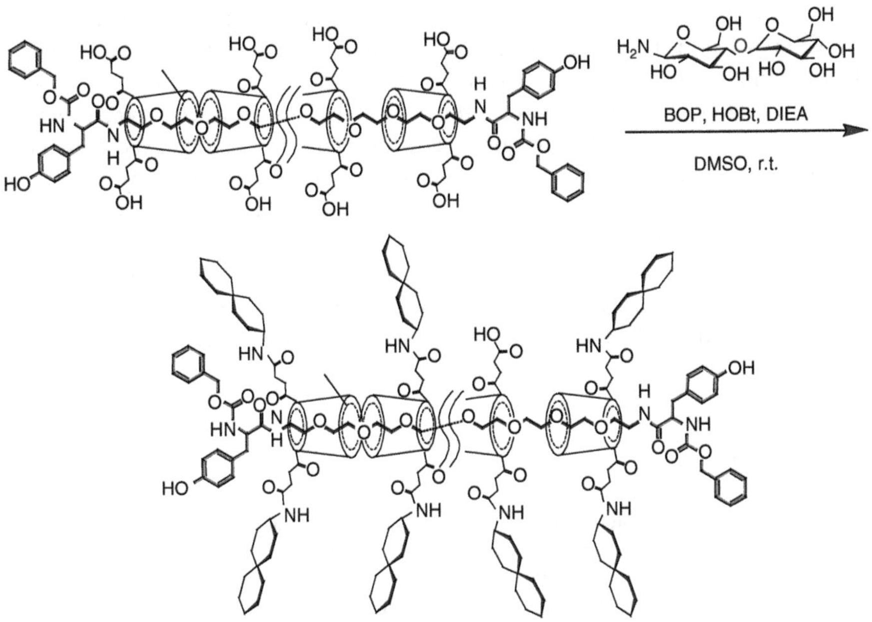

FIGURE 14.10 Synthetic scheme of maltose–polyrotaxane conjugates.

relative potency of the inhibitory effect was over 3000 times as high as the potency of maltose alone.

A ^{1}H-NMR signal of the maltose-polyrotaxane conjugates with the 38% α-CD threading was very sharp although those of the other conjugates with higher (53%) and lower (22%) α-CD threadings were broader. The sharpening may have been due to the high mobility of maltose-introduced α-CDs in the mechanically locked structure of the polyrotaxane backbone that has shorter correlation time. The spin–spin relaxation time (T_2) of C(1)H (δ, 5.1 ppm) of maltose groups in the conjugates with the 38% α-CD threading was much longer (0.23 s) than the times of the 53% (0.08 s) and 22% (0.12 s) compounds. In addition, the conjugates with the 38% α-CD threading exhibited almost the same T_2 as maltose-induced α-CD (0.24 s). This finding strongly suggests that the mobility of maltose groups along polyrotaxane backbones including their sliding and rotation along the PEG chain contributes much to enhancing binding with Con A.

CONCLUDING REMARKS

The sliding motion observed in polypseudorotaxane formation, stimuli-responsive [2]-rotaxanes, and polyrotaxanes is recognized as a dynamic function of supramolecular materials. As described in this chapter, the most important point to achieve fast sliding motion is to control intramolecular interaction between cyclic molecules and linear polymer chains, including π–π stacking, electrostatic pole–dipole attraction, hydrogen bonding, and hydrophobic interaction.

In typical cases, the strong intramolecular interactions in polypseudorotaxane formation result in crystallization that could be utilized to form hydrogels. Reducing the crystallinity of polyrotaxanes by some chemical modification provides another idea for developing polyrotaxanes for biomedical devices. However, some technical hurdles in terms of fast sliding in aqueous conditions must still be resolved. Researchers are now trying to design supramolecular assemblies and directly detect the molecular motion of fast sliding. Development of analytical methods such as cross-saturation NMR,[55] coldspray ionization mass,[56] light scattering, and stopped-flow[57] spectroscopies will enable us to obtain *in situ* data of supramolecular complexes without chemical labeling. Therefore, more detailed fast sliding in supramolecular materials system will be found and lead to designs of supramolecular assemblies as artificial muscles.

REFERENCES

1. Percec, V. and Holerca, M.N., Detecting the shape change of complex macromolecules during their synthesis with the aid of kinetics: a new lesson from biology, *Biomacromolecules*, 1, 6–16, 2000.
2. Noji, H., Yasuda, R., Yoshida, M., and Kinoshita, K., Direct observation of the rotation of F1-ATPase, *Nature*, 386, 299–302, 1997.
3. Balzani, V., Gómez-López, M., and Stoddart, J.F., Molecular machines, *Acc. Chem. Res.*, 31, 405–414, 1998.
4. Sqauvage, J.P., Transition metal-containing rotaxanes and catenanes in motion: toward molecular machines and motors, *Acc. Chem. Res.*, 31, 611–619, 1998.
5. Gibson, H.W., Liu, S., Lecavalier, P., Wu, C., and Shen, Y.X., Synthesis and preliminary characterization of some polyester rotaxanes, *J. Am. Chem. Soc.*, 117, 852–874, 1995.
6. Yui, N. and Ikeda, T., Interlocked molecules, in *Supramolecular Design for Biological Applications*, Yui, N., Ed., CRC Press, Boca Raton, FL, 2002, pp. 137–165.
7. Harada, A. and Kamachi, M., Complex formation between poly(ethylene glycol) and α-cyclodextrin, *Macromolecules*, 23, 2821–2833, 1999.
8. Harada, A., Preparation and structures of supermolecules between cyclodextrins and polymers, *Coord. Chem. Rev.*, 148, 115, 1996.
9. Wenz, G. and Keller, B., Speed control for cyclodextrin rings on polymer chains, *Macromol. Symp.*, 87, 11–16, 1994.
10. Weickenmeir, M. and Wenz, G., Threading of cyclodextrins onto a polyester of octanedicarboxylic acid and polyethylene glycol, *Macromol. Rapid. Commun.*, 18, 1109–1115, 1997.
11. Herrmann, W., Keller, B., and Wenz, G., Kinetics and thermodynamics of the inclusion of ionene-6,10 in α-cyclodextrin in an aqueous solution, *Macromolecules*, 30, 4966–4972, 1997.
12. Ceccato, M., Nostro, P.L., and Baglioni, P., α-Cyclodextrin/polyethylene glycol polyrotaxanes: a study of the threading process, *Langmuir*, 13, 2436–2439, 1997.
13. Nostro, P.L., Lopes, J.R., and Cardelli, C., Formation of cyclodextrin-based polypseudororaxanes: solvent effect and kinetic study, *Langmuir*, 17, 4610–4615, 2001.
14. Nostro, P.L., Lopes, J.R., Ninham, B.W., and Baglioni, P., Effects of cations and anions on the formation of polypseudorotaxanes, *J. Phys. Chem. B*, 106, 2166–2174, 2002.

15. Becheri, A., Nostro, P.L., Ninham, B.W., and Baglioni, P., The curious world of polypseudorotaxanes: cyclodextrins as probes of water structure, *J. Phys. Chem. B,* 107, 3979–3987, 2003.

16. Li, J., Ni, X., Zhou, Z., and Leong, K.W., Preparation and characterization of polypseudorotaxanes based on block-selected inclusion complexation between poly(propylene oxide)-poly(ethylene oxide)-poly(propylene oxide) triblock copolymers and α-cyclodextrin, *J. Am. Chem. Soc.,* 125, 1788–1795, 2003.

17. Harada, A. and Kamachi, M., Complex formation between poly(ethylene glycol) and α-cyclodextrin, *Macromolecules,* 23, 2821–2823, 1990.

18. Laidler, K.Y., *Chemical Kinetics,* McGraw Hill, New York, 1965.

19. Kawaguchi, Y. and Harada, A., A cyclodextrin-based molecular shuttle containing energetically favored and disfavored portions in its dumbbell component, *Org. Lett.,* 2, 1353–1356, 2000.

20. Anelli, P.L., Spencer, N., and Stoddart, J.F., A molecular shuttle, *J. Am. Chem. Soc.,* 113, 5131–5133, 1991.

21. Sutherland, I.O., The investigation of the kinetics of conformational changes by nuclear magnetic resonance spectroscopy, *Annu. Rep. NMR Spectrosc.,* 4, 71–235, 1971.

22. Harada, A. and Okada, M., Complex formation between hydrophobic polymers and methylated cyclodextrins. oligo(ethylene) and poly(propylene) *Polym. J.,* 31, 1095–1096, 1999.

23. Harada, A., Okada, M., and Kamachi, M., Preparation and characterization of inclusion complexes of poly(alkyl vinyl ether) with cyclodextrins, *Bull. Chem. Soc. Jpn.,* 71, 535–542, 1998.

24. Wenz, G., Cyclodextrins as building blocks for supramolecular structures and functional units, *Angew. Chem. Int. Ed. Engl.,* 33, 803–822, 1994.

25. Huh, K.M., Tomita, H., Ooya, T., Lee, W.K., and Sasaki, S., pH dependence of inclusion complexation between cationic poly(ε-lysine) and α-cyclodextrin, *Macromolecules,* 35, 3775–3777, 2002.

26. Shin, I.D., Huang, L., and Tonelli, A.E., NMR observation of the conformations and motions of polymers confined to the narrow channels of their inclusion compounds, *Macromol. Symp.,* 138, 21–40, 1999.

27. Lu, J., Mirau, P.A., and Tonelli, A.E., Dynamics of isolated polycaprolactone chains in their inclusion complexes with cyclodextrins, *Macromolecules,* 34, 3276–3284, 2001.

28. Okumura, H., Okada, M., Kawaguchi, Y., and Harada, A., Complex formation between poly(dimethylsiloxane) and cyclodextrins: new *pseudo*-polyrotaxanes containing inorganic polymers, *Macromolecules,* 33, 4297–4298, 2000.

29. Porbeni, F.E., Edeki, E.M., Shin, I.D., and Tonelli, A.E., Formation and characterization of the inclusion complexes between poly(dimethylsiloxane) and polyacrylonitrile with γ-cyclodextrin, *Polymer,* 42, 6907–6912, 2001.

30. Kamitori, S., Matsuzaka, O., Kondo, S., Muraoka, S., Okuyama, K., Noguchi, K., Okada, M., and Harada, A., A Novel pseudo-polyrotaxane structure composed of cyclodextrins and a straight-chain polymer: crystal structures of inclusion complexes of β-cyclodextrin with poly(trimethylene oxide) and poly(propylene glycol), *Macromolecules,* 33, 1500–1502, 2000.

31. Hummer, G., Garde, S., and García, A.E., New perspective on hydrophobic effects, *Chem. Phys.,* 258, 349–370, 2000.

32. Ikeguchi, M., Nakamura, S., and Shimizu, K., Molecular dynamics study on hydrophobic effects in aqueous urea solutions, *J. Am. Chem. Soc.,* 123, 677–682, 2001.

33. Cao, J., Fyfe, M.C.T., Stoddart, J.F., Cousins, G.R.L., and Glink, P.T., Molecular shuttles by the protecting group approach, *J. Org. Chem.*, 65, 1937–1946, 2000.

34. Chiu, S.H., Elizarov, A.M., Glink, P.T., and Stoddart, J.F., Translational isomerism in a [3] catenane and [3] rotaxanes, *Org. Lett.*, 4, 3561–3564, 2002.

35. Lane, A.S., Leigh, D.A., and Murphy, A., Peptide-based molecular shuttle, *J. Am. Chem. Soc.*, 119, 11092–11093, 1997.

36. Zhao, X., Jiang, X.K., Shi, M., Yu, Y.H., Xia, W., and Li, Z.T., Self-assembly of novel [3]- and [2] rotaxanes with two different ring components: donor–acceptor and hydrogen bonding interactions and molecular-shuttling behavior, *J. Org. Chem.*, 66, 7035–7043, 2001.

37. Hunter, C.A. and Sanders, K.M., The nature of interactions, *J. Am. Chem. Soc.*, 112, 5525–5534, 1990.

38. Murakami, H., Kawauchi, A., Kotoo, K., Kunitake, M., and Nakashima, N., Light-driven molecular shuttle based on rotaxane, *J. Am. Chem. Soc.*, 119, 7605–7606, 1997.

39. Fujita, H., Ooya, T., and Yui, N., Thermally induced localization of cyclodextrins in a polyrotaxane consisting of β-cyclodextrins and poly(ethylene glycol)-poly(propylene glycol) triblock copolymer, *Macromolecules*, 32, 2534–2541, 1999.

40. Ikeda, T., Watabe, N., Ooya, T., and Yui, N., Study on the solution properties of thermo-responsive polyrotaxanes with different numbers of cyclic molecules, *Macromol. Chem. Phys.*, 202, 1338–1344, 2001.

41. Harada, A. and Kamachi, M., Complex formation between cyclodextrin and poly(propylene glycol), *J. Chem. Soc. Chem. Commun.*, 1322–1323, 1990.

42. Harada, A., Okada, M., Li, J., and Kamachi, M., Preparation and characterization of inclusion complexes of poly(propylene glycol) with cyclodextrins, *Macromolecules*, 28, 8406–8411, 1995.

43. Panova, I.G., Gerasinov, V.I., Grokhovskaya, T.E., and Topchieva, I.N., Novel nanostructures based on block copolymers: inclusion complexes of proxanols with cyclodextrins, *Doklaady Chem.*, 347, 61–65, 1996.

44. Jiao, H., Goh, S.H., and Valiyaveetti, S., Inclusion complexes of multiarm poly(ethylene glycol) with cyclodextrins, *Macromolecules*, 35, 1980–1983, 2002.

45. Li, J., Harada, A., and Kamachi, M., Sol–gel transition during inclusion complex formation between α-cyclodextrin and high molecular weight poly(ethylene glycol)s, *Polymer J.*, 26, 1019–1026, 1994.

46. Huh, K.M., Ooya, T., Lee, W.K., Sasaki, S., Kwon, I.C., Jeong, S.Y., and Yui, N., Supramolecular-structured hydrogel showing a reversible phase transition by inclusion complexation between poly(ethylene glycol) grafted dextran and α-cyclodextrin, *Macromolecules*, 34, 8657–8662, 2001.

47. Choi, H.S., Kontani, K., Huh, K.M., Sasaki, S., Ooya, T., Lee, W.K., and Yui, N., Rapid induction of thermoreversible hydrogel formation based on poly(propylene glycol)-grafted dextran inclusion complexes, *Macromol. Biosci.*, 2, 298–303, 2002.

48. Li, J., Li, X., Zhou, Z., Ni, X., and Leong, K.W., Formation of supramolecular hydrogels induced by inclusion complexation between pluronics and α-cyclodextrin, *Macromolecules*, 34, 7236–7237, 2001.

49. Alexandridis, P., Holzwarth, J.F., and Hatton, T.A., Micellization of poly(ethylene oxide)-poly(propylene oxide)-poly(ethylene oxide) triblock copolymers in aqueous solutions: thermodynamics of copolymer association, *Macromolecules*, 27, 2414–2425, 1994.

50. Ooya, T., Eguchi, M., and Yui, N., Supramolecular design for multivalent interaction: maltose mobility along polyrotaxane enhanced binding with concanavalin A, *J. Am. Chem. Soc.*, 125, 13016–13017, 2003.

51. Ooya, T. and Yui, N., Multivalent interactions between biotin–polyrotaxane conjugates and streptavidin as a model of new targeting for transporters, *J. Control. Rel.*, 80, 219–228, 2002.

52. Ooya, T., Kawashima, T., and Yui, N., Synthesis of polyrotaxane–biotin conjugates and surface plasmon resonance analysis of streptavidin recognition, *Biotechnol. Bioprocess Eng.*, 6, 293–300, 2001.

53. Yui, N., Ooya, T., Kawashima, T., Saito, Y., Tamai, I., Sai, Y., and Tsuji, A., Inhibitory effect of supramolecular polyrotaxane–dipeptide conjugates on digested peptide uptake via intestinal human peptide transporter, *Bioconjugate Chem.*, 13, 582–587, 2002.

54. Ooya, T., Eguchi, M., Ozaki, A., and Yui, N., Carboxyethylester polyrotaxanes as a new calcium chelating polymer: synthesis, calcium binding and mechanism of trypsin inhibition, *Int. J. Pharm.*, 242, 47–54, 2002.

55. Nakanishi, T., Miyazawa, M., Sakakura, M., Terasawa, H., Takahashi, H., and Shimada, I., Determination of the interface of a large protein complex by transferred cross-saturation measurements, *J. Mol. Biol.*, 318, 245–249, 2002.

56. Sakamoto, S., Fujita, M., Kim, K., and Yamaguchi, K., Characterization of self-assembling nano-sized structures by means of coldspray ionization mass spectrometry, *Tetrahedron*, 56, 955–964, 2000.

57. Choi, H.S., Huh, K.M., Ooya, T., and Yui, N., pH- and thermosensitive supramolecular assembling system: rapidly responsive properties of β-cyclodextrin-conjugated poly(ε-lysine), *J. Am. Chem. Soc.*, 125, 6350–6351, 2003.

15 Light-Induced Molecular Orientations

Kunihiro Ichimura

CONTENTS

INTRODUCTION

Orientation alterations of organic and polymeric thin films responsive to light irradiation are induced by both structural changes and by the rearrangement of orientation directions of photosensitive molecules to generate optical anisotropy. As revealed by extensive studies on photoorientation behavior of azobenzenes exhibiting reversible geometrical isomerization carried out in molecular[1] and polymeric films,[2,3] the orientation direction of their molecular axis is modified as a result of photoselected isomerization of photochromic molecules.

When a film of a polymer bearing azobenzene side chains with a random orientation is exposed to linearly polarized light for photoisomerization, the incident light is absorbed angular-selectively by thermodynamically more stable E-isomers of azobenzene residues with an electronic transition moment in parallel with the electric vector of the light, producing Z-isomers that can regenerate E-isomers photochemically and thermally. As a consequence of the reversions of the Z-isomers, the distribution of the molecular axis is changed and induces dichroism of the film that comes from the predominant distribution of azobenzene moieties with the transition moment perpendicular to the electric vector of actinic light.

An overall level of optical anisotropy is optionally influenced by orientation relaxation, which is closely related with free volumes of the film. Since the molecular axis of the E-isomer of the azobenzene is shifted more or less after exposure to linearly polarized light, this phenomenon is reasonably referred to as photoinduced reorientation or photoreorientation.

Note the difference between photoorientation and photoreorientation. Photoreorientation is defined somewhat differently by Natansohn and Rochon.[2] According to their proposal, the term *photoinduced orientation* is used when a photosensitive material is either amorphous or disordered before photoirradiation. *Photoreorientation* corresponds to the alteration of orientation direction of a preoriented film of a liquid–crystalline polymer that suffers from the treatment of a substrate plate such as rubbing of a plate surface for uniaxial alignment of mesogenic units.

Films of liquid–crystalline polymers with azobenzene side chains cast from solution on substrates without surface treatment are nonoriented and isotropic at ambient temperature when the glassy-mesophasic transition temperature is higher than room temperature. In this respect, the term *photoreorientation* defined by the Canadian authors is applicable for a specified material state. Consequently, *photoreorientation* is used when a molecular axis is evidently changed by photoirradiation, whereas *photoorientation* is a phenomenon that exhibits photoinduced generation of optical anisotropy or dichroism and possesses a wider meaning when compared with *photoreorientation*. Accordingly, photoorientation is workable without any photoreorientation.

Consider a film of a polymer exhibiting an irreversible photoreaction such as photodecomposition. Linearly polarized irradiation of the film leads to an angular-selective decomposition of photosensitive moieties generating optical anisotropy, even though no change of molecular orientation occurs. This kind of destructive photoorientation phenomenon[4] has been known since 1921 as the Weigert effect and is considered rather trivial.[5]

One reason why photoorientation phenomena have attracted extensive interest is that the photoinduced generation of optical anisotropy is markedly enhanced by a combination with liquid crystal (LC) systems as a result of their self-organizing nature to exhibit the so-called command effect.[2–9] The amplification of photoorientation by

LCs can be performed in two ways. The first is for systems consisting of LCs doped with photoactive molecules, and, in particular, of liquid–crystalline polymers bearing photoactive moieties. This topic has been discussed in review articles.[2–4] The second methodology is the transfer of photogenerated orientation of surface molecules or polymer thin films called command surfaces or layers to nematic LCs[8,9] so that the alignment of tremendous numbers of LCs is controllable by photosensitive topmost surfaces.

The other reason that photoorientation phenomena attract attention arises from practical applicabilities. While rewritable optical memory devices are operable by using photoorientation of LC systems, the surface-mediated photoalignment control of nematic LCs is of practical significance because the procedure allows the production of LC-aligning films that are fabricated for assembling LC flat panel display devices.[10]

Based on increasing interest in photoorientation phenomena from both fundamental and practical views, this chapter deals predominantly with recent advancements achieved by the author's group in order to minimize overlaps with the descriptions from previous review articles. In this context, photoreorientation modes of azobenzene moieties tethered to polymer main chains are described first by focusing on thin films of liquid–crystalline and crystalline polymers under various irradiation conditions to list factors affecting photoorientation and photoreorientation. Surface-mediated photoorientation of LC systems is presented to show that the command surface technique is now applied not only to conventional low-mass nematic LCs, but also to other LC systems including cholesteric (chiral nematic) LCs, discotic LCs, and even lyotropic LCs. Finally, the surface-mediated transfer of photoorientation in polymer ultrathin films is mentioned for self-organized materials other than LCs to illustrate novel photofunctional materials.

PHOTOORIENTATION OF POLYMERS

PHOTOGENERATED DICHROISM OF POLYMER THIN FILMS

Light-induced molecular orientation modes as illustrated in Figure 15.1 and the orientation photocontrols between them are multifarious. The in-plane and out-of-plane orientations take place as consequences of changes of molecular axes in azimuthal and polar angles, respectively, whereas the tilted orientation arises from the combination of both. The helical orientation occurs three-dimensionally so that there are right-handed and left-handed helical senses. A helical axis is usually perpendicular to the xy-plane, although the axis can be tilted or in parallel with the xy-plane.

Among these modes, the in-plane orientation has been extensively investigated by using irradiation with linearly polarized light. As mentioned in a review article,[2] Teitel[11] probably first achieved the exposure of a viscous solution of Congo Red to linearly polarized light to observe birefringence. Progress was accelerated by reports by Todorov[12] and Wendorff,[13,14] who employed polymer films physically doped with and covalently attached with azobenzenes to demonstrate rewritable holographic

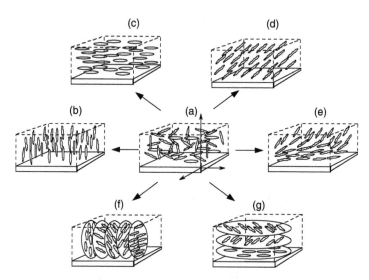

FIGURE 15.1 Photoalignment modes exhibiting (a) random, (b) homeotropic (perpendicular), (c) homogeneous (planar), (d) tilted, (e) hybrid, (f) helical with parallel axes and (g) helical with perpendicular axes orientations.

recording. Systematic studies of photoorientation of amorphous and liquid–crystalline polymers bearing azobenzene side chains continued throughout the early 1990s.[2–4,15]

When compared with azobenzene-containing polymers, angular-selective photochemical events have not been studied extensively for polymers with photosensitive side chains other than azobenzenes. Accordingly, we looked into the generation of optical anisotropy in thin films of polymethacrylates with photoisomerizable and/or photodimerizable moieties in their side chains including azobenzene,[16,17] benzylidenephthalimidine,[18,19] styrylpyridine,[20,21] cinnamate,[22–24] diphenylacetylene,[25] and coumarin.[26,27] The compounds were classified into three groups. Only azobenzene exhibited reversible E–Z photoisomerization. The benzylidenephthalimidine, styrylpyridine, and cinnamate chromophores, having conjugated C = C bonds displayed both E–Z photoisomerization and photodimerization. Diphenylacetylene and coumarin produced only photodimerization.

Films of these polymers were exposed to linearly polarized light and subjected to measurements of linearly polarized absorption spectroscopy to estimate levels of dichroism defined as $DR = (A_\perp - A_{//})/(A_\perp + A_{//})$. The results are summarized in Table 15.1. It is worth noting that the DR values were estimated specifically on the basis of remaining chromophoric units and provided no information about the anisotropy of photoproducts because monitored absorbances arose from unreacted chromophores. The polymethacrylates listed in Table 15.1 are all amorphous since dichroism induced by linearly polarized light is markedly enhanced by liquid crystallinity of polymers, as shown below. DR values are independent of photochemical reactions and are similar to each other, implying that levels of photogenerated dichroism (photodichroism) are determined by orientation relaxation due to micro-Brownian motions within free volumes of polymer films.

TABLE 15.1
Photogenerated Dichroism and Molecular Reorientation

Photochemistry		DR[a]	Ref.
		0.03–0.05	16
	dimers	0.04–0.05	18
	dimers	0.02–0.04	23
	dimers	0.02–0.04	20,21
	dimers	0.025–0.03	25
	dimers	0.02–0.04	27

[a] Dichroic ratio.

IN-PLANE PHOTOORIENTATION OF AZOBENZENE UNDER ILLUMINATION WITH LINEARLY POLARIZED LIGHT

Background

DR values for typical azobenzene-containing polymers are 0.03 to 0.05, as shown in Table 15.1. Care must be taken that levels of photodichroism are considerably influenced by various factors including irradiation conditions, phases of polymer solids, post-exposure treatment, etc.[2–4] This section reviews the ways photoorientation phenomena are influenced by these factors and by employing polymers — predominantly those with azobenzene side chains.

The choice of employing azobenzenes as photosensitive units was based on the following facts:

1. Azobenzene-containing polymers are extensively used for photoorientation studies.
2. Structural modifications are achieved easily because azobenzene derivatives are readily available.

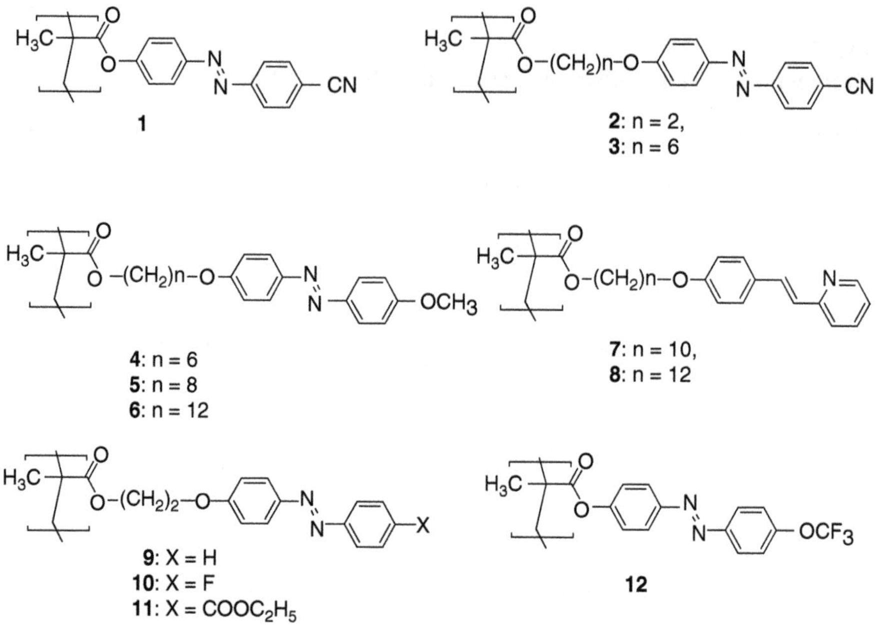

FIGURE 15.2 Chemical structures of polymers with azobenzene side chains cited in this chapter.

3. The photochemistry involves the reversible E–Z isomerization and excellent photofatigue resistance so that spectral analysis can be performed conveniently.
4. Because the π–π* transition moment is approximately in line with the molecular axis, orientation directions of the chromophore can be readily and distinctly identified by means of absorption spectral analysis.
5. The rod-shaped chromophore acts as a mesogen to produce a variety of liquid–crystalline polymers that display unique command effects in photoreorientation behavior.

The chemical structures of the polymers cited in this chapter are shown in Figure 15.2.

Excitation Wavelength

Because isomer ratios of azobenzenes in photostationary states are well known to be wavelength-dependent, thin films of the polymers were exposed to 365-nm light for E-to-Z photoisomerization and 436-nm light for Z-to-E photoisomerization. Polymethacrylates tethering p-cyanoazobenzene through different spacer lengths[28] used in this section and material properties are summarized in Table 15.2. While Polymer 1 is semicrystalline, Polymer 2 and Polymer 3 are liquid–crystalline.

As observed for the other azobenzene-containing polymers, excitation with linearly polarized 436-nm light brought about monotonous increases of DR values

TABLE 15.2
Properties of Polymethacrylates with
***p*-Cyanoazobenzene Side Chains**

Polymer	T_g (°C)	T_{CL} (°C)	$M_w \times 10^{-4}$	M_w/M_n
1	185	—	4.3	3.3
2	109	160	2.6	2.9
3	61	168	3.4	3.6

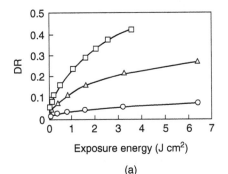

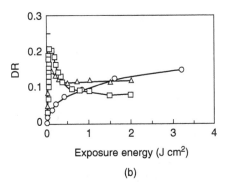

(a)   (b)

FIGURE 15.3 Photogeneration of dichroism for spin-cast thin films of **1** (circles), **2** (triangles), and **3** (squares) under irradiation with linearly polarized (a) 436-nm and (b) 365-nm light at ambient temperature as a function of exposure doses.

due to the molecular reorientation process (Figure 15.3a). The longer the spacer, the higher the DR, supporting a significant role of azobenzene assisted by spacers in molecular mobility. After irradiation with linearly polarized 365-nm light, **2** and **3** exhibited maximum DR values at an exposure energy of about 0.1 mJ cm^{-2} and leveled off finally upon prolonged photoirradiation (Figure 15.3b).

These results can be interpreted as follows. Angular-selective excitation with the 365-nm light resulted in the consumption of azobenzene with a transition moment parallel with the polarization plane of the light, leading to the reduction of absorbance with monitoring light of the electric vector in parallel with that of the actinic light ($A_{//}$). The decreases of $A_{//}$ values contributed predominantly to the generation and subsequent changes of DR values because the extinction coefficient of the Z-isomer at λ_{max} = 360 nm of the monitoring light is much smaller than that of E-isomer and the E-to-Z photoisomerization of the azobenzene with a transition moment perpendicular to the polarization plane of the light is effectively retarded.[16] In other words, the abrupt increase of DR at the early stage corresponds to the angular-selective photochemistry.

The subsequent process after the appearance of the DR maximum may be ascribed to the following events. Because the probability of light absorption is proportional to the cosine square of the angle between the transition moment and the polarization of the light, azobenzene residues with nonparallel transition moments undergo gradual photoisomerization. The second event is the excitation of the Z-isomer with light to produce the E-isomer. The combination of the two events results in repetition of photoisomerization, leading to molecular reorientation, the level of which is saturated to give a constant DR value upon prolonged irradiation. The appearance of maximum DR values suggests that the photoreorientation follows the angular-selective photoisomerization.

On the other hand, no DR maximum was observed for Polymer **1**. The reason may be that the rate and level of E-to-Z photoisomerization were low because of the restricted mobility of the side chains without spacers when compared with **2** and **3**, so that the contribution of the angular-selective photochemistry at the early stage was practically hidden. The fact that DR increased monotonously at 436-nm light irradiation was due to the minute contribution of absorbances at 360 nm of E-isomer, because the photostationary state contained Z-isomer as a major component so that DR values were insensitive to changes of $A_{//}$.

Irradiation of films of liquid–crystalline polymers with azobenzene side chains at 365-nm light for π–π^* transition makes them isotropic because the rod-shaped mesogenic E-isomer is converted into the bent and nonmesogenic Z-isomer that destroys the mesophases.[29–31] Irradiation of their spin-cast films with linearly polarized 436-nm light of n–π^* transition gives rise to marked enhancement of optical anisotropy due to the so-called command effect[2–4,32–35] that arises from the self-assembling nature of mesogenic moieties and the major involvement of mesogenic E-isomer under the irradiation conditions.

It is interesting to know aspects of the photogeneration of dichroism when the irradiation of their films is performed with linearly polarized 365-nm light.[36] Properties of liquid–crystalline polymers (**4**, **5**, and **6**) used for this study are summarized in Table 15.3. When films of these types of polymers are subjected to linearly polarized 365-nm light, optical anisotropy hikes considerably at the early stage, followed by an abrupt decrease that levels off. A typical example for Polymer **4** is shown in Figure 15.4. Note that the spin-cast films display no optical anisotropy before irradiation and are consequently thermodynamically unfavorable on account of their liquidity–crystallinity.

An order parameter defined as $S = (A_{\perp} - A_{//})/(A_{\perp} + 2A_{//})$ was employed to evaluate levels of optical anisotropy and displayed the maximum at a dose of about 30 mJ cm^{-2}, followed by a sudden reduction that leveled off around 200 mJ cm^{-2}, leading to a constant value of about 0.05 — not far from the levels of amorphous

TABLE 15.3
Properties of Liquid–Crystalline Polymers

Polymer	M_w	M_w/M_n	Phase Transition (°C)[a]	Refractive Index
4	1.25×10^5	2.8	G 76 S 95 N 137 I	1.64
5	5.4×10^4	2.5	G 69 S 114 N 132 I	1.64
6	5.9×10^4	2.8	G 68 S 131 I	1.64

[a] G = Glassy; S = smectic; N = nematic; I = isotropic.

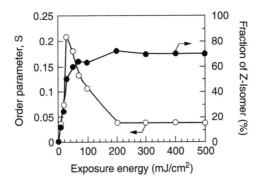

FIGURE 15.4 Changes in order parameters (S) and fractions of Z-isomer of a film of Polymer **4** as a function of exposure doses of linearly polarized 365-nm light. (Adapted from Han, M. and Ichimura, K., *Marcomolecules*, 34, 90, 2001. With permission of The American Chemical Society.)

azobenzene polymers (Table 15.1). The exposure dose required to produce the maximum caused the formation of about 50% Z-isomer, which enhanced the molecular mobility in the glassy state of the film. Further irradiation resulted in the disappearance of the mesophase because of the reduction of E-isomer fractions.

One of the characteristic features of liquid–crystalline azobenzene polymers is that their films exposed to linearly polarized light exhibit prominent enhancement of optical anisotropy upon postexposure annealing at temperatures below a mesophasic-to-isotropic transition.[32–35] The enhancement of photodichroism upon exposure to linearly polarized 365-nm light is critically influenced by exposure doses, because the Z-isomer involved plays dual and opposite roles in improving molecular mobility leading to enhancing the self-organization of the mesogenic E-isomer at its lower fraction and destroying the mesophase at its higher fraction. This suggests the existence of an optimum exposure dose for sufficient optical anisotropy after postultraviolet exposure baking.

This is the case, as presented in Table 15.4. For both polymers (**4** and **5**), exposures less than about 20 mJ cm^{-2} brought about a considerable boost of S values after annealing at 78°C — sufficiently lower than their mesophasic-to-isotropic transition temperature. Optical anisotropy decreases or disappears completely upon heat treatment when the exposure gives rise to more than 50% of E-to-Z photoconversion. Exposure doses of a few joules per square centimeter are necessary to produce the same order of optical anisotropy when irradiation is carried out at 436 nm so that excitation energies for the photogeneration of optical anisotropy are significantly reduced by using 365-nm light and subsequent annealing.

The role of liquid crystallinity in enhancing photoinduced optical anisotropy was observed for azobenzene-containing polymers and also for liquid–crystalline polymers with styrylpyridine side chains (**7**, **8**) even though the chromophore possesses no substituent owing to its rod-like shape with a relatively large dipole moment (Table 15.5).[20,21] As shown in Table 15.1, polymers with photodimerizable units including **7** and **8** showed the generation of photodichroism under irradiation with

TABLE 15.4
Thermal Amplification of Photodichroism of Liquid–Crystalline Polymers (4 and 5)

| | | Polymer 4 | | | | Polymer 5 | |
| | | Order Parameter | | | | Order Parameter | |
Exp. Dose (mJ cm^{-2})	Z-Fraction (%)	Before Annealing	After Annealing	Z-Fraction (%)	Before Annealing	After Annealing
10	13	0.036	0.57	20	0.075	0.43
20	24	0.074	0.61	33	0.13	0.34
30	50	0.055	0.26	nm	nm	nm
40	nm	nm	nm	54	0.15	0.0019
70	64	0.001	0.0077	67	0.067	0.0005
200	72	0.038	0.0000	73	0.015	0.0000

nm = Not measured.

Source: Adapted from Han, M. and Ichimura, K., *Marcomolecules*, 34, 90, 2001. With permission of The American Chemical Society.

TABLE 15.5
Properties of Polymethacrylates with Styrylpyridine Side Chains

Polymer	M_w	M_w/M_n	Phase Transition
7	8.6×10^4	2.6	G 47 N 78 I
8	1.76×10^4	3.5	G 86 S 105

linearly polarized 313-nm light. Figure 15.5 shows that annealing of films of **7** and **8** was accompanied by changes of dichroism. Because the E-to-Z photoisomerization deteriorated the liquid crystallinity of **7** and **8** as occurred with azobenzene-containing polymers subjected to 365-nm light irradiation, there were optimum exposure doses for demonstrating the thermal enhancement of photodichroism. Accordingly, the optimum exposure doses are 3 mJ cm^{-2} and 60 mJ cm^{-2} for **7** and **8**, respectively.

As seen in Figure 15.5, the dichroism of **7** increases considerably at about 50°C and subsequently declines around 70°C. Optical anisotropy disappears because the mesophase is converted into an isotropic phase. Polymer **8** displays a heat-assisted enhancement of optical anisotropy, although its behavior upon further heating is quite different from that of **7**. After a moderate decrease, essentially no marked change is observed until the film is heated above about 230°C, indicating that the optical anisotropy is very thermostable. Evidently, this comes from the photodimerization to form a crosslinked structure.

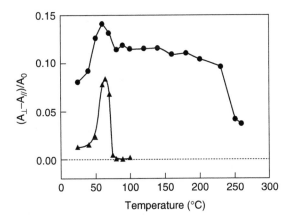

FIGURE 15.5 Changes in photodichroism of films of **7** (▲) and **8** (●) exposed to linearly polarized 313-nm light of 3 and 60 mJ cm^{-2}, respectively, as a function of annealing temperature.

Sample Temperatures

As described above, the photoreorientation of azobenzenes induced by irradiation with linearly polarized light occurs in such a way that the molecular axis approximately parallel to a transition moment moves to the azimuthal direction perpendicular to the polarization of the light to result in an in-plane reorientation. This is because photon absorption takes place only when the transition moment of a molecule lies in parallel with the electric vector of the actinic light. This section deals with the novel phenomenon that involves conventional in-plane reorientation followed by out-of-plane reorientation under prolonged irradiation with linearly polarized light.[37,38]

Figure 15.6a shows the temperature dependence of photogeneration of optical anisotropy of liquid–crystalline Polymer **4** under irradiation with linearly polarized 436-nm light. For comparison, the results for amorphous Polymer **9** are also shown in Figure 15.6b. Order parameters (S) for the amorphous polymer increased as increments of a sample temperature below the T_g glass transition temperature, and optical anisotropy was not generated at an elevated temperature above the T_g (Figure 15.6b). More complicated behavior is obtainable for the liquid–crystalline Polymer **4** (Figure 15.6a). Whereas S values increase very slowly in the glassy state at room temperature, the growth of S occurs monotonously and outstandingly in smectic phase at 76°C. On the other hand, when irradiation is achieved at 90°C (near the smectic-to-nematic transition temperature), S values boost rapidly at low exposure doses, then gradually decline. A similar pattern was observed for an experiment at 120°C, though S values were much reduced because of accelerated relaxation in the nematic phase. In order to trace the generation of optical anisotropy in more detail, polarized absorbances perpendicular to (A) and parallel to (A$_{//}$), the electric vector of the linearly polarized light, were plotted against exposure doses. Since changes in photogenerated S were more pronounced at 90°C when compared with those at

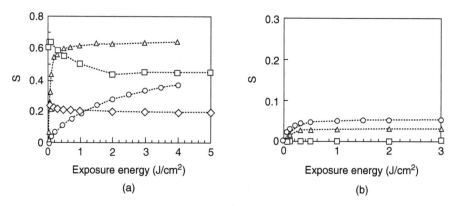

FIGURE 15.6 Changes in order parameters (S) of films of Polymers **4** (a) and **9** (b) during irradiation with linearly polarized 436-nm light. Sample temperatures for **4** are room temperature (circles), 76°C (triangles), 90°C (squares), and 120°C (diamonds). Those for **9** are room temperature (circles), 70°C (triangles), and 105°C (squares). (From Han, M., Morino, S., and Ichimura, K., *Macromolecules*, 33, 6360, 2000. With permission of The American Chemical Society.)

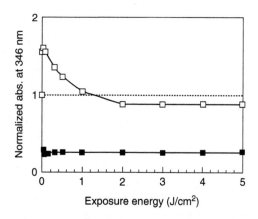

FIGURE 15.7 Changes of normalized absorbances at 346 nm of a film of **4** monitored by linearly polarized light with the electric vector perpendicular to $A_\perp$ (open squares) and parallel with $A_{//}$ (closed squares) and polarized 436-nm light as a function of exposure doses. Film was exposed to the light at 90°C. (From Han, M., Morino, S., and Ichimura, K., *Macromolecules*, 33, 6360, 2000. With permission of The American Chemical Society.)

120°C, spectral analysis was carried out for the 90°C experiment. The results shown in Figure 15.7 reveal that $A_{//}$ decreased rapidly at a dose of 20 mJ cm^{-1} to give a constant S value, whereas $A_\perp$ reached maximum value at the exposure dose, followed by a gradual decrease later leveled off.

It should be stressed that averaged absorbances defined as $A_{av} = (2A_\perp + A_{//})/3$ decreased simultaneously to give a much smaller constant value at doses of 2 J cm^{-2} or more with respect to absorbance before photoirradiation, suggesting an out-of-plane reorientation of azobenzene. Measurement of electronic absorption spectra of

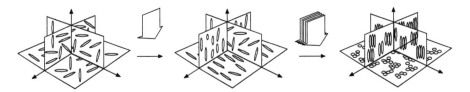

FIGURE 15.8 Successive in-plane and out-of-plane reorientations upon exposure to linearly polarized light. (From Han, M., Morino, S., and Ichimura, K., *Macromolecules*, 33, 6360, 2000. With permission of The American Chemical Society.)

the film with *p*-polarized probe lights at various incident angles (θ_m) was an unequivocal way to confirm the perpendicular orientation of the chromophore.[37,38]

The spectra were essentially independent of θ_m for a film at a 0.05 J cm^{-2} exposure dose, suggesting no perpendicular orientation. The larger θ_m was for a film illuminated at a 5 J cm^{-2} dose, the larger were the absorbances for the π–π* transition, in particular, the blue-shifted absorbance at 320 nm, supporting the suggestion that (1) the azobenzene reoriented perpendicularly and (2) the perpendicular reorientation was accompanied by the formation of H aggregates of azobenzene having λ_{max} values of 320 nm.

These results led to the conclusion that biaxial molecular reorientations took place consecutively when a film of the liquid–crystalline polymer **4** was subjected to irradiation with linearly polarized light at 90°C. At the early stages of irradiation, the in-plane reorientation occured in the *xy* plane, followed by gradual out-of-plane reorientation in the *yz* plane, as seen in Figure 15.8. Because exposure doses to achieve both reorientations are quite different, it is possible to make photoimages simply by controlling exposure periods to give rise to differences in refractive indices of a film due to the orientation directions of the azobenzene.

Somewhat different photoreorientation behavior was observable when the irradiation was conducted at 120°C and produced a nematic phase. Changes of S as functions of exposure doses displayed the maximum at an early stage, followed by a gradual decrease to give a constant value, similar to irradiation at 90°C, as seen in Figure 15.6a. The levels of S at the maximum and after leveling off were much lower when compared with the 90°C experiments. The *p*-polarized absorption spectra were not influenced by incident angles (θ_m) of the probe light, indicating that no out-of-plane reorientation was involved. No blue-shifted absorption band due to the H aggregate was detected, suggesting that the face-to-face aggregation was suppressed thoroughly in the nematic phase. Accordingly, the contrasting behavior at 120°C came from nematic phase with a larger free volume when compared with the smectic phase to enhance the molecular mobility.

Thermal Enhancement

The photoinduced optical anisotropy of films of liquid–crystalline polymers with azobenzene side chains intensified remarkably via thermal treatment at temperatures below a mesophasic-to-isotropic transition temperature.[32–35] Figure 15.9 shows examples.[28]

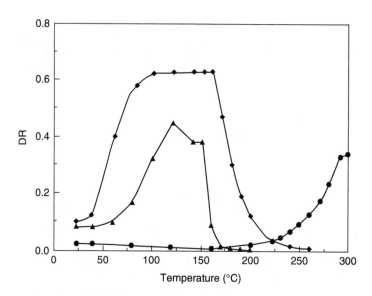

FIGURE 15.9 Thermal alterations of photoinduced dichroism of films of **1** (circles), **2** (tri-angles), and **3** (diamonds) irradiated with linearly polarized 436-nm light at a 0.2 J cm^{-2} dose at room temperature. DR values were estimated from polarized absorption spectra taken after annealing at each temperature for 3 min.

The photodichroism of liquid–crystalline polymers **2** and **3** increased consider-ably upon heating and abruptly decreased at temperatures that led to the isotropic phase. Outstanding results were observed for Polymer **1**. The DR increased gradually at temperatures above about 200°C and increased sharply above 250°C. The DR remained at a high level even when the film was heated at 300°C. Prolonged heating at this temperature caused partial decomposition.[39,40]

Thermal alterations of the photogenerated optical anisotropy of the polymers were conveniently followed by monitoring changes of birefringence (Δn) by means of an ellipsometer equipped with a hot stage to perform *in situ* observation at a heating rate of 6°C min^{-1}. Figure 15.10 shows changes in photobirefringence of films of the three polymers upon heating after exposure to linearly polarized lights of various doses. For the liquid–crystalline polymers, Δn increased above the temper-atures corresponding glassy-to-mesophasic transition and disappeared suddenly due to the conversion to the isotropic phase (Figure 15.10b and Figure 15.10c).

The levels of thermally enhanced birefringence were not much influenced by exposure doses. On the other hand, the degree of thermal enhancement was rather sensitive to exposure doses for Polymer **1**, whereas the optical anisotropy was extremely thermostable. Such unique behavior of **1** may be ascribed to its crystalline nature. A similar result was reported for a polyester with azobenzene side chains[41] that displayed a considerable increment of optical anisotropy by elevating temper-atures after linearly polarized photoirradiation because the polymer is crystalline.

In summary, alterations of photoinduced optical anisotropy upon heating depend drastically on the nature of polymers when films are cast from solutions. When a

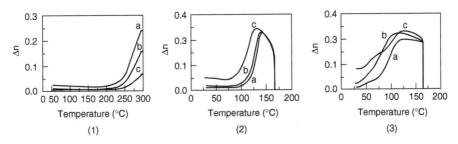

FIGURE 15.10 Changes of photoinduced birefringence of films of (1) **1**, (2) **2**, and (3) **3** irradiated with linearly polarized 436-nm light at doses of 0.05 (a), 0.2 (b), and 1 (c) J cm^{-2}, respectively, upon heating at 6°C min^{-1}.

polymer is amorphous, photogenerated dichroism is thoroughly removed at temperatures above its T_g, as expected. Photodichroism is considerably enhanced at temperatures produces mesophases for liquid–crystalline polymers and disappears above the temperature of the corresponding mesophasic-isotropic transition. Crystalline polymers exhibit the marked enhancement of photodichroism which is extremely thermally stable even at high temperatures. Films obtained by spin coating from solutions were amorphous for all polymers with T_g values much higher than ambient temperatures.

PHOTOORIENTATION INDUCED BY IRRADIATION WITH NONPOLARIZED LIGHT

Background

While in-plane reorientations of azobenzenes under irradiation with linearly polarized light were reported to produce birefringent films, few reports have covered the generation of optical anisotropy by nonpolarized light irradiation. Molecular reorientation induced by irradiation with nonpolarized light was reported for the first time by achieving oblique irradiation of a cell surface modified with azobenzene groups filled with a nematic liquid crystal (LC) to produce a homogeneous (uniaxially aligned) texture.[42]

The results indicate that in-plane molecular orientation is achievable by oblique irradiation even though the light is not linearly polarized. In other words, the Weigert effect may be obtained by nonpolarized light irradiation when irradiation is performed obliquely.

Clear-cut results for molecular photoreorientation induced by nonpolarized light irradiation show that azobenzene chromophores reorient toward the propagation direction of nonpolarized actinic light in amorphous[43] and liquid–crystalline[44–46] polymethacrylates with azobenzene side chains. As described earlier, the photoreorientation of azobenzene side chains is remarkably enhanced by the liquid crystallinity of polymers so that liquid–crystalline polymers are very suitable for this type of research investigating the relationship of propagation direction of actinic light and photoinduced molecular orientation direction.

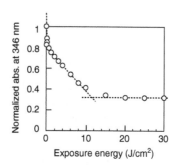

FIGURE 15.11 Changes of normalized absorbances at 346 nm as a function of exposure dose of light. (From Han, M., Morino, S., and Ichimura, K., *Macromolecules*, 33, 6360, 2000. With permission of The American Chemical Society.)

Tilted Photoreorientation

Irradiation of a film of a conventional (amorphous) azobenzene-containing polymer with 436-nm light from surface normal immediately gave rise to a photostationary state containing E-isomer as a major component so that no further change in absorption spectrum was observed. The situation was quite different for a film of a liquid–crystalline polymer, however. Figure 15.11 shows the results.

The λ_{max} decreased rapidly at an exposure dose of about 0.2 J cm^{-2}, followed by a gradual decrease that leveled off at about 10 J cm^{-2} so that the spectral changes were divided into three zones. The early stage corresponded to E-to-Z photoisomerization that led to a photostationary state. The subsequent slow process was due to the spatial reorientation of the E-isomer toward the propagation direction of the light in order to minimize light absorption. The perpendicular reorientation was saturated finally upon prolonged irradiation.[45]

Because the perpendicular orientation originated from the irradiation condition achieved from surface normal, it appears that tilted reorientation occurs upon oblique irradiation with nonpolarized light.

In order to determine tilted directions of the azobenzene, both the azimuthal (in-plane; φ_{azi}) and polar (out-of-plane; φ_{pol}) angles of its molecular axis with respect to the incidence direction of the light should be identified (Figure 15.12a). The geometry for estimating photodichroism is illustrated in Figure 15.12b. A_1 and A_2 denote absorbances at λ_{max} determined by using a polarized probe light with the electric vectors perpendicular to and parallel to the plane of incidence of the actinic light to estimate the level of photodichroism defined as $DR_{np} = (A_2 - A_1)/(A_2 + A_1)$. Note that a positive DR_{np} value means that azobenzene orients preferentially in parallel with the incident direction of light ($\varphi_{azi} = 0$). The results for films of Polymer **4** summarized in Figure 15.12c show that DR_{np} became larger with increases of exposure doses and did not level off even after prolonged irradiation. DR_{np} is markedly dependent on and enhanced by increases in incident angles (θ_a), confirming that photodichroism is determined by the tilt reorientation of the azobenzene.

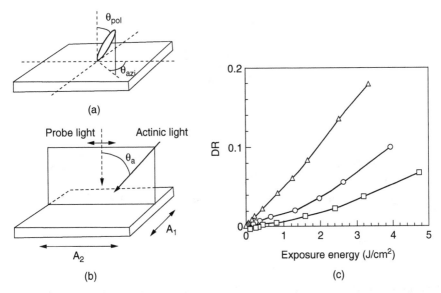

FIGURE 15.12 Geometries of (a) tilted orientation of a molecule and (b) incidence of nonpolarized actinic light and polarized probe light to give absorbances (A_1 and A_2) perpendicular to and parallel with the incidence plane. (c) Changes of $DR = (A_2 - A_1)/(A_2 + A_1)$ of a film of Polymer **4** exposed to nonpolarized 436-nm light at incident angles (θ_a) of 30° ($\square$), 45° ($\bigcirc$), and 60° ($\triangle$) as a function of exposure doses. (From Han, M., Morino, S., and Ichimura, K., *Macromolecules*, 33, 6360, 2000. With permission of The American Chemical Society.)

Tilt angles (φ_{pol}) can be determined by spectral measurements with p-polarized probe light at various incident angles (θ_m) in the plane parallel to the azimuthal orientation of azobenzene ($\varphi_{azi} = 0$), as seen in Figure 15.13a. In order to examine the orientation direction of the azobenzene molecular axis, the parameter Ap_{346}/As_{346} was plotted as a function of θ_m. Ap_{346} and As_{346} denoted p-polarized and s-polarized absorbances at 346 nm, respectively. The absorbances were corrected, taking the reflection of probe light and the refractive index of the polymer into consideration.[45]

The λ_{max} was blue-shifted due to the H aggregation and λ_{max} values for all p-polarized absorption spectra were plotted as functions of θ_m. The results for incident angles of the actinic light (θ_a) at 0, 20, and 45° are summarized in Figure 15.13b through Figure 15.13d. The fact that θ_m gives minimum Ap_{346}/As_{346} values in accordance with θ_a for every case unequivocally supports the premise that the molecular axis of the azobenzene lies in parallel with the propagation direction of the actinic light. This was confirmed by conoscopic observation to identify the directions of optical axes of the films. Figure 15.13 indicates that λ_{max} at 360 nm for monomeric azobenzene appears at θ_m centered at θ_a, implying that H-aggregated azobenzene orients in line with θ_a. In conclusion, nonpolarized irradiation results in the reorientation of azobenzene in a direction parallel to the propagation direction of the actinic light accompanied by H aggregation.

The inconsistency of directions between the photoinduced orientation of azobenzene and the propagation direction occurs more or less under certain conditions.

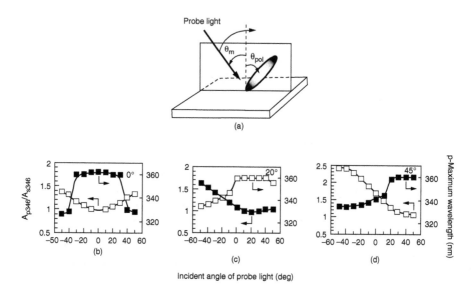

FIGURE 15.13 The geometry of determining the orientation direction of azobenzene. (a) Incident angles of polarized monitoring light (θ_m) are changed in such a way that the directions are contained in the polarization plane of azimuthal direction of the photooriented azobenzene. Changes in Ap_{346}/As_{346} and λ_{max} taken by p-polarized probe light (see text) as a function of θ_m after irradiation of films of **4** at incident angles (θ_a) of (b) 0° (c) 20°, and (d) 45°. (From Han, M. et al., *Macromolecules*, 33, 6360, 2000. Reproduced by permission of The American Chemical Society.)

When films of Polymer **4** are exposed at θ_a = 20 and 45° at 80°C, respectively, the azobenzene tilts toward the propagation direction of the light at θ_m = 10 and 30°. Such disagreement very likely arises from enhanced molecular mobility at temperature, resulting in thermal reorientation to minimize surface energy.

Spacer lengths tethering the azobenzene to polymethacrylate backbone chains also influence the relationship between θ_a and θ_m. The results are summarized in Table 15.6. It is noteworthy that no tilted reorientation is induced since **6**, with the longest C_{12} spacer, is generated even at θ_a = 45°. As shown in Table 15.6, surface energies taken as advancing contact angles are irrespective of the chemical structures of the polymers and not changed by photoirradiation. The interface between the surface and the air plays no role in this case. On the other hand, spectral analysis reveals that H aggregation takes place extraordinarily fast for Polymer **6** so that it is likely that H aggregation suppresses tilted reorientation.

On the basis of this kind of tilted photoreorientation under nonpolarized irradiation, sunshine-induced reorientation of the azobenzene was achieved, leading to the novel hypothesis that the absolute chirality on Earth is generated by sunlight as a moving light source that changes both azimuthal and polar angles continuously.[47] Several hypotheses for the chirality problem in relation to the origin of life have been put forth since the last century when Louis Pasteur found that bacteria can grow only on one enantiomer, tartaric acid.[48] The hypotheses include, for instance,

TABLE 15.6
**Tilt Angles of Azobenzene Residues of Polymers 4, 5, and 6
with Different Spacer Lengths Induced by Oblique Irradiation
with 436-nm Light at Various Incident Angles (θ_a)**

	Polymers								
	4			**5**			**6**		
Incident angle (θ_a/deg)	5	20	45	5	20	45	5	20	45
Tilt angle of azobenzene	0	20	50	0	10	30	0	0	0
Contact angle (deg)[a]	86.9	—	86.5	85.7	—	86.0	82.5	—	83.7

[a] Advancing contact angles after photoirradiation. Films of polymers before irradiation exhibited
contact angles of 87.0, 85.3, and 83.4°, respectively.

radioactive decay on the basis of the parity violation,[49] asymmetric adsorption at the
surfaces of chiral crystals such as quartz and clay minerals,[50] extraterrestrial transport
of chiral molecules to Earth,[51] and selective photochemical reactions induced by
circularly polarized light.[52,53] Most of them are not persuasive or conclusive.

The intensity of sunshine is enough to trigger the reorientation of azobenzene
units in a film of Polymer **4**. It is possible that sunshine from noon to evening leads
to the helical arrangement on film of the moieties with larger polar angles, as
illustrated in Figure 15.14. Accordingly, the helical sense is absolutely determined
by the orbital motion of the sun to be left-handed, at least in the Northern hemisphere.
Because prolonged exposure to the sun gives rise to the H aggregation which in turn
suppresses continuous photoreorientation, distinct observation of photoinduced
chirality has not been achieved for the polymer. The hypothesis for the origination
of homochirality appears attractive because it is based on the orbital motion of the
Earth and should be universal. Needless to say, chromophores other than azobenzenes may have acted as photoreceptors for sunshine-induced reorientation in organized layers on the primitive Earth, and further studies are required.

To summarize, tilted reorientation is induced by oblique irradiation with nonpolarized light in such a way that the molecular direction is in line with the propagation direction of the light, whereas the tilt angles are influenced by sample temperatures and the chemical structures of polymers.

PHOTOALIGNMENT OF LOW-MASS LIQUID
CRYSTALS BY AZOBENZENE POLYMER NETWORKS

As described in the preceding sections, liquid crystallinity of polymers plays a critical
role in photoreorientation phenomena when compared with amorphous compounds,
reflecting the command effects of photooriented azobenzenes to enhance levels of
optical anisotropy. The photoreorientation of azobenzene units of liquid–crystalline
azobenzene-containing copolymers triggered reorientation of photoinactive
mesogenic comonomer units.[54] It is interesting from both fundamental and practical

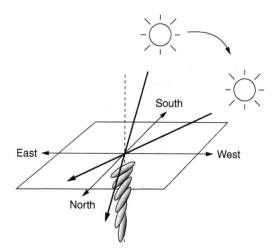

FIGURE 15.14 Hypothetical formation of a helical arrangement of azobenzene in a polymer film exposed to sunshine from noon to evening. (From Ichimura, K. and Han, M., *Chem. Lett.*, 286, 2000. Reproduced by Permission of the Chemical Society of Japan.)

viewpoints to study the control of alignment of photochemically inactive low-mass nematic liquid crystals (LCs) by azobenzene molecules, the orientations of which are determined photochemically.

Because of the fluidity of LC bulk, photoinduced orientation of a low-mass azobenene dissolved in an LC layer is readily relaxed. Azobenzene units were tethered to crosslinked polymer networks to give photoresponsive hybrid composites by the thermal radical copolymerization of an azobenzene acrylate (Az) with a diacrylate (Ac) as a crosslinker in a nematic LC layer initiated by benzoyl peroxide (BPO) in a cell.[55] A typical mixing ratio of Az:Ac:LC:BPO in weight was 5:30:60:5; the LC was the major component. While a mixture may be anisotropic during thermal polymerization because of the lower nematic-to-isotropic transition, a hybrid composite thus prepared exhibits a polymer-dispersed mesophase. When the cell is irradiated with linearly polarized 436 nm, the LC shows a uniaxial texture with the orientation direction perpendicular to the electric vector of the light, indicating that the homogeneous alignment of the LC is originated by the in-plane photoreorientation of the azobenzene (Figure 15.15b). Irradiation with nonpolarized light resulted in the reorientation of LC molecules to enable us to control their three-dimensional orientation, as in cases of films of liquid–crystalline azobenzene polymers (Figure 15.15c).[56]

This type of photoresponsive composite contains azobenzene as a phototrigger for LC alignment in much lower concentrations when compared with liquid–crystalline polymers with azobenzene side chains so that the penetration depth of actinic light is far larger. Accordingly, thick cells filled with composites are applicable for rewritable volume-type holographic recordings.[57]

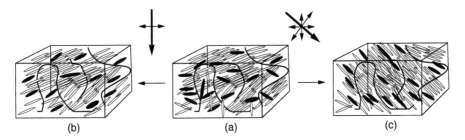

FIGURE 15.15 Cells filled with a nematic LC in a crosslinked azobenzene network (a) before irradiation, (b) after irradiation with linearly polarized light to give in-plane orientation, and (c) after oblique irradiation with nonpolarized light to lead to tilt orientation.

SURFACE-MEDIATED PHOTOORIENTATION OF LIQUID CRYSTALS

BACKGROUND

Since our observation that the alignment of a nematic LC changes reversibly between homeotropic (perpendicular) and planar (parallel) orientations by the E-to-Z photo-isomerization of monolayered azobenzenes,[58] numerous works have contributed to developing various types of photoresponsive LC systems displaying the transfer of molecular photoorientations of topmost surfaces of thin layers to LC bulk layers.[5–10]

One reason for the extensive interest is the fact that photochemical events of monomolecular layers trigger the reorientations of numerous LC molecules, exhibiting outstanding degrees of molecular amplification.[59] An alternative reason stems from practical significance; this phenomenon is applicable to production of LC-aligning films for assembling LC flat-panel display devices in a noncontact way.[10] The three modes of achieving surface-mediated alignment control of LCs include operations of out-of-plane and in-plane and tilted orientations of LC molecules.

The out-of-plane LC alignment (Figure 15.1b) is usually performed by geometrical photoisomerization of surface molecules or residues, whereas the in-plane control of LC alignment is achievable by irradiation with linearly polarized light (Figure 15.1c). The tilted LC alignment is induced by oblique photoirradiation of actinic light (Figure 15.1d). Accordingly, surface-assisted LC alignment control is closely related to molecular photoorientation in thin films, as discussed above.

The transfer of photoorientation of topmost surfaces to LC layers is definitely an interfacial phenomenon and it is important to reveal the working mechanisms of command surfaces at molecular levels. Azobenzenes are again very suitable for shedding light on this problem because their molecular orientation can be identified spectroscopically even when they are settled as monolayers on substrate surfaces. Randomly oriented monolayered p-hexylazobenzene units tethered to a silica surface displayed the reorientation of their molecular axes perpendicular to the surface upon contact with an LC layer, leading to homeotropic alignment.[8,9]

This section deals first with advanced studies on the working mechanisms of command surfaces to control alignment of low-mass nematic LCs, followed by

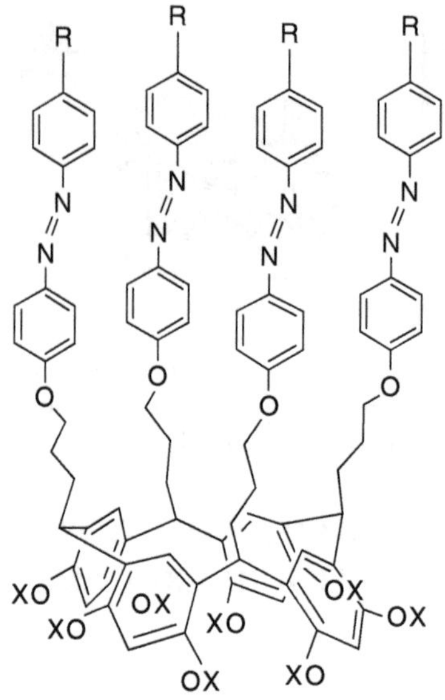

CRA-H: R = C_8H_{17}; X = CH_2COOH
CRA-F: R = C_8F_{17}; X = CH_2COOH

FIGURE 15.16 Calix[4]resorcinarene derivatives substituted with azobenzene residues.

extension of the procedure to versatile LC systems including cholesteric, discotic, and lyotropic LCs.

MECHANISTIC STUDIES

In order to determine the mechanism for orientation transfer from a surface to a bulk LC layer[60] to elucidate molecular interactions at the interface of a photoresponsive surface and an LC layer, calix[4]resorcinearene (CRA) derivatives substituted with four p-octyl- and p-perfluorooctylazobenzenes (CRA-H and CRA-F) were designed to give self-assembled monolayers (SAMs) by adsorption from a dilute solution onto a silica surface (Figure 15.16).[61]

The multisite formation of hydrogen bonds between carboxyl groups of the molecules and a silica surface produced SAMs. The cylindrical skeletons of the CRAs in the SAMs thus fabricated were packed tightly enough to cover efficiently a bare surface of the substrate.[62,63] The E-to-Z photoisomerization proceeded smoothly because free space for the isomerization was ensured by the larger occupied area of the cyclic skeleton when compared with cross-sectional areas of the four azobenzenes.[64] Surface energies can be finely modulated by mixing ratios of both CRA-H and CRA-F, whereas fractions of both compounds in SAMs are just in line with their mixing ratios. Consequently, it is possible to study the relationship between surface energies and alignment behavior of nematic LCs by using such well-defined azobenzene monolayers.

Figure 15.17 shows photogenerated pretilt angles of nematic LCs in cells that were surface-modified beforehand with mixed monolayers of CRA-F and CRA-H

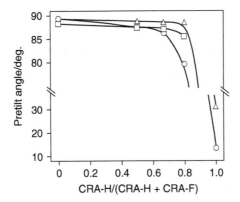

FIGURE 15.17 Pretilt angles of LCs generated by mixed monolayers of the two CRAs after oblique irradiation with nonpolarized ultraviolet light at an incident angle of 30° from surface normal as a function of fractions of CRA-F. (From Oh, S.-K., Nakagawa, M., and Ichimura, K., *J. Mater. Chem.*, 11, 1563, 2001. With permission of The Royal Society of Chemistry.)

after oblique irradiation with nonpolarized ultraviolet light. The LCs used were 5CB (4-cyanobiphenyl type), NPC-02 (aliphatic ester type), and MLC-6608 (Schiff-base type). They have positive, nearly zero, and negative dielectric anisotropies (directions of dipole moments with respect to longitudinal molecular axes), respectively. Pretilt angles started to decline at a CRA-F:CRA-H ratio of 1:4, whereas homogeneous alignment was induced for a Z-isomer surface of CRA-H. Because the generation of pretilt angles as a function of mixing ratios is relatively independent of the level and sign of dielectric anisotropy of the LCs, the results suggest that dipole–dipole interactions between LC molecules and the alkylazobenzene residues at the outer-most surface are not responsible for the alignment transition.

To obtain further information about the relationship of surface energies and photoalignment modes of LCs, contact angle measurements were achieved as a function of mixing ratios of the two. Because the dipole moment of the Z-isomer is much larger than that of the E-isomer, contact angles for water on a surface covered with an azobenzene monolayer became smaller upon E-to-Z photoisomerization. The contact angle hysteresis defined as a difference between advancing (θ_{adv}) and receding (θ_{rec}) contact angles for water depended markedly on mixing ratio, as shown in Figure 15.18. The hysteresis for a nematic LC, NPC-02, on E-isomer surfaces was little influenced by the mixing ratio, but a critical change was observable when the fraction of CRA-H (f_H = CRA-H/(CRA-H + CRA-F)) was switched from 0.8 to 1.0. A comparison of Figure 15.17 and Figure 15.18 indicates that the drastic change in pretilt angles of NPC-02 was coupled with a change in contact angle hysteresis in the range of f_H from 0.8 to 1.0, implying that LC photoalignment is closely related with hysteresis, not with contact angles.

It has been suggested that contact angle hysteresis reflects the molecular-level topography and rigidity of a surface tethering long-chain alkyl residues; a surface exhibits a small hysteresis when covered with a monolayer consisting of flexible molecular chains to form a smooth surface, whereas hysteresis becomes larger when

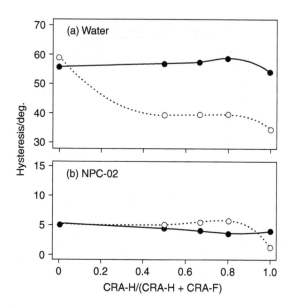

FIGURE 15.18 Contact angle hysteresis ($\theta_{adv} - \theta_{rec}$) for (a) water and (b) NPC-02 before (●) and after (○) ultraviolet exposure. (From Oh, S.-K., Nakagawa, M., and Ichimura, K., *J. Mater. Chem.*, 11, 1563, 2001. With permission of The Royal Society of Chemistry.)

molecular chains are so rigid to form an uneven surface with "pin holes," into which fluid molecules can penetrate.[65–67] If this is the case for the CRA surfaces, it is assumed that monolayers of $f_H < 0.8$ covered with Z-isomers form uneven surfaces at a molecular level because the contribution of the E-isomer of CRA-F at a photo-stationary state was not negligible owing to the rigidity of perfluorooctyl chains coupled with rod-shaped azobenzene moiety. Consequently, pin-hole surfaces are formed to give large hysteresis values and filled by LC molecules, leading to homeotropic alignment. Conversely, Z-isomer chains of CRA-H at $f_H = 1.0$ may be so flexible as to result in a smooth surface with a small hysteresis so that homogeneous alignment is generated.

Our conclusion is that LC alignment modes are determined reasonably by contact angle hysteresis, although they have been discussed on the basis of surface critical energies, i.e., contact angles.[60]

Pretilt Angle Photocontrol of Low-Mass LCs

The oblique irradiation of films of azobenzene-containing polymers with nonpolarized light results in the generation of tilt orientation of chromophores. It is possible to modulate pretilt angles of LCs (tilt angles of LC molecules from a surface) when cells filled with LCs are assembled by coating their substrate surfaces with this kind of polymer film to be subjected to oblique photoirradiation. This phenomenon is of practical significance for applying the production of LC-aligning films for LC flat-panel display devices. Consequently, it is important to reveal conditions for surface-assisted LC pretilt angle generation by using polymers with azobenzene side

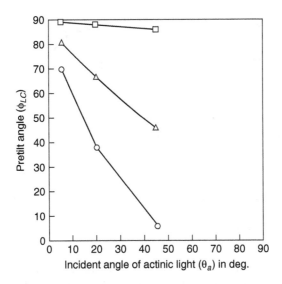

FIGURE 15.19 Pretilt angles (ϕ_{LC}) of an LC, NPC-02, as a function of incident angles (θ_a) of nonpolarized 436-nm light. Films of **4** (circles), **5** (triangles), and **6** (squares) on substrate plates were exposed to the light before cell assembly.

chains because the three-dimensional tilt orientations of azobenzene side chains can be unequivocally identified, as shown above.[45]

The inclination of azobenzene chromophores is controllable by incident angles of nonpolarized light in such a way that a tilting direction is in line with the propagation direction of the light at least for the Polymer **4** LC. It is important to understand the relationship of photoinduced tilt angles of azobenzene and the pretilt angles of nematic LCs when cells are assembled with substrates covered with photooriented films of LC polymers. Figure 15.19 shows pretilt angles (ϕ_{LC}) of an LC, NPC-02, on photoirradiated thin films of three polymers (**4**, **5**, and **6**) as functions of incident angles (θ_a) of 436-nm light. The ϕ_{LC} is an angle from surface normal whereas ϕ_{LC} is a tilting angle of the molecular axis of LC from a substrate surface so that $\phi_{LC} = 90° - \theta_a$ if the orientation direction of the LC is just in agreement with the propagation direction of the light. Pretilt angles induced by **5** are relatively in line with $90° - \theta_a$, whereas **4** and **6** give much smaller and larger pretilt angles than expected values, respectively, suggesting that spacer length influences ϕ_{LC} values. The larger ϕ_{LC} generated by **6** stems from the hydrophobicity of the longest C_{12} spacer and probably dense packing of the azobenzene to give rise to a rigid and uneven surface at a molecular level, leading to high pretilt angles even at high incident angles, as discussed in the section about working mechanisms of LC photoalignment. The fact that the *p*-methoxyazobenzene side chains of Polymer **6** display H aggregation on a film supports this interpretation.

The *p*-substituent effect on ϕ_{LC} is also critical.[68] Figure 15.20 shows changes of ϕ_{LC} of the LC filled in cells surface-modified with thin films of three types of

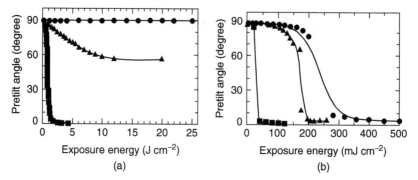

FIGURE 15.20 Changes in pretilt angles of a nematic LC, NPC-02, filled in cells, the surfaces of which are covered with thin films of Polymers **9** (squares), **10** (triangles), and **11** (circles), respectively, as a function of exposure doses of nonpolarized (a) 436-nm and (b) 365-nm light at an incident angle of 45° from surface normal.

polymethacrylates (**9**, **10**, and **11**) upon oblique irradiation with 436-nm and 365-nm light at an incident angle of 45°. Regarding conditions for pretilt angle generation:

1. The dependence of ϕ_{LC} on p-substituents was remarkable. The ϕ_{LC} generated by irradiation of Polymer **9** with 436 nm of light with unsubstituted azobenzene decreased suddenly to be leveled off at a minute level of ϕ_{LC}, whereas essentially no pretilt angle was generated by the Polymer **11** with a p-CO$_2$Et substituent that underwent self-aggregation. The F-substituent produced moderately high ϕ_{LC}.
2. The 365-nm light irradiation caused drastic decreases of pretilt angles for each polymer to yield small ϕ_{LC}, although exposure doses required for the sudden decrease were dependent on polymer structure.

Because LC alignment comes from molecular interactions at the interface between an LC-aligning film and an LC layer, it is anticipated that levels of photo-generated ϕ_{LC} are affected by the nature of LCs,[68] as shown in Figure 15.21. The NPC-02, RDP-60716, and MLC-6608 LCs have different dielectric anisotropies (Δε) of −0.1, +4.8, and −4.2, respectively. The two latter compounds have benzene rings in mesogens. Consequently, pretilt angles are settled not only by orientation directions of the azobenzene, but also by the nature of substituents at the chromophores and Δε.

Efforts have concentrated on generating high pretilt angles in order to fabricate twisted, vertically aligned LC flat panel displays exhibiting wide-view angles. The photoalignment technique required to produce an inclined homeotropic LC orientation is very important. An LC-photoaligning film must demonstrate reasonable thermostability of the photoorientation. Based on the results shown above, it is anticipated that the substitution of a fluoro-containing residue at the p-position of the azobenzene chromophore results in a high pretilt angle.

The optimization of the chemical structures of polymers led to the preparation of Polymer **12** with p-trifluoromethylazobenzene side chains tethering main chains

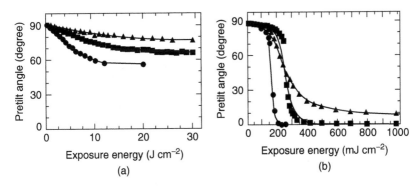

FIGURE 15.21 Changes in pretilt angles of nematic LCs of NPC-02 (●), RDP-60716 (▲), and MLC-6608 (■) the cells assembled with substrate plates coated by thin films of Polymer **10** as a function of exposure doses of nonpolarized (a) 436-nm and (b) 365-nm light for oblique irradiation at an incident angle of 45°.

without a spacer.[69] Similar to Polymer **1**, photogenerated optical anisotropy of a film of **12** was enhanced by annealing at an elevated temperature to yield LC-aligning films with high pretilt angles that were reasonably thermostable.

CHIRAL NEMATIC (CHOLESTERIC) LCs

Liquid crystalline materials are classified into four categories on the basis of (1) presence or absence of solvent, (2) nature of mesophase, (3) molecular shape of mesogen, and (4) molecular weight. Numerous reports have discussed photoalignment of nematic LCs by using photosensitive molecular and polymeric layers, but major LCs employed for photoalignment research comprise a group of thermotropic (solvent-free), nematic, calamitic, and low molecular weight LCs.

Accordingly, conventional nematic LCs (NLCs) occupy only a small part of the vast LC world, although NLCs have practical importance because of their applications for LC flat-panel displays. It is very attractive to verify the applicability of the command surface technique to LC systems other than conventional NLCs.[5,6] It has been reported, for instance, that a liquid–crystalline polymer exhibiting a nematic phase was photoalignable on a film of an azopolymer in a way similar to low-mass counterparts.[70]

Chiral nematic LCs (CNLCs) with helical supramolecular arrangements displayed multifarious alignment modes when inserted in cells: a focal conic texture with random orientation of the helix axes, a Grandjean texture in which the helix axes were perpendicular to the surface, and a fingerprint texture with the helix axes parallel to the surface.[71] The surface-mediated alignment control of CNLCs was achievable only when the orientation of the helix axes was homogeneously determined by the surface. The surface buffing technique generally accepted for the alignment of NLCs gave rise to the Grandjean texture of CNLC. A focal conic texture was obtained by rapid cooling from the isotropic phase without particular surface treatment. The fingerprint texture was generated by surfaces for homeotropic alignment of CNLCs, but the helix axes had no preferred orientation direction.

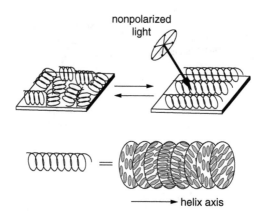

FIGURE 15.22 Oblique irradiation with nonpolarized light for CNLC photoalignment control.

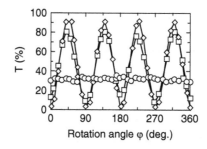

FIGURE 15.23 Normalized transmission (T) of probing He–Ne laser beam of a cell of 10 μm thickness filled with a CNLC with a pitch of 1.2 μm as a function of azimuthal angle φ after exposure to nonpolarized 436-nm light at an incident angle of 35°.

Consequently, no general way to control alignment of CNLCs has been found although some have been proposed.

CNLCs are photoalignable on films of azobenzene polymers under specific conditions.[72] The conventional method for NLC photoalignment by using thin films of photosensitive polymers exposed to linearly polarized light generated Grandjean textures only.

The situation was different when irradiation was performed obliquely. Among the polymers with azobenzene side chains tested, a thin film of polymethacrylate with *p*-fluoroazobenzene side chains (**10**) played a crucial role in the photoalignment of CNLCs.[39,40] Figure 15.22 shows the geometry of the photoalignment and the photooriented directions of the helix axes perpendicular to the incident plane of the light. One of the representative results of a CNLC derived from a NLC doped with a chiral agent is shown in Figure 15.23. Uniaxial orientation was demonstrated by recording transmitted light intensity of a linearly polarized probe He–Ne laser beam as a function of rotation angle of the cell around the optical axis. While no angular dependence was observed before irradiation because of a fonal conic texture, the oblique irradiation of the cell led to the generation of birefringence, indicating CNLC photoalignment that can be confirmed by ellipsometry measurements and polarized optical microscope observation. Detailed studies of CNLC photoalignment revealed:

1. Oblique photoirradiation with nonpolarized light was a necessary condition.
2. The level of photoalignment depended considerably on the chemical structures of azobenzene polymers, suggesting that thin films of the polymers giving rise to high pretilt angles upon oblique nonpolarized irradiation were favorable. The polymer with the *p*-fluoro substituent (**10**) generated a high pretilt angle of NLC, as noted earlier (Figure 15.20 and Figure 15.21), when compared with polymers with non-substituted or *p*-hexyl-azobenzene side chains.
3. Both cholesteric pitch and cell thickness markedly influenced the level of photoalignment to produce optimal conditions for cell assembly.

Because CNLCs provide potential applicability to electrooptical devices, the present photoalignment technique presents a promising way to fabricate novel types of CNLC-based cells.

Discotic LCs

Conventional LCs used for flat-panel displays are rod-shaped and discotic LCs (DLCs) have molecular structures of disk-shaped aromatic cores substituted at their peripheral positions with flexible alkyl chains. Their unique structures have attracted increasing interest from both fundamental and practical viewpoints[51] since they can be applied to novel devices exhibiting electric conductivity, photoconductivity, photovoltaic properties, anisotropic optical properties, etc.

These types of physical properties are very sensitive to molecular orientations and arrangements and alignment control plays an essential role in DLC science and technology. While some reports have covered DLC alignment based on mechanically buffed polymer films and surface-deposited inorganic materials, the command surface technique has potential value because of the versatility of alignment modes and the ability to form lithographic patterning.

One problem in DLC photoalignment stems from certain characteristics including higher transition temperatures required to exhibit the nematic phase and higher viscosity due to strong molecular interactions when compared with conventional rod-shaped calamitic LCs. Excellent stability of photosensitive states toward head and solvent is necessary for photosensitive polymers to achieve DLC photoalignment. This is because an oriented DLC layer is usually prepared by coating a solution of DLC on an LC-aligning film, followed by heating to generate nematic mesophase at an elevated temperature.

Polymer **1** was very suitable for this purpose because of the high thermostability of photooriented states and excellent resistance to solvent treatment.[73,74] The crucial prerequisite for DLC photoalignment is oblique exposure of the film to nonpolarized light, followed by heat treatment for enhancing the photooriented state. When a film is irradiated with linearly polarized light from surface normal, DLC molecules display only homeotropic alignment in which the disk-shaped molecules align parallel with a surface, as shown in Figure 15.24a, and no optical anisotropy is generated.

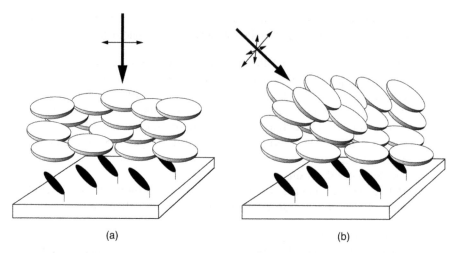

FIGURE 15.24 (a) Homeotropic and (b) tilting alignment of DLC molecules on films of **1** exposed to linearly polarized light and obliquely to nonpolarized light, respectively.

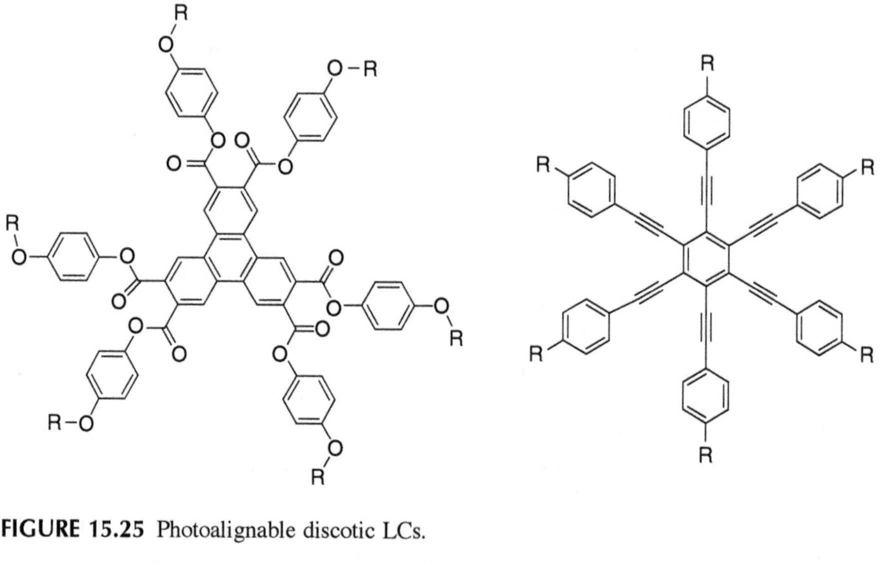

FIGURE 15.25 Photoalignable discotic LCs.

The oblique irradiation results in a tilting orientation of DLC molecules, as illustrated in Figure 15.24b, to give an optically anisotropic DLC film. Consequently, the general procedure for photoaligment of DLCs (Figure 15.25) involves the following steps. A thin film of **1** is subjected to oblique irradiation and postexposure baking at 240°C for 30 min, followed by fabricating a DLC layer by coating it with a DLC solution and annealing to generate a discotic nematic (ND) phase.[75] DLC molecules in an orientation-controlled layer displayed hybrid alignment. Pretilt angles changed continuously to show the largest angle at the topmost surface due to molecular interactions at the air/layer interface. A polymer with cinnamate side chains was also suitable for DLC photoalignment according to the same procedure.[76]

Since a tilting direction of a fluorescent DLC is controllable reversibly by an incidence direction of the light, anisotropic fluorescent photoimages are easily formed by altering incidence direction of the light.[77] For example, a film of **1** was first subjected to oblique flood exposure with nonpolarized light and subsequently to oblique irradiation through a photomask after changing the direction of light incidence. These steps were followed by annealing at an elevated temperature to transfer latent photoimages to a coated DLC film.

LYOTROPIC LCS

LCs are classified by whether they contain solvents. Conventional LCs are thermotropic (TLCs) that do not contain solvents. Lyotropic LCs (LLCs) are solutions of particular molecules or polymers.[78] Although LLCs are of great significance in biological systems, they have been out of the mainstream of LC science when compared with TLCs; no systematic studies have focused on alignment control of LLCs.

LLCs are categorized as amphiphilic, polymeric, or chromonic.[79] Amphiphilic and polymeric LLCs are derived from solutions of amphiphilic low-mass compounds and polymeric materials of specified concentrations, respectively. Chromonic LLCs consist usually of aqueous solutions of molecules with rigid electronic aromatic cores substituted with hydrophilic groups at their periphery positions, leading to self-assemblies due to face-to-face interactions of the core moieties to form stacked columnar aggregates. While reports on LLCs are limited, water-soluble derivatives of xanthones,[80,81] azo dyes,[82,83] cyanines,[84,85] perylenes,[86,87] and some others have been known to display mesophases in their aqueous solutions. Because of the involvement of π-electronic systems in self-assembled aggregates, they possess potential applicability to fabrication of versatile supramolecular devices exhibiting optical, electronic, and photoconductive functionalities. Procedures for controlling the orientation of LLCs are critical.

Our studies revealed that LLCs are photoalignable by the command surface technique when they show nematic phases. Aqueous solutions of disodium chromoglycate (DSCG in Figure 15.26) are LLCs that have been well studied as antiasthmatic drugs.[88] They exhibit middle mesophase in aqueous solutions and are

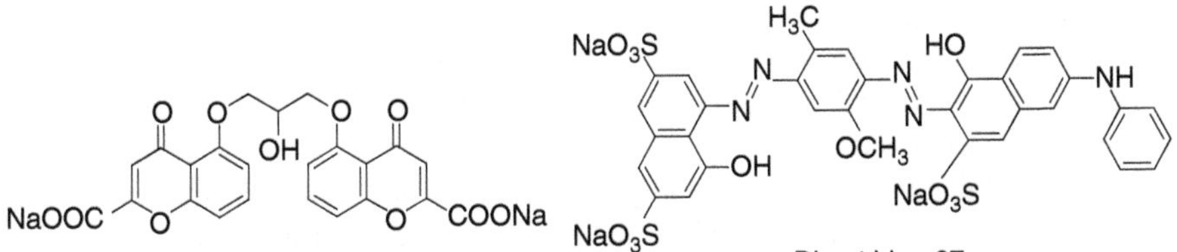

FIGURE 15.26 Water-soluble compounds giving lyotropic mesophases.

converted to nematic phase by adding small amounts of nonionic surfactants.[89,90] As with conventional TLCs, aqueous solutions of DSCG with nematic phases show homogeneous alignments when placed into cells, the inside walls of which are coated with thin films of an azobenzene polymer and exposed to linearly polarized light in advance.[91]

Another compound subjected to LLC photoalignment experiments is a diazodye known as C.I. Direct Blue 67 (Figure 15.26).[92] Aqueous solutions of the water-soluble dye gave rise to a lyotropic mesophase able to be changed into a nematic phase in the presence of a small amount of a surfactant in a way similar to DSCG. Detailed studies on molecular aggregates of the dye in aqueous solutions revealed that dye molecules are tightly stacked to form columnar supramolecular structures that result in mesophases. Aqueous solutions of the dye can be aligned uniaxially on films of azobenzene polymers exposed to linearly polarized light. The photo-alignment of the LLC derived from the dye is of practical significance because the orientation direction of dye molecules is controlled by the electric vector of actinic linearly polarized light for the reorientation of azobenzene moieties in polymer thin films to give dichroic dye films providing polarizer sheets.[93,94]

The procedure for the fabrication of oriented dye films involves linearly polarized light irradiation of a thin film of an azobenzene polymer and coating of an aqueous dye solution, followed by the evaporation of water to fix the orientations of the dye molecules. Since optically anisotropic photoimages can be conveniently recorded on polymer film by imagewise exposure to light through a photomask, this technique to obtain oriented dye films is applicable to production of multiaxis dye films that are suitable for color filters for three-dimensional LC display devices.

OTHER SELF-ORGANIZED MATERIALS

The surface-mediated orientation control of molecules described above covers versatile types of LCs. This method has opened the way to novel research and practical applications. If this kind of orientation transfer is achievable from command surfaces to molecular bulks other than LCs, it is anticipated that versatile functional materials for electronic and photonic applications can be developed because the control of molecular orientation of organic compounds plays a critical role in achieving optimum performance.

Polysilanes have been extensively investigated because of their unique physical properties, in particular, optoelectronic characteristics arising from the delocalized σ electronic conjugation of their Si main chains. The conformation of the main chains in a spin-cast polysilane film was altered upon storage due to crystallization stemming from the formation of all-*trans* zigzag conformations of Si chains. These types of conformational changes can be monitored conveniently by following ultra-violet absorption bands.

The crystallization behavior of a spin-cast film of poly(dihexylsilane) exhibiting a disordered state was influenced by the nature of the substrate surface, implying that the orientation of polymer main chains was influenced by the nature of the substrate surface. When a thin film of polysilane was fabricated by spreading its hexane solution on a film of an azobenzene polymer exposed to linearly polarized

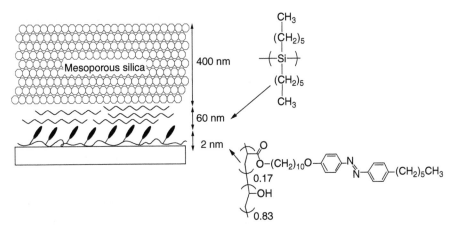

FIGURE 15.27 Orientation photocontrol of a mesoporous silica deposited on a doubled layer consisting of a monolayer of a photoaligned azobenzene-polymer and a thin film of poly(hexylsilane).

light in advance, a disordered state of the polymer was gradually converted to a uniaxially aligned state during crystallization.[95] Annealing of the film enhanced the main chain orientation. This means that photooriented states of azobenzene groups were transferred to the main chain orientations in the film. The orientation directions were in line with those of photocontrolled azobenzene moieties. Thus, orientation direction was determined by the electric vector of the actinic light for azobenzene isomerization.

Since levels of main chain orientation are relatively high, these types of films are applicable for aligning nematic LCs conveniently.[96] A more interesting feature of oriented polysilane films is their capability of demonstrating orientation control of mesostructured sol–gel silica films. Such films are quite stiff, whereas the materials subjected to the photoalignment technique described above are rather soft. The first step of the procedure to achieve orientation control of mesoporous materials[97] is photoorientation of a thin film of an azobenzene polymer by irradiation with linearly polarized light, followed by spincasting and annealing of a film of the polysilane as the second step. The third step consists of coating an acidic aqueous solution of tetraethoxysilane and cetyltrimethylammonium to produce a surfactant-templated mesoporous film of an organic–inorganic hybrid (Figure 15.27). The photochemical removal of surfactant template molecules by irradiation with deep ultraviolet light generates novel silica materials with orientation-controlled microchannels.

OUTLOOK

Studies of photoorientation, defined as photogenerated optical anisotropy, were pioneered by Weigert in 1921. Systematic efforts to understand and apply this phenomenon were initiated only about two decades ago. The motivation to expand this research field arises from combinations with liquid–crystalline materials,

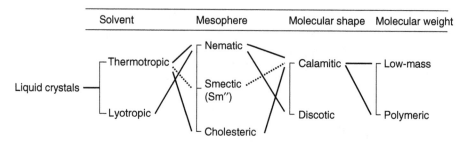

FIGURE 15.28 Surface-assisted photoalignment control of various types of LCs.

because photogenerated optical anisotropy is markedly amplified by the self-assembling nature of LCs to provide practical applications to rewritable optical recording materials, LC-aligning films for LC flat display devices, and various types of optical elements with optical anisotropies. The late 1990s saw significant advancement in this research field that revealed the mechanisms of photoorientation and relaxation of photooriented states in polymer solids and provided novel procedures for controlling orientation directions of molecules including oblique irradiation with nonpolarized light to achieve tilting photoorientation.

Azobenzene photochemistry played a crucial role in revealing photoorientation phenomena from fundamental and practical standpoints. This progress was made possible by certain characteristic features of azobenzenes. First, azobenzene suffers from single and fatigue-resistant photoisomerization, as a result of which kinetic analysis is easy to perform and reuse of the same samples under different irradiation conditions is possible. Also, because the electric dipole transition moment of azobenzene for $\pi-\pi^*$ transition is approximately in accordance with the longitudinal molecular axis, the identification of the molecular axis can be carried out accurately by determining polar and azimuthal angles of azobenzene by ultraviolet visible absorption spectral measurements.

Geometrical isomers of azobenzene are quite different in molecular shape and in dipole moment so that photoisomerization can be coupled with other molecular events, as typified by the photoalignment of LCs triggered by command surfaces. Also, azobenzene derivatives are readily available and suitable to clarify structure–function relationships, as noted in this chapter.

On the basis of the photoorientation behavior of azobenzenes in molecular and polymeric films, the working principle of the photoinduced generation of optical anisotropy was determined and led to exploring diverse molecular and polymeric materials exhibiting tailor-made optical anisotropy by incorporating various photosensitive units other than azobenzenes. One typical example illustrating this scenario is the development of photogenerated LC-aligning films suitable for LC flat-panel display devices by employing various types of photochemical reactions.[8–10]

The command surface technique is applicable to conventional nematic LCs and to other types of LCs. The results of photoalignments of LC systems are summarized in Figure 15.28,[98] indicating that wide ranges of LC materials can allow photoinduced alignment control. Considering that industrial significance has been restricted to low-mass nematic LCs and that fundamental studies have concentrated on other types of LCs, we believe that the surface-assisted photoorientation technique provides novel and efficient ways to promote LC technologies.

An alternative advancement of photoorientation can be expected by combinations with self-organized materials other than LCs. A clue has been found in systems consisting of crystalline materials such as polysilane, as noted above. Finally, levels of photoorientation are relatively low for anisotropic materials such as amorphous polymers — even below glass transition temperatures — owing to the involvement of thermal micro-Brownian motions. In this respect, the amplification of molecular photoorientation is required by adopting materials displaying molecular self-organization that may be triggered by photoorientation exhibiting marked molecular amplification.[98]

REFERENCES

1. Sekkat, Z. and Knoll, W., Eds., *Photoreactive Organic Thin Films*, Academic Press, Amsterdam, 2002.
2. Natansohn, A. and Rochon, P., Photoinduced motions of azo-containing polymers, *Chem. Rev.* 102, 4139, 2002.
3. Sekkat, Z., Photoisomerization and photoorientation of azo dye in films of polymers: molecular interaction, free volume, and polymer structural effects, in *Photoreactive Organic Thin Films*, Sekkat, Z. and Knoll W., Eds., Academic Press, Amsterdam, 2002, chap. II-4.
4. Ichimura, K., Photochromic polymers, in *Organic Photochromic and Thermochromic Compounds*, Vol. 2, Crano, J.C. and Guglielmetti, R.J., Eds., Kluwer Academic/Plenum, New York, 1999, chap. 1.
5. Michl, J., Photochromism by orientation, in *Photochromism: Molecules and Systems*, Dürr, H. and Bouas-Laurent, H., Eds., Elsevier, Amsterdam, 1990, chap. 27.
6. Michl, J. and Thulstrup, E.W., in *Spectroscopy with Polarized Light*, VCH Publishers, New York, 1995, p. 198.
7. Weigert, F., Über einen neuen Effekt der Strahlung, *Naturwissenschaften*, 29, 583, 1921.
8. Ichimura, K., Photoregulation of liquid crystal alignment by photochromic molecules and polymeric thin films, in *Polymers as Electrooptical and Photooptical Active Media*, Shibaev, V., Ed., Springer, Berlin, 1996, chap. 4.
9. Ichimura, K., Photoalignment of liquid crystal systems, *Chem. Rev.*, 100, 1847, 2000.
10. O'Neill, M. and Kelly, S.M., Photoinduced surface alignment for liquid crystal displays, *J. Phys. D Appl. Phys.*, 33, R67, 2000.
11. Teitel, A., Über eine besondere mechanische Wirkung des polarisierten Lichts. *Naturwissenschaften*, 44, 370, 1957.
12. Todorov, T., Nikolova, L., and Tomova, N., Polarization holography: a new high-efficiency organic material with reversible photoinduced birefringence, *Appl. Opt.*, 23, 4309, 1984.
13. Eich, M. et al. Reversible digital and holographic optical storage in polymeric liquid crystals, *Makromol. Chem.*, 8, 59, 1987.
14. Eich, M. and Wendorff, J., Erasable holograms in polymeric liquid–crystalline side chain polymers, *Makromol. Chem.*, 8, 467, 1987.
15. Xie, S., Natansohn, A., and Rochon, P., Recent developments in aromatic azo polymer research, *Chem. Mater.*, 5, 403, 1993.

16. Akiyama, H., Kudo, K., and Ichimura, K., Command surfaces. 10. Novel polymethacrylates with laterally attached azobenzene groups displaying photoinduced optical anisotropy, *Macromol. Chem. Rapid Commun.*, 16, 35, 1995.

17. Akiyama, H. and Ichimura, K., Photochromic behavior in thin films of polymethacrylates substituted with side-on and head-on type azobenzenes, *Mol. Cryst. Liq. Cryst.*, 315, 47, 1998.

18. Suh, D.-H. et al., Polymethacrylates with benzylidenephthalimidine side chains. 1. Photochemical characterstics of model compounds and polymers, *Macromol. Chem. Phys.*, 199, 363, 1998.

19. Suh, D.-H. et al., Polymethacrylates with benzylidenephthalimidine side chains. 2. Photocontrol of alignment of a nematic liquid crystal, *Macromol. Chem. Phys.*, 199, 375, 1998.

20. Yamaki, S. et al., Photochemical behavior and the ability to control liquid crystal alignment of polymethacrylates with styrylpyridine side chains, *Macromol. Chem. Phys.*, 202, 325, 2001.

21. Yamaki, S. et al., Effect of methylene spacers of poly(methacrylates) bearing styrylpyridine side chains on the ability to control liquid crystal alignment, *Macromol. Chem. Phys.*, 202, 354, 2001.

22. Ichimura, K. et al., Role of E/Z photoisomerization of cinnamate side chains attached to polymer backbones in the alignment photoregulation of nematic liquid crystals, *Jpn. J. Appl. Phys.*, 35, L996, 1996.

23. Ichimura, K. et al., Reactivity of polymers with regioisomeric cinnamate side chains and their ability to regulate liquid crystal alignment, *Macromolecules*, 30, 903, 1997.

24. Obi, M., Morino, S., and Ichimura, K., Reversion of photoalignment direction of liquid crystals induced by cinnamate polymer films, *Jpn. J. Appl. Phys.*, 38, L145, 1999.

25. Obi, M., Morino, S., and Ichimura, K., Photocontrol of liquid crystal alignment by polymethacrylate with diphenylacetylene side chains, *Chem. Mater.*, 11, 1293, 1999.

26. Obi, M., Morino, S., and Ichimura, K., The reversion of photoalignment direction of a liquid crystal induced by a polymethacryalte with coumarin side chains, *Macromol. Rapid Commun.*, 19, 643, 1998.

27. Obi, M., Morino, S., and Ichimura, K., Factors affecting photoalignment of liquid crystals induced by polymethacrylates with coumarin side chains, *Chem. Mater.*, 11, 656, 1999.

28. Kidowaki, M. et al., Thermal amplification of photoinduced optical anisotropy of *p*-cyanoazobenzene polymer films monitored by temperature scanning ellipsometry, *Appl. Phys. Lett.*, 76, 1377, 2000.

29. Ikeda, T. et al., Photochemically induced isothermal phase thransition in polymer liquid crystals with mesogenic phenyl benzoate side chain. I. Calorimetric studies and order parameters, *Macromolecules*, 23, 36, 1990.

30. Ikeda, T. et al., Photochemically induced isothermal phase transition in polymer liquid crystals with mesogenic phenyl benzoate side chains. 2. Photochemically induced isothermal phase transition behaviors, *Macromolecules*, 23, 42, 1990.

31. Ikeda, T. and Tsutsumi, O., Optical switching and image storage by means of azobenzene liquid–crystal films, *Science*, 268, 1873, 1995.

32. Stumpe, J. et al., Photoreaction in mesogenic media. 5. Photoinduced optical anisotropy of liquid–crystalline side chain polymers with azo chromophores by linearly polarized light of low intensity, *Makromol. Chem. Rapid Commun.*, 12, 81, 1991.

33. Fischer, T. et al., Photoinduced optical anisotropy in films of photochromic liquid crystalline polymers, *J. Photochem. Photobiol. A*, 80, 453, 1994.

34. Geue, T., Ziegler, A., and Stumpe, J., Light-induced orientation phenomena in Langmuir–Blodgett multipairs, *Macromolecules*, 30, 5729, 1997.
35. Wu, Y. et al., Photoinduced alignment of polymer liquid crystals containing azobenzene moieties in the side chain. 2. Effect of spacer length of the azobenzene unit on alignment behavior, *Macromolecules*, 31, 1104, 1998.
36. Han, M. and Ichimura, K., In-plane and tilt orientation of *p*-methoxyazobenzene side chains tethered to liquid crystalline polymethacrylates by irradiation with 365 nm light, *Macromolecules*, 34, 90, 2001.
37. Han, M., Morino, S., and Ichimura, K., Photochemistry determined by light propagation. 1. Three-dimensional photomanipulation of self-organized azobenzenes in liquid–crystalline polymers, *Chem. Lett.*, 645, 1999.
38. Han, M., Morino, S., and Ichimura, K., Factors affecting in-plane and out-of-plane photoorientation of azobenzene side chains attached to liquid crystalline polymers induced by irradiation with linearly polarized light, *Macromolecules*, 33, 6360, 2000.
39. Kidowaki, M., Fujiwara, T., and Ichimura, K., Extraordinarily thermostable photodichroism of poly(4-cyano-4′-methacryloyloxyazobenzene) films, *Chem. Lett.*, 641, 1999.
40. Ichimura, K., Kidowaki, M., and Fujiwara, T., Thermally stable photaligned *p*-cyanoazobenzene moieties in polymer thin films, *Macromol. Symp.*, 137, 129, 1999.
41. Natansohn, A. et al., Azo polymers for reversible optical storage. 4. Cooperative motion of rigid groups in semicrystalline polymers, *Macromolecules*, 27, 2580, 1994.
42. Kawanishi, Y., Tamaki, T., and Ichimura, K., Photoregulation of liquid–crystalline orientation by anisotropic photochromism of surface azobenzenes, *ACS Symp. Ser.*, 537, 453, 1994.
43. Ichimura, K., Morino, S., and Akiyama, H., Three dimensional orientational control of molecules by slantwise photoirradiation, *Appl. Phys. Lett.*, 73, 921, 1998.
44. Ichimura, K., Han, M., and Morino, S., Photochemistry determined by light propagation. 1. Three-dimensional photomanipulation of self-organized azobenzenes in liquid–crystalline polymers, *Chem. Lett.*, 85, 1999.
45. Han, M., Morino, S., and Ichimura, K., Tilt orientation of *p*-methoxyazobenzene side chains in liquid crystalline polymer films by irradiation with non-polarized light, *Macromolecules*, 34, 82, 2001.
46. Wu, Y., Ikeda, T., and Zhang, Q., Three-dimensional manipulation of an azo polymer liquid crystal with unpolarized light, *Adv. Mater.*, 11, 300, 1999.
47. Ichimura, K. and Han, M., Molecular reorientation induced by sunshine suggesting the generation of absolute chirality, *Chem. Lett.*, 286, 2000.
48. Keszthelyi, L., Origin of the homochirality of biomolecules, *Q. Rev. Biophys.*, 28, 473, 1995.
49. Ulbricht, T.L.V., Asymmetry: non-conservation of parity and optical activity, *Q. Rev.*, 13, 48, 1959.
50. Bonner, W.A., The origin and amplification of biomolecules, *Origins Life Evol. Biosphere*, 21, 59, 1991.
51. Oró, J., Comets and the formation of biochemical compounds on the primitive Earth, *Nature*, 190, 389, 1961.
52. Balavoine, G., Moradpour, A., and Kagan, H.B., Preparaton of chiral compounds with high optical purity by irradiation with circularly polarized light: a model reaction for the prebiotic generation of optical activity, *J. Am. Chem. Soc.*, 96, 5152, 1974.
53. Norden, B., Was photoresolution of amino acids the origin of optical activity of life? *Nature*, 266, 567, 1977.
54. Anderle, K. et al., Molecular addressing? Studies on light-induced reorientation in liquid–crystalline side chain polymers, *Liq. Cryst.*, 9, 691, 1991.

55. Morino, S., Kaiho, A., and Ichimura, K., Photoinduced generation of birefringence of liquid crystal/polymer composites, *Appl. Phys. Lett.*, 73, 1317, 1998.

56. Yoshimoto, N., Morino, S., and Ichimura, K., Photochemistry determined by light propagation. 3. Three-dimensional orientational photocontrol of liquid–crystalline molecules in photoresponsive polymer networks, *Chem. Lett.*, 711, 1999.

57. Yoshimoto, N. et al., Holographic Bragg gratings in a photoresponsive cross-linked polymer–liquid–crystal composite, *Opt. Lett.*, 27, 182, 2002.

58. Ichimura, K. et al., Reversible change in alignment mode of nematic liquid crystals regulated photochemically by "command surfaces" modified with an azobenzene monolayer, *Langmuir*, 4, 1214, 1988.

59. Ichimura, K., Surface-assisted photoregulation of molecular assemblage as commander–soldier molecular systems, *Supramol. Sci.*, 3, 67, 1996.

60. Jérôme, B., Surface alignment, in *Handbook of Liquid Crystals*, Vol. 1, Demus, D. et al., Eds., Wiley-VCH, Weinheim, 1998, p. 535.

61. Oh, S.-K., Nakagawa, M., and Ichimura, K., Relationship between the ability to control liquid crystal alignment and wetting properties of calix[4]resorcinarene monolayers, *J. Mater. Chem.*, 11, 1563, 2001.

62. Kurita, E. et al., Macrocyclic amphiphiles. 2. Multi-point adsorptivity of crown conformer of calix[4]resorcinarenes and their derivatives on surfaces of amorphous polar substrates, *J. Mater. Chem.*, 1998, 8, 397.

63. Ichimura, K. et al., Convenient preparation of self-assembled monolayers derived from calix[4]resorcinarene derivatives exhibiting resistance to desorption, *J. Inclusion Phenom. Mol. Recognition*, 35, 173, 1999.

64. Fujimaki, M. et al., Macrocyclic amphiphiles. 3. Monolayers of O-octacarboxyl-methoxylated calix[4]resorcinarenes with azobenzene residues exhibiting efficient photoisomerizability, *Langmuir*, 14, 4495, 1998.

65. DiMilla, P.A. et al., Wetting and protein adsorption of self-assembled monolayers of alkanethiolates supported on transparent films of gold, *J. Am. Chem. Soc.* 116, 2225, 1994.

66. Jin, W., Koplik, J., and Banavar, J.R., Wetting hysteresis at the molecular level, *Phys. Rev. Lett.*, 78, 1520, 1997.

67. Fadeev, A.Y. and McCarthy, T.J., Trialkylsilane monolayers covalently attached to silicone surfaces: Wettability studies indicating that molecular topography contributes to contact angle hysteresis, *Langmuir*, 15, 3759, 1999.

68. Furumi, S., Morino, S., and Ichimura, K., unpublished results.

69. Furumi, S. et al., Photogeneration of high pretilt angles of nematic liquid crystals by azobenzene-containing polymer films, *Appl. Phys. Lett.*, 74, 2438, 1999.

70. Kidowaki, M., Fujiwara, T., and Ichimura, K., Surface-assisted photomanipulation of orientation of a polymer liquid crystal, *Chem. Lett.*, 1999, 643.

71. Coles, H.J., Chiral nematics: physical properties and applications, in *Handbook of Liquid Crystals*, Vol 2A, Demus, D. et al., Eds., Wiley-VCH, Weinheim, 1998, p. 335.

72. Ruslim, C. and Ichimura, K., Photocontrolled alignment of chiral nematic liquid crystals, *Adv. Mater.*, 2001, 13, 641.

73. Kawata, K., Orientation control and fixation of discotic liquid crystals, *Chem Rec.*, 2, 59, 2002.

74. Chandrasekhar, S., Columnar, discotic nematic and lamellar liquid crystals: their structures and physical properties, in *Handbook of Liquid Crystals*, Vol. 2B, Demus, D. et al., Eds., Wiley-VCH, Weinheim, 1998, p. 749.

75. Ichimura, K. et al., Photocontrolled orientation of discotic liquid crystals, *Adv. Mater.*, 12, 950, 2000.

76. Furumi, S. et al., Photochemical manipulation of discotic liquid crystal alignment by a poly(vinyl cinnamate) thin film, *Appl. Phys. Lett.*, 77, 2689, 2000.

77. Furumi, S. et al., Polarized photoluminescence from photo-patterned discotic liquid crystal films, *Chem. Mater.* 13, 1434, 2001.

78. Attwood, T.K. and Lydon, J.E., The chromonic phases of dyes, *Liq. Cryst.*, 1, 499, 1986.

79. Boden, N. et al., Designing new lyotropic amphiphilic mesogens to optimize the stability of nematic phases, *Liq. Cryst.*, 1, 109, 1986.

80. Attwood, T.K. and Lydon, J.E., A new model for the molecular arrangements in chromonic mesophases, *Mol. Cryst. Liq. Cryst. Lett. Sect.*, 4, 9, 1986.

81. Perahia, D., Wachtel, E.J., and Luz, Z., NMR and x-ray studies of the chromic lyomesophases formed by some xanthone derivatives, *Liq. Cryst.*, 9, 479, 1991.

82. Sadler, D.E. et al., Lyotropic liquid–crystalline mesophases and a novel, solid physical form of some water-soluble reactive dyes, *Liq. Cryst.*, 1, 509, 1986.

83. Loewenstein, A. and Brenman, M., Study of the liquid crystalline phases of benzopurpurin in water, *Liq. Cryst.*, 17, 499, 1994.

84. Tiddy, G.J.T. et al., Highly ordered aggregates in dilute dye–water systems, *Langmuir*, 11, 390, 1995.

85. Harrison, W.J., Mateer, D.L., and Tiddy, G.J.T., Liquid–crystalline J-aggregates formed by aqueous ionic cyanine dyes, *J. Phys. Chem.*, 100, 2310, 1996.

86. Iverson, I.K. and Tam-Chang, S.-W., Cascade of molecular order by sequential self-organization, induced orientation, and order transfer processes, *J. Am. Chem. Soc.*, 121, 5801, 1999.

87. Iverson, I.K. et al., Controlling molecular orientation in solid films via self-organization in the liquid–crystalline phase, *Langmuir*, 18, 3510, 2002.

88. Attwood, T.K. and Lydon, J.E., Lyotropic mesophase formation by anti-asthmatic drugs, *Mol. Cryst. Liq. Cryst.*, 108, 349, 1984.

89. Lydon, J.E., New models for the mesophases of disodium chromoglycate (INTAL), *Mol. Cryst. Liq. Cryst.*, 64, 19, 1980.

90. Attwood, T.K. and Lydon, J.E., The distinction between chromic and amphiphilic lyotropic mesophases, *Liq. Cryst.*, 7, 657, 1990.

91. Fujiwara, T. and Ichimura, K., Surface-assisted photoalignment control of lyotropic liquid crystals. 2. Photopatterning of aqueous solutions of a water-soluble anti-asthmatic drug as lyotropic liquid crystals, *J. Mater. Chem.*, 12, 3387, 2002.

92. Fujiwara, T. et al., Surface-assisted photoalignment control of lyotropic liquid crystals. 1. Characterisation and photoalignment of aqueous solutions of a water-soluble dye as lyotropic liquid crystals, *J. Mater. Chem.*, 12, 3380, 2002.

93. Ichimura, K. et al., Surface-assisted photolithography to form anisotropic dye layers as a new horizon of command surfaces, *Langmuir*, 11, 2341, 1995.

94. Matsunaga, D. et al., Photofabrication of micro-patterned polarizing elements for stereoscopic liquid crystal displays, *Adv. Mater.*, 14, 1477, 2002.

95. Seki, T., Fukuda, K., and Ichimura, K., Photocontrol of polymer chain organization using a photochromic monolayer, *Langmuir*, 15, 5098, 1999.

96. Fukuda, K., Seki, T., and Ichimura, K., Photocontrol of poly(dihexylsilane) chain organization using a photochromic monolayer, *Mol. Cryst. Liq. Cryst.*, 2001, 368, 461.

97. Kawashima, Y. et al., Photo-orientation of mesostructured silica via hierarchical multiple transfer, *Chem. Mater.*, 14, 2842, 2002.

98. Ichimura, K., Molecular amplification of photochemical events, *J. Photochem. Photobiol. A Chem.*, 158, 205, 2003.

16 Fast Responsive Liquid Crystalline Polymer Systems

Seiji Kurihara

CONTENTS

INTRODUCTION

Thermotropic liquid crystalline side chain polymers with photochromic molecules have been widely studied in the field of optical devices.[1–17] Liquid crystalline side chain polymers combine the properties of side chain polymeric materials and low molecular weight liquid crystals. Polymeric materials exhibit self-standing properties and good processing ability; low molecular weight liquid crystals possess physical properties that are intermediate between a liquid and a crystal, that is, fluidity and anisotropy properties such as refractive index and dielectric constant.

Anisotropic molecular shapes (e.g., rod-like and disc-like) are generally required for liquid crystallinity and the appearance of liquid crystalline phases. Therefore, if we can change the molecular shapes of molecules in liquid crystalline polymers photochemically, we will be able to switch liquid crystalline properties photochemically. Consequently, we can manufacture various optical devices by simple methods such as casting and coating from solutions containing photoresponsive liquid crystal polymers.

Many types of photochromic compounds have been reported and explored for application to optical devices, including azobenzenes,[18,19] stilbenes,[20] spiropyrans,[21]

0-8493-1487-9/04/$0.00+$1.50

diarylethens,[22] flugides,[23] and thioindigos.[24] Some azobenzene compounds show liquid crystalline phases because of their molecular shapes. The azobenzene compounds are well known to show reversible photoisomerization between the *trans* and *cis* forms. The *trans* azobenzene molecules with rod shapes can convert into *cis* forms with bent shapes by ultraviolet irradiation, and return thermally or photochemically to their *trans* forms. The *cis* forms of azobenzenes do not show liquid crystallinity, because of diminished anisotropy in their molecular shapes. Therefore, it is expected that azobenzene molecules are suited to act as trigger molecules to modulate the molecular orientations and optical properties of liquid crystalline systems.

The *trans* to *cis* photoisomerization of the azobenzene molecules disorganizes the structure of the liquid crystalline phase and causes a depression of phase transition temperatures from the liquid crystalline phase to other phases.[25] Consequently, an isothermal phase transition known as the photochemical phase transition can be induced photochemically. The photoresponsive liquid crystalline polymers can be prepared by doping and copolymerizing with appropriate azobenzene compounds.

Ikeda et al. extensively explored the photochemical phase transition of polymer liquid crystalline systems by the use of the liquid crystalline polymers having only azobenzenes as the mesogenic side groups. The time required to achieve phase transition, resolution, and stability of the data stored are important factors for optical storage systems, whereas the rate of repetition cycle is also significant for data processing, display, and so on. The major aim of this chapter will be to describe the photochemical switching of polymeric liquid crystalline materials with azobenzene compounds in fast repetition systems.

LIQUID CRYSTALLINE POLYMER NETWORKS

LIGHT CROSSLINKING OF LIQUID CRYSTALLINE POLYMERS

Liquid crystals tend to form turbid films without monodomain treatment. Therefore, the formation of a macroscopically anisotropic molecular orientation is required for the application of liquid crystals to optical devices. Although the formation of the macroscopically anisotropic molecular orientation of low molecular weight liquid crystals can be achieved easily by various alignment treatments such as rubbing, the molecular orientations of polymeric materials are hard to control because of their high viscosity.

One effective method of accomplishing macroscopically anisotropic molecular orientations of liquid crystalline polymers is polymerization of liquid crystals having polymerizable groups (liquid crystalline monomers) in a unidirectional orientation. Many studies on the preparation and application of liquid crystalline monomers to provide the anisotropic polymer films and optical materials have been widely reported by the Phillips' group and others.[26–40]

We prepared lightly crosslinked polymer networks and explored the effects of crosslinking on the stability of macroscopically anisotropic molecular orientations[16,41] in order to prepare liquid crystalline networks possessing both stability of macroscopic molecular orientation and the ability to respond to external stimuli. Scheme 16.1 shows liquid crystalline monomers **APB6** and **A6PB6A**.

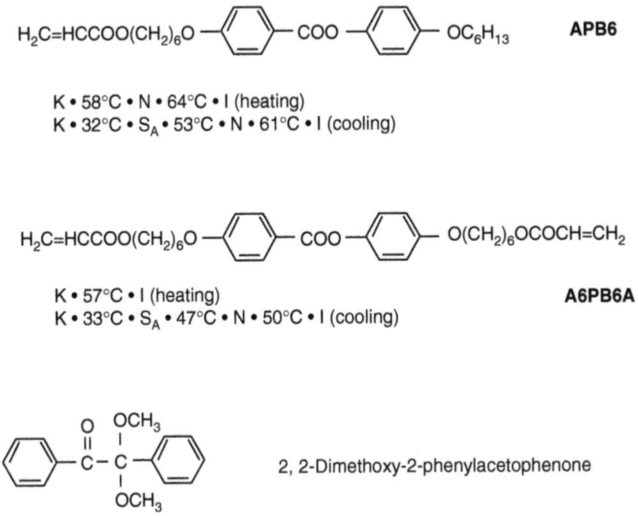

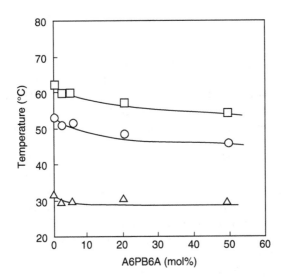

SCHEME 16.1 Structures of liquid crystal monomers APB6 and A6PB6A and 2,2-dimethoxy-2-phenylacetophenone.

FIGURE 16.1 Phase diagram of binary mixtures of APB6 and A6PB6A.

Monoacrylate **APB6** exhibits only a nematic (N) phase on heating, whereas smectic (SA) and N phases were observed on cooling. Diacrylate **A6PB6A** had two polymerizable groups in the molecule and was used as crosslinking agent. **A6PB6A** is a monotropic liquid crystal, both N and SA phases were observed only on cooling.

Figure 16.1 is a phase diagram of binary mixtures of **APB6** and **A6PB6A** in which **A6PB6A** is in a concentration range from 0 to 50 mol%. Phase separation of each monomer in the mixtures was not recognized in all mixtures studied, although

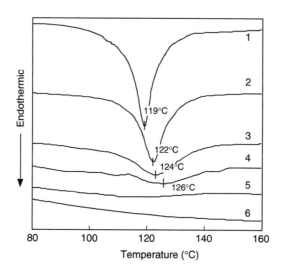

FIGURE 16.2 DSC thermograms of poly(APB6/A6PB6A) on heating. 1 = p(100:0). 2 = p(98:2). 3 = p(95:5). 4 = p(90:10). 5 = p(85:15). 6 = p(80:20). p(m:n) = composition of poly(APB6/A6PB6A); m and n are the contents of APB6 and A6PB6A in mol%, respectively.

a little depression in the transition temperatures was observed with the increase in the concentration of **A6PB6A**. Similarly, the structures of both monomers resulted in good mutual solubility.

Polymerizable mixtures were prepared by adding 2 mol% of 2,2-dimethoxy-2-phenylacetophenone to **APB6/A6PB6A** mixtures as a photoradical initiator. The amount of **A6PB6A** in the **APB6/A6PB6A** mixtures was varied from 0 to 20 mol%. Into two glass plates, 2 mg of each **APB6/A6PB6A** mixture containing the photo-radical initiator were loaded and irradiated at 55°C (N phase). The conversion was higher than 90% by ultraviolet (UV) irradiation longer than 10 min.

Figure 16.2 shows DSC thermograms of poly(**APB6/A6PB6A**) containing various amounts of **A6PB6A** obtained on heating. Although the crosslinking density of the poly(**APB6/A6PB6A**)s was not determined exactly, the amounts of **A6PB6A** fed in the monomer mixtures were roughly equal to the crosslinking density because of the high polymerization conversion. The result shown in Figure 16.2 indicates the effect of crosslinking density on the phase transition behavior of the poly(**APB6/A6PB6A**)s.

The crosslinking density clearly has an influence on phase transition behavior. An endothermic peak at 119°C was observed for poly(**APB6**) without **A6PB6A**. It has been reported that the poly(**APB6**) showed the S phase as a liquid crystalline phase.[42] Therefore, the peak can be assigned to the S-to-I phase transition.

The endothermic peak was shifted to higher temperatures and broadened by increasing the crosslinking density. To clarify the effect of the crosslinking density on phase transition behavior, the change in the phase transition temperature and enthalpy change were plotted as functions of crosslinking density (Figure 16.3). The phase transition temperature was increased and the enthalpy change was decreased with the increase in crosslinking density. The effect of the crosslinking density was

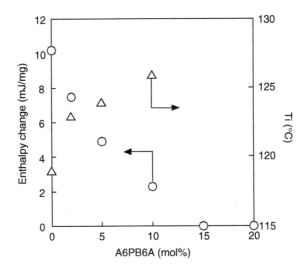

FIGURE 16.3 Effect of crosslinking density on enthalpy change and nematic–isotropic phase transition temperature (Ti) of poly(APB6/A6PB6A).

interpreted in terms of extreme depression in the molecular motion of the polymer segments in the polymer network. The higher the crosslinking density increases, the less the molecular motion becomes. No peak was observed on DSC thermograms for poly(**APB6/A6PB6A**)s containing **A6PB6A** above 15% due to the depression of molecular motion.

The poly(**APB6/A6PB6A**) networks having crosslinking densities lower than 15 mol% still had enough molecular motion to show the transitions to the I phase. In order to explore the effect of crosslinking on both stability and thermal reversibility of the macroscopic molecular orientation, transmittance, and birefringence of the polymer networks with various crosslinking densities were measured as function of temperatures.

Figure 16.4 shows changes in both birefringence (Δn) and transmittance of a poly(**APB6/A6PB6A**) 95:5 mol% network by heating and subsequent cooling. The network was prepared by polymerization of a mixture of 95 mol% of **APB6** and 5 mol% of **A6PB6A** in a 50-μm homogeneous cell at the N phase. The value of Δn was determined by measuring the number of interference lines of the poly(**APB6/A6PB6A**) network in the Cano-wedge cell between two crossed polarizers by the use of a probe light from a laser diode. Before polymerization, the Δn of the (**APB6/A6PB6A**) mixture was 0.08 at 57°C — roughly equal to the value of Δn measured with an Abbe refractometer. Although a little increase in Δn was observed by polymerization, as can be seen in Figure 16.4, the value of the poly(**APB6/A6PB6A**) network was around 0.1 and remained constant up to 120°C. Above that temperature, Δn was decreased rapidly due to the transition to the I phase. After cooling, Δn was increased again and restored to its initial value. The results clearly demonstrate that the poly(**APB6/A6PB6A**) network shows a reversible phase transition between the uniaxial liquid crystalline and I phases (Figure 16.5).

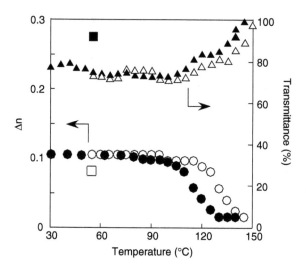

FIGURE 16.4 Changes in birefringence (Δn).

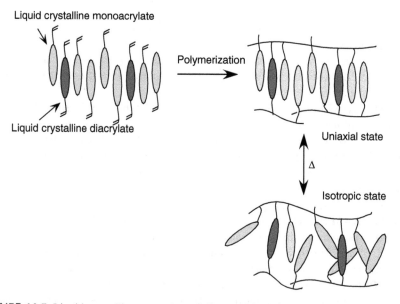

FIGURE 16.5 Liquid crystalline networks and the transition between uniaxial and isotropic phases.

On the other hand, the polymerization of **APB6** without **A6PB6A** affected the temperature dependence of both Δn and transmittance in a different way from the poly(**APB6/A6PB6A**) network. A significant decrease in transmittance was observed by polymerization, as can be seen in Figure 16.6. Polarized optical microscopic

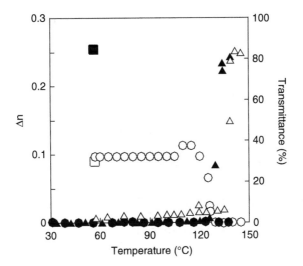

FIGURE 16.6 Changes in birefringence (Δn).

observation revealed that the polymerization resulted in the transformation from a uniaxial monodomain structure to a multidomain structure. Poly(**APB6**) remains in the S phase below 119°C, whereas **APB6** is in the N phase at the irradiation temperature (55°C).

The macroscopically structural transformation to the multidomain structure may be related to the transformation from the N phase to the S phase during polymerization. The multidomain structure may be responsible for the significant decrease in transmittance due to strong light scattering. Although the Δn of poly(**APB6**) was about 0.9 and remained at 0.9 during heating up to 110°C, no restoration of the Δn of poly(**APB6**) was caused by heating above 130°C and subsequent cooling after a single transition to the I phase. After the transition to the I phase, the size of the multidomain structure became smaller than that immediately after polymerization. The comparison of results obtained for poly(**APB6/A6PB6A**) and poly(**APB6**) implies that the crosslinking of polymer networks with a few mol% of **A6PB6A** is enough to sustain their macroscopically uniaxial molecular orientations and is responsible for the thermal reversible changes in the macroscopic molecular orientation of the uniaxial liquid crystalline phase and the I phase.

To explore the effects of monomer structures, **APB6** was copolymerized with other monomers such as 4,4′-diacryloyloxybiphenyl (**ABA**), tetraethyleneglycol dimethacrylate (**4G**), methylene bisacrylamide (**MBA**), and hexamethylene diacrylate (**HA**) (Scheme 16.2). The copolymer of **APB6** and **ABA** showed stable macroscopic molecular orientation, while the copolymers of **APB6** and **4G**, **MBA**, or **HA** did not. The result can be interpreted in terms of the structures of the monomers. Both **A6PB6A** and **ABA** monomers have mesogenic core moieties; the others do not. The intermolecular interaction between mesogenic moieties is one of the most important factors influencing properties of resulting polymer networks.

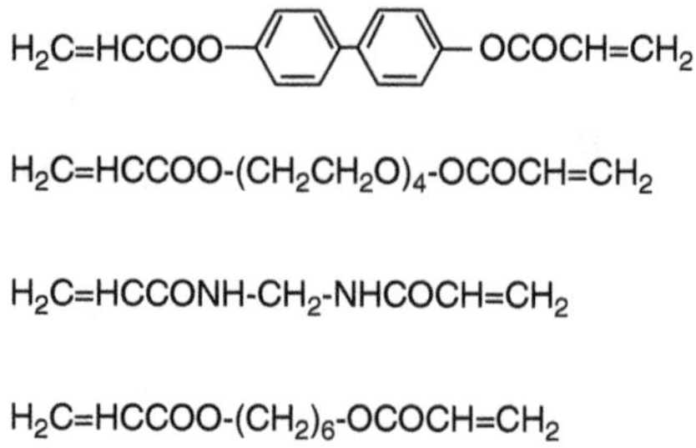

H₂C=HCCOO—⟨◯⟩—⟨◯⟩—OCOCH=CH₂ **ABA**

$H_2C=HCCOO-(CH_2CH_2O)_4-OCOCH=CH_2$ **4G**

$H_2C=HCCONH-CH_2-NHCOCH=CH_2$ **MBA**

$H_2C=HCCOO-(CH_2)_6-OCOCH=CH_2$ **HA**

SCHEME 16.2 Structures of ABA, 4G, MBA, and HA.

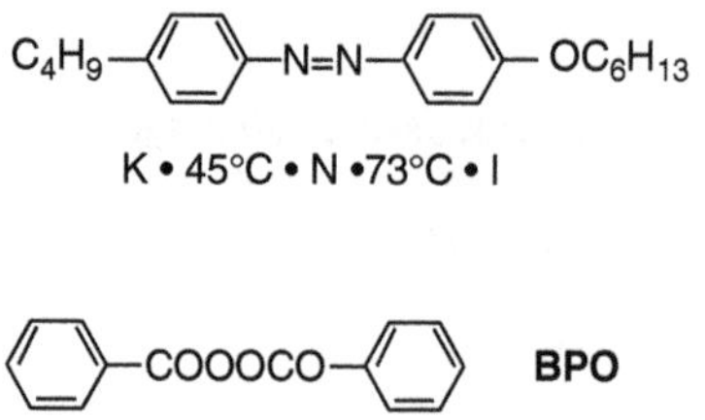

C_4H_9—⟨◯⟩—N=N—⟨◯⟩—OC_6H_{13} **BHAB**

K • 45°C • N •73°C • I

⟨◯⟩—COOOCO—⟨◯⟩   **BPO**

SCHEME 16.3 Structures of BHAB and BPO.

PHOTORESPONSIVE BEHAVIORS OF NETWORKS DOPED WITH AZOBENZENE MOLECULES

Lightly crosslinked liquid crystalline networks were found to hold stable uniaxial molecular orientation and also show the phase transition from the anisotropic molecular orientation to the I phase. Therefore, the same responses to external stimuli may be expected from low molecular weight liquid crystals and liquid crystalline polymers without crosslinking.

Photoresponsive liquid crystalline networks were prepared by polymerization of mixtures of **APB6**, **A6PB6A**, and **BHAB** (Scheme 16.1 and Scheme 16.3) containing 3 mol% of benzoyl peroxide (BPO) as a radical initiator at the nematic phase (57°C) for 1 h in a homogeneous glass cell.[16,17,41,43] The conversion of the mixtures was higher than 80%. Figure 16.7 shows the temperature dependence of both Δn and transmittance for the poly(**APB6/A6PB6A/BHAB**) 90:5:5 network and poly(**APB6/BHAB**) (95:5 mol%). As mentioned, the lightly crosslinked network exhibited a stable uniaxial molecular orientation and a reversible phase transition between the liquid crystalline and I phases. Azobenzene molecules doped in the network exerted no influence on the stability of the macroscopic molecular orientation or the phase transitions of the liquid crystalline networks.

Changes in the birefringence of the poly(**APB6/A6PB6A/BHAB**) (90:5:5 mol%) and the poly(**APB6/BHAB**) (95:5 mol%) by UV irradiation at T_{red} (T/Ti) of 0.98 (around 100°C for both samples) are shown in Figure 16.8. The networks in a homogeneous glass cell with a 5-μm gap were placed between two crossed polarizers and thermostatted. The directions of the two polarizers were set at angles of 45° with respect to the orientation axis of the cell. The transmitted light intensity through

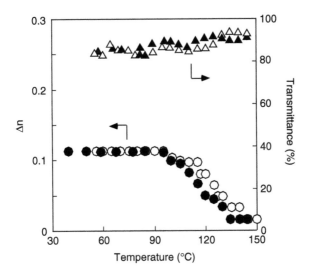

FIGURE 16.7 Changes in birefringence (Δn) and transmittance (%).

each network was monitored while irradiating with a Xe lamp to cause a *trans–cis* photoisomerization of **BHAB** in the networks. The transmitted light intensity of the probe light was decreased by the UV irradiation and restored in the dark. The restoration of the transmitted light intensity is related to the rapid thermal *cis–trans* reverse isomerization at higher temperature (Figure 16.9). The estimated values of Δn before and after irradiation were 0.034 and 0.027 for the poly(**APB6/A6PB6A/BHAB**) and 0.015 and 0.010 for the poly(**APB6/BHAB**).

The changes in the transmittance are large enough to detect, but the photochemical phase transition of the liquid crystalline networks could not be induced completely. The initial value of Δn for the poly(**APB6/A6PB6A/BHAB**) network was higher than that for the poly(**APB6/BHAB**) network. In addition, it is likely that the time required for restoration of Δn for the poly(**APB6/A6PB6A/BHAB**) network is slightly shorter than that for the poly(**APB6/BHAB**) network. The results indicated that the crosslinking affected the stability of the macroscopic molecular orientation and also the photochemical switching behavior.

Time-resolved measurements of the photochemical change in birefringence were carried out by means of pulse irradiation in order to explore the crosslinking effects on the photochemical switching behaviors of the liquid crystalline networks. The time-resolved measurements were performed for the crosslinked networks and those without crosslinking by irradiation with a third harmonic single pulse of a Nd:YAG laser. As shown in Figure 16.10, the transmittance of the poly(**APB6/A6PB6A/BHAB**) network was found to decrease and reach minimum value upon pulse irradiation. Subsequently, the transmittance increased and returned to the initial level.

To discuss the switching behavior, the response time and decay time were defined as the time required to decrease to the minimum value and the time required to increase to 90% of the initial value, respectively. The response time was in a range of a few microseconds. The decay time was much longer than the response time,

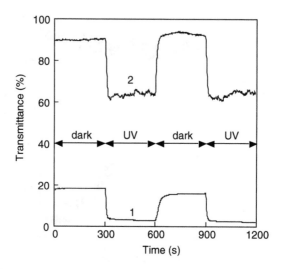

FIGURE 16.8 Changes in transmittance of liquid crystalline networks between two crossed polarizers by ultraviolet radiation at $T_{red} = 0.98$. Bottom (1) = APB6/BHAB = 95:5. Top (2) = APB6/A6PB6A/BHAB = 90:5; 5.5 mol%. Reference light intensity (I_0) for transmittance measurement was defined as transmitted light intensity through two parallel polarizers.

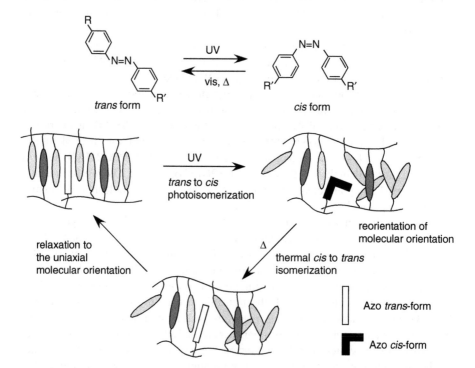

FIGURE 16.9 Photoresponses of liquid crystalline networks by photoisomerization of azo dye.

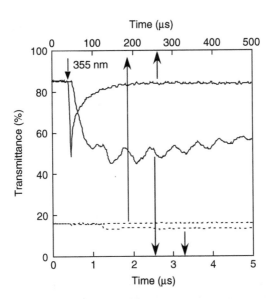

FIGURE 16.10 Time-resolved measurements of changes in transmittance of poly(APB6/A6PB6A/BHAB) 90:5:5 (solid line) and poly(APB6/BHAB) 95:5 (dotted line) networks between two crossed polarizers on pulse irradiation (355 nm, 15 ns FWHM, 10 mJ/cm).

and was in a range of a few hundred microseconds. Little change in transmittance was observed for the network without crosslinking by pulse irradiation, contrary to the change in transmittance by UV irradiation with a Xe lamp (Figure 16.8). The light scattering due to the transformation from the uniaxial monodomain structure to a multidomain may be one of the factors in the poor response of the network without light crosslinking.

Figure 16.11 shows the time-resolved measurements of changes in Δn of the networks crosslinked with different amounts of **A6PB6A** and poly(**APB6/A6PB6A/BHAB**) 90:5:5 and 93:2:5 mol% networks. The amount of **A6PB6A** corresponded to the crosslinking density because of the high polymerization conversion. The optical switching behavior was clearly dependent on the amounts of **A6PB6A** in the liquid crystalline networks, indicating the effect of the crosslinking density.

The change in Δn of the liquid crystalline network crosslinked with 2 mol% of **A6PB6A** was larger than that of the network crosslinked with 5 mol% of **A6PB6A,** that is, the sensitivity was depressed by the crosslinking. On the other hand, the switching time, defined as the sum of the response and decay times, was decreased by crosslinking. The decay time was assumed to be related to the thermal *cis–trans* isomerization.[44] The measurements were carried out at almost the same temperature (120 and 119°C) so that the temperature dependence of thermal *cis–trans* isomerization could be neglected. The result implies that crosslinking leads to enhancement of the switching rate.

The thermal motion of the network chains in mesogenic resins was significantly suppressed by crosslinking.[45] In addition, studies on the dynamic thermomechanical behavior of liquid crystalline polymers revealed that the relaxation of liquid crystalline

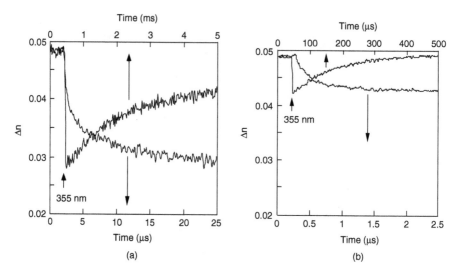

FIGURE 16.11 Time-resolved measurements of changes in Δn of (A) poly(APB6/A6PB6A/BHAB) 93:2:5 network at 120°C and (B) poly(APB6/A6PB6A/BHAB) 90:5:5 network at 119°C by pulse irradiation (355 nm, 15 ns FWHM, 10 mJ/cm).

networks associated with the relaxation of the whole network was shifted to higher temperatures with increasing crosslinking density.[33–34,46] The photochemical change in Δn was considered to arise from the transient deformation of uniaxial molecular orientation by *trans–cis* photoisomerization. Thus, motions of the liquid crystalline network chains including mesogenic side chains are required for the photochemical switching of Δn. The crosslinking effect on the optical switching behavior may be interpreted in terms of facility of the molecular motion of the mesogenic moieties in the liquid crystalline networks. The higher the motion of the network chains increases, the higher the sensitivity becomes. However, the facile motion of the chains gives a negative effect on the restoration of the uniaxially molecular orientation from the transiently disorganized state, resulting in a decrease in the switching rate.

EFFECTS OF STRUCTURES OF AZOBENZENES

Properties of liquid crystalline materials are often influenced by the structures of their side chains, aromatic rings, linking groups, terminal groups, and dopants. Therefore, it can be expected that the photoresponsive behaviors of liquid crystalline networks will be dependent on the structures of the azobenzene compounds.

Two types of photoresponsive liquid crystalline networks with macroscopically uniaxial molecular orientations were prepared by polymerizing mixtures of liquid crystalline monoacrylates and diacrylates and an azobenzene compound in a homogeneous glass cell at a nematic (N) phase. One group of networks was doped with azobenzene molecules and the other was copolymerized with azobenzene monomers as shown in Scheme 16.4.[47] The optical switching behavior of the liquid crystalline networks was examined with respect to the molecular structures of the azobenzene

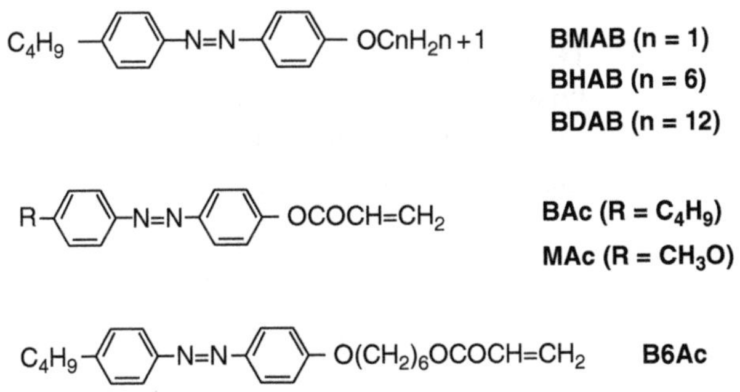

C_4H_9 —⟨benzene⟩—N=N—⟨benzene⟩— $OCnH_{2n+1}$ **BMAB (n = 1)**
                                                      BHAB (n = 6)
                                                      BDAB (n = 12)

R—⟨benzene⟩—N=N—⟨benzene⟩— $OCOCH=CH_2$ **BAc (R = C_4H_9)**
                                            MAc (R = CH_3O)

C_4H_9—⟨benzene⟩—N=N—⟨benzene⟩— $O(CH_2)_6OCOCH=CH_2$ **B6Ac**

SCHEME 16.4 Structures of azobenzene compounds.

TABLE 16.1
Properties of Liquid Crystalline Monomers and Azobenzene Compounds

Compound	λ_{max} (nm) in MeOH	$\varepsilon_{max} \times 10^{-4}$ in MeOH	Phase Transition Temperature (°C)[a]
APB6	—	—	K 32 S 53 N 61 I
A6PB6A	—	—	K 33 S 47 N 50 I
BMAB	345	3.1	K 33 N 48 8
BHAB	350	3.0	K 45 N 73 I
BDAB	355	2.1	K 65 S 76 I
BAc	336	4.0	K 47 N 52 I
MAc	352	3.1	K 46 N 117 I
B6Ac	355	3.1	K 64 I

[a] K, crystalline phase; S, smectic phase; N, nematic phase; I, isotropic phase. Transition temperatures were measured on cooling.

compounds by using a Xe lamp and a single pulse light from a Nd:YAG laser as light sources.

Thermotropic properties of liquid crystalline monomers and azobenzenes are shown in Table 16.1. Liquid crystalline diacrylate **A6PB6A** was also used as a crosslinking agent to hold uniaxial molecular orientation. A network crosslinked with 5 mol% of **A6PB6A** was prepared because the photochemical response was found to depend strongly on the crosslinking density as noted above. The networks with uniaxial molecular orientations were prepared by polymerization of the mixtures of **APB6** (90 mol%), **A6PB6A** (5 mol%) and azobenzenes (5 mol%) in a 5-μm homogeneous glass cell. All mixtures before polymerization showed the N phase and polymerization was carried out by heating for 2 h at the N phase (50 to 60°C).

The polymerization conversion was higher than 75%. All the networks were transparent above room temperature due to stable uniaxial molecular orientation. The phase transition temperature to the I phase (isotropization temperature, Ti) was determined by measuring temperature dependence of the transmitted light intensity

TABLE 16.2
Phase Transition Temperatures of the (APB6/A6PB6A/Az) (90:5:5 mol%) Networks

Az	Phase Transition Temperature (°C)[a]
BMAB	LC 136 I
BHAB	LC 135 I
BDAB	LC 136 I
BAc	LC 142 I
MAc	LC 139 I
B6Ac	LC 143 I

[a] Phase transition temperature was defined as the temperature to reduce the transmittance intensity through crossed polarizers to 10% of the maximum value.

of the probe light through the networks between crossed polarizers and defined as the temperature to reduce the transmittance to 10% of the maximum value. The reduction temperature was defined as T/Ti, where T was the experimental temperature. The Ti values of the networks containing **BMAB, BHAB,** or **BDAB** were lower than those of the networks prepared by polymerization with azobenzene monomers as can be seen in Table 16.2. It is likely that the doping of azobenzene molecules in the networks disorganized the anisotropic molecular orientation.

Figure 16.12 shows a change in Δn of the liquid crystalline networks containing **BMAB, BHAB,** or **BDAB** by UV irradiation as a function of irradiation temperature. The birefringence (Δn) is one parameter for judging uniaxial molecular orientation. In a comparison of Δn values of three liquid crystalline networks prepared by doping **BMAB, BHAB,** and **BDAB,** Δn in the dark tended to decrease with the length of alkoxy groups at the 4' position of 4-butyl azobenzene. The longer the molecular shape of the azobenzenes becomes, the larger the influence on the macroscopic molecular orientation in the dark becomes. The values of Δn of the liquid crystalline networks prepared by copolymerization with **MAc, BAc,** and **B6Ac** were higher than those of the liquid crystalline networks doped with azobenzene molecules, although the results are not given here.[47]

To clarify the temperature dependence of the optical switching, changes in Δn before and after UV irradiation ($\Delta(\Delta n)$) were plotted as functions of irradiation temperatures in Figure 16.13. The value of $\Delta(\Delta n)$ increased with irradiation temperature, but decreased rapidly near isotropization temperature. The maximum $\Delta(\Delta n)$ were roughly in the range of 0.02 to 0.04 at T_{red} of 0.98 for the doped-type networks. On the other hand, the copolymerized networks gave maximum $\Delta(\Delta n)$ values in a temperature range from 0.94 to 0.96 of T_{red}. At lower temperatures, the copolymerized-type networks showed larger $\Delta(\Delta n)$s than the doped-type networks. Although the

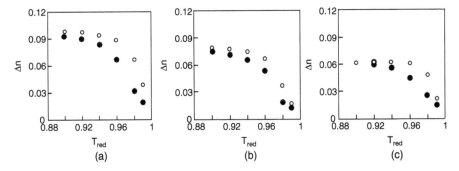

FIGURE 16.12 Changes in birefringence of (a) poly(APB6/A6PB6A/BMAB), (b) poly(APB6/A6PB6A/BHAB), and (c) poly(APB6/A6PB6A/BDAB) networks (90:5:5 mol%) by ultraviolet (366 nm, 10 mW) irradiation. o = Before irradiation. • = After irradiation.

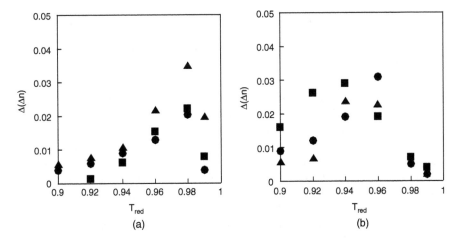

FIGURE 16.13 Changes in birefringence before and after ultraviolet irradiation of (a) liquid crystalline networks doped with azo dyes and (b) liquid crystalline networks copolymerized with azo dyes.

different temperature dependencies of $\Delta(\Delta n)$ between doped-type and copolymerized-type networks are not clear, one factor may be an interaction through the bonds between azobenzene molecules and mesogenic molecules formed by copolymerization.

The value of $\Delta(\Delta n)$ is large enough to detect, although the photochemical phase transition of the liquid crystalline networks can not be induced completely. The switching rate is an important property of an optical material. To explore the structural effects of azobenzene molecules on switching rates, time-resolved measurements of photochemical changes in the transmittance between two crossed polarizers were carried out.

Figure 16.14 shows results of measurements of three doped-type liquid crystalline networks at 126°C (T_{red} of 0.98). The light intensity ($I_\perp$) through a liquid crystal between two crossed polarizers is expressed as $I_\perp = \sin^2(\pi \cdot \Delta n \cdot d/\lambda)$. Therefore, it

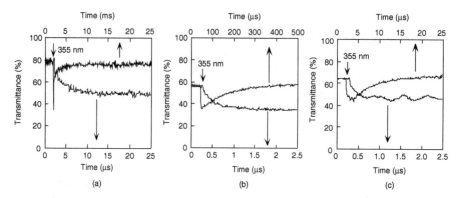

FIGURE 16.14 Time-resolved measurements of photochemical changes in transmittance of (a) poly(APB6/A6PB6A/BM), (b) poly(APB6/A6PB6A/BH), and (c) poly(APB6/A6PB6A/BD) networks (90:5:5 mol%) between two crossed polarizers induced by single-pulse irradiation from a Nd:YAG laser (355 nm, 10 mJ/pulse, 15 ns FWHM) at T_{red} of 0.98 (126°C).

can be assumed that the photochemical change in Δn is proportional to the decrease in $I_\perp$ by pulse irradiation. The decreases in $I_\perp$ were 31% at 15 μs, 23% at 1.5 μs, and 18% at 1.0 μs for liquid crystalline networks doped with **BMAB**, **BHAB**, and **BDAB**, respectively. The times to recover the initial transmittance (decay times) were about 5 ms for **BMAB**, 300 μs for **BHAB**, and 15 μs for **BDAB**, respectively. It is likely that the time required to reach minimum $I_\perp$ (response time) and decay time become shorter by increasing the lengths of the alkoxy groups. However, the changes in Δn decreased with increasing lengths of alkoxy groups, that is, the longer alkoxy groups attached to the same azobenzene skeleton become, the less the disordering effect due to *trans–cis* photoisomerization becomes.

The smectic (S) phase is often observed for liquid crystals having long side substituents such as alkyl and alkoxy groups. Actually, **BMAB** and **BHAB** show the N phase, while **BDAB** shows the S phase as liquid crystalline phases. This means that the laterally intermolecular interaction of **BDAB** is stronger than those of **BMAB** and **BHAB**. Therefore, the *trans–cis* photoisomerization of **BDAB** molecules is considered to be influenced strongly by the molecular orientation compared to **BMAB** and **BHAB** molecules. Both smaller changes in Δn and rapid optical switching are closely related to the restriction of *trans–cis* photoisomerization of **BDAB** due to strong lateral interaction.

Results of time-resolved measurements of liquid crystalline networks copolymerized with **MAc** at a T_{red} of 0.96 are shown in Figure 16.15. Two other networks copolymerized with **BAc** and **B6Ac** gave similar results to those of the network copolymerized with **MAc**. The response times were a few microseconds and the decay times were in a range of a few milliseconds.

GRATING SWITCHING OF LIQUID CRYSTALLINE NETWORKS

Holography is one of the intriguing applications of photoresponsive polymer systems.[11,14,48–51] In particular, dynamic holography offers an attractive potential for

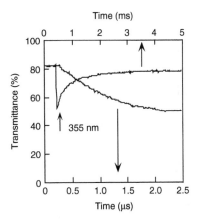

FIGURE 16.15 Time-resolved measurement of photochemical changes in transmittance of a poly(APB6/A6PB6A/MAc) network (90:5:5 mol%) between two crossed polarizers induced by single-pulse irradiation from a Nd:YAG laser (355 nm, 10 mJ/pulse, 15 ns FWHM) at T_{red} of 0.96.

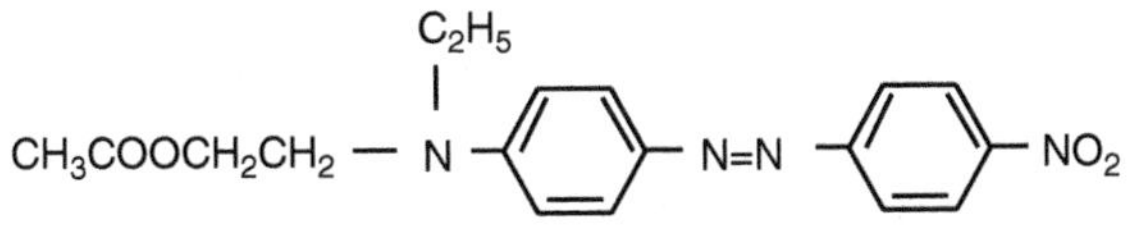

$$CH_3COOCH_2CH_2 - \underset{\underset{\displaystyle C_2H_5}{|}}{N} - \!\!\!\bigcirc\!\!\! - N\!\!=\!\!N - \!\!\!\bigcirc\!\!\! - NO_2$$

DR1A $\lambda max = 470$ nm, $\varepsilon = 4 \times 10^4 (MeOH)$

SCHEME 16.5 Structure of DR1A.

optical applications such as real-time image processing. To achieve real-time image processing, the recording, reading, and erasing of optical information should be performed at real time. The photoisomerization of azobenzene compounds in liquid crystalline networks caused changes in optical properties. The change in birefringence was in the range of 0.005 to 0.02, and the response and restoration times were in the ranges of a few microseconds and a few milliseconds, respectively. Therefore, lightly crosslinked liquid crystalline networks are suited for dynamic grating because of their quick responsiveness and repetition reliability.

Mixtures for polymerization were prepared by addition of 3 mol% of 2,2-dimethoxy-2-phenylacetophenone as a photo-initiator to mixtures of **APB6**, **A6PB6A**, and **DR1A** (Scheme 16.5). Figure 16.16 shows absorption spectra of **DR1A** and the photoradical initiator used in methanol. It is clear that the absorption maximum of the photoradical initiator and the absorption minimum of **DR1A** overlapped around 350 nm. Thus, the polymerization of mixtures consisting of **APB6**, **A6PB6A**, and **DR1A** was successfully achieved by UV irradiation. The mixtures were injected into a homogeneous glass cell with a 5-μm cell gap at an isotropic phase and polymerized by UV irradiation (366 nm) with a 500-W high pressure Hg lamp for 3 min. The polymerization conversion was higher than 80% with UV irradiation for 3 min.

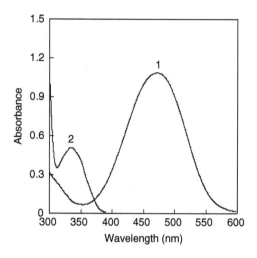

FIGURE 16.16 Absorption spectra of (1) DR1A and (2) 2,2-dimethoxy-2-phenylacetophe-none in MeOH.

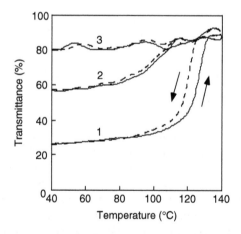

FIGURE 16.17 Changes in transmittance of poly(APB6/A6PB6A/DR1A) networks as functions of temperature on heating (solid line) and cooling (dotted line). 1 = 94:1:5 mol%. 2 = 92:3:5%. 3 = 90:5:5 mol%.

Figure 16.17 shows temperature dependence of the transparencies of three poly(**APB6/A6PB6A/DR1A**) networks containing different amounts of **A6PB6A**. The liquid crystalline networks were prepared by photopolymerization of the monomer mixtures containing 1, 3, and 5 mol% of **A6PB6A** in a homogeneous glass cell at the nematic phase to produce the uniaxial molecular orientation. A marked decrease in the transmittance was caused by photopolymerization of the monomer mixtures containing 1 and 3 mol% of **A6PB6A**. The crosslinking with **A6PBA** required more than 5 mol% to hold stable macroscopic molecular orientation.

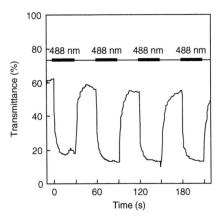

FIGURE 16.18 Change in transmittance of liquid from a diode laser (670 nm) through a poly(APB6/A6PB6A/DR1A) 90:5:5 mol% network between two crossed polarizers by 488 nm irradiation (Ar$^+$ laser, 0.8 W/cm^2) at T_{red} of 0.98 (111°C). Plane of polarization of Ar$^+$ laser beam was parallel to the direction of uniaxial molecular orientation.

Prior to study formation and removal of grating, the effect of direction of light polarization on the molecular orientation of the liquid crystalline networks was clarified in terms of the photoisomerization of **DRIA**. Figure 16.18 shows photo-chemical changes in the transmittance through a poly(**APB6/A6PB6A/DR1A**) 90:5:5 mol% network between two crossed polarizers by irradiation of an Ar$^+$ beam at 488 nm and a T_{red} of 0.98. No change in transmittance was observed when the direction of polarization of light was normal to the rubbing direction, that is, no change in the birefringence. The reversible change in the transmittance was brought about by turning on and off the irradiation of the Ar$^+$ beam at 488 nm with polar-ization parallel to the rubbing direction. The increase in the transmittance by turning off the irradiation took place rapidly. The reversible change in the transmittance was explained as a result of the disorganization and the recovery of the uniaxial molecular orientation of the liquid crystalline networks by *trans–cis* photoisomerization and subsequent rapid thermal *cis–trans* back isomerization of **DR1A**.[23,52,53]

Figure 16.19 shows the set-up of the holographic experiments. The Ar$^+$ laser was used as the source. The beam passed through a pinhole and was divided into two by means of a beam splitter. Two writing beams with equal intensities were overlapped in the sample through the adjustments of mirrors. A grating spacing (d) was varied by control of an incident angle (θ) of the two writing beams. The grating spacing is:

$$d = \lambda(2 \cdot \sin\theta)$$

where λ is the wavelength of the writing beam. A linearly polarized He–Ne laser light (633 nm) was used to monitor first-order diffraction efficiency. The beam from the He–Ne laser was incident at normal to the surface of the sample. The first-order diffraction efficiency (η) was determined by the ratio of intensities between the

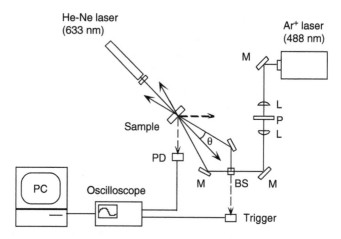

FIGURE 16.19 Experimental set-up for dynamic grating.

impinging probe beam (I_0) from the He–Ne laser and the first-order diffracted beam (I_1):

$$\eta = I_1/I_0$$

In order to study formation and removal of the dynamic grating, the diffracted beam was detected with a laser power meter and recorded on a digital oscilloscope. Figure 16.20 shows the formation and removal of the first-order diffraction signal of the poly(**APB6/A6PB6A/DR1A**) 90:5:5 mol% network by turning on and off two Ar$^+$ beams at a T_{red} of 0.98 (111°C). The grating spacing was 2.0 μm. The diffraction signal was induced by turning on the writing beams, and disappeared rapidly when the beams were turned off. As shown in Figure 16.18, the irradiation led to disorganization of the uniaxial molecular orientation of the liquid crystalline networks, resulting in a decrease in the birefringence. The reversible change of the first-order diffraction signal was interpreted in terms of disorganization and reorientation of the uniaxial molecular orientation by the reversible photoisomerization of **DR1A**. The diffraction efficiency of the networks doped with **DR1A** was found to depend on the irradiation temperature, fringe spacing, crosslinking density, and film thickness. However, the efficiency was smaller than 1%. In addition, the diffracted light intensity was not stable as shown in Figure 16.20.

To improve response performance, liquid crystalline networks were prepared by photopolymerization of **APB6**, **A6PB6A**, and **DR1ac** (Scheme 16.6) in a homogeneous glass cell. The transparent films could be obtained by crosslinking with **A6PB6A** above 3 mol%. Figure 16.21 shows the effect of crosslinking on diffraction efficiency. The diffraction efficiency increased with decreasing concentration of **A6PB6A**, indicating the lowering of the crosslinking density. The networks crosslinked with 1 mol% exhibited significant decreases in diffraction efficiency due to strong light scattering. Figure 16.22 shows dependence of the concentration of **DR1ac** in the networks crosslinked with 3 mol% **A6PB6A**. Significant enhancement

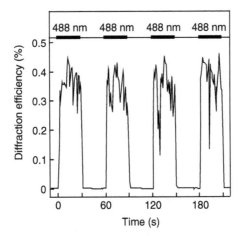

FIGURE 16.20 Change in diffraction efficiency of a poly(APB6/A6PB6A/DR1A) 90:5:5 mol% network induced by turning on and off two writing beams (each at 0.4 W/cm² intensity) at T_{red} of 0.98 (111°C); fringe spacing was 2.0 μm.

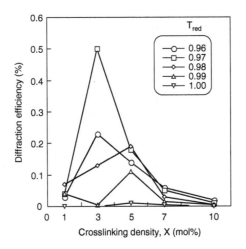

FIGURE 16.21 Change in diffraction efficiency of poly(APB6/A6PB6A/DR1ac) 95:X:X:5 (X = 1, 3, 5, 7, 10) induced by turning on and off two writing beams (total light intensity = 5 mW) with fringe spacing of 2.0 μm at various temperatures. $T_{red} = T/T_c$ where T_c is a clearing temperature.

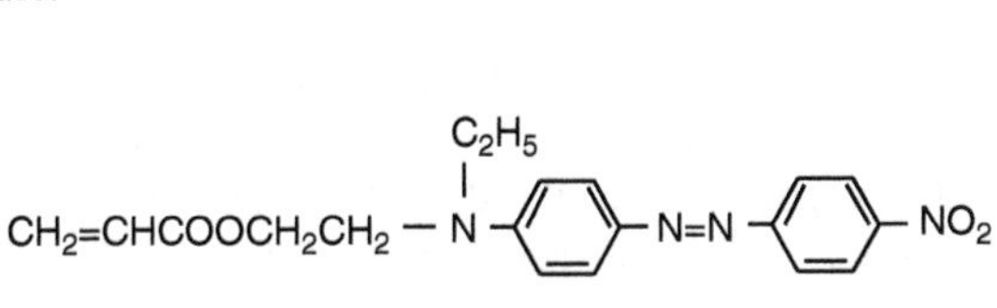

$$CH_2=CHCOOCH_2CH_2 - \overset{\overset{\displaystyle C_2H_5}{|}}{N} - \!\!\!\!\bigcirc\!\!\!\! - N=N - \!\!\!\!\bigcirc\!\!\!\! - NO_2$$

DR1ac

SCHEME 16.6 Structure of DR1ac.

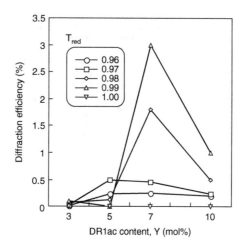

FIGURE 16.22 Change in diffraction efficiency of poly(APB6/A6PB6A/DR1ac) 97-Y:3:Y) network induced by turning on and off two writing beams (total light intensity = 5 mW) with fringe spacing of 2.0 μm at various temperatures.

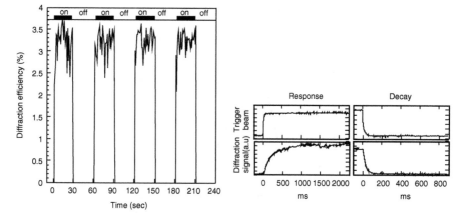

FIGURE 16.23 Change in diffracted light intensity of poly(APB6.A6PB6A/DR1ac) 90L:3:7 mol% network induced by turning on and off two writing beams with fringe spacing of 2.0 μm at T_{red} of 0.99.

of the diffraction efficiency was brought about by adjusting the concentration of **DR1ac**.

Image processing should be performed at real time and it is important to explore the formation and removal of the grating of the liquid crystalline networks. Figure 16.23 shows the time dependence of the diffraction efficiency of the poly(**APB6/A6PB6A/DR1ac**) 90:3:7 mol% network at a T_{red} of 0.99. The time dependence measurements were performed by turning on and off the two Ar^+ beams with a mechanical shutter with a response time of a few milliseconds. The grating spacing was adjusted at 2.0 μm. The formation of the grating was required for 500 ms, while the grating disappeared in 100 ms. The times required for the formation and the removal of the grating are dependent on crosslinking density. The time was decreased by increasing the crosslinking density. In other words, the repetition rate was improved by increasing the crosslinking density. The response and decay times were 50 and 30 ms, respectively, for poly(**APB6/A6PB6A/DR1ac**) 90:5:5 mol%. However, the diffraction efficiency was also reduced by the increase in the crosslinking density.

LIQUID CRYSTALLINE TELOMERS

Fluidity and molecular motions of low molecular weight liquid crystals are higher than those of liquid crystalline polymers. Therefore, the response of the low molecular weight liquid crystals to external stimuli can be brought about rapidly compared to polymeric materials. However, a cell is usually required for low molecular weight liquid crystals to manufacture optical devices such as liquid crystalline flat display panels. On the other hand, liquid crystalline polymers exhibit self-standing abilities.

Liquid crystalline oligomers having lower molecular weights can be expected to combine the properties of low molecular weight liquid crystals and liquid crystalline polymers, that is, fast response to external stimuli and self-standing abilities. A few studies have focused on the effects of the molecular weight and distribution of polymer liquid crystals on their liquid crystalline properties.[54] Atom-transfer radical polymerization (ATRP)[55–57] and controlled (living) radical polymerization[58] have been used to synthesize liquid crystalline side chain polymers in order to control their molecular weight and distribution. The molecular weights of the polymers can be controlled easily by polymerization (telomerization) in the presence of a chain transfer reagent or telogen (Scheme 16.7).[59]

Telomers were synthesized by telomerization of acrylate with a mesogenic side group in the presence of AIBN (2,2′-azobisisobutyronitrile) and dodecane thiol as radical initiator and telogen as shown in Scheme 16.8 and Table 16.3. The homopolymer and telomers showed the nematic phase as a liquid crystalline phase. Table 16.4 shows the averaged molecular weights and isotropization temperatures. The increases in the concentrations of telogens in the monomer mixtures caused depression of the molecular weights and isotropization temperatures. Films containing **BHAB** were prepared by spin coating from the solution containing the homopolymer or telomer and 10 mol% of **BHAB** on a glass plate. The thicknesses of the films ranged from 200 to 400 nm. The *trans–cis* isomerization of **BHAB** can be achieved by UV and visible light irradiation as shown in Figure 16.24. Similar results were obtained for all the films prepared.

The photoresponsive behaviors of the films composed of the homopolymer or telomers and 10 mol% of **BHAB** were then studied via the set-up shown in Figure 16.25. The transmitted light intensity through the samples was measured by irradiating UV light (365 nm) and/or visible light (488 nm) from an Ar⁺ laser. Both UV and visible light irradiations were performed on the films at the same time in order to explore whether the in-plane reorientation of liquid crystalline molecules took place.

Initiation

$$I \longrightarrow 2R^{\bullet}$$

$$R^{\bullet} + AH \longrightarrow A^{\bullet} + RH$$

$$A^{\bullet} + M \longrightarrow AM^{\bullet}$$

Propagation

$$AM^{\bullet} + (n-1)M \longrightarrow A(M)\,n-1M^{\bullet}$$

Termination

$$A(M)\,n-1M^{\bullet} + AH \longrightarrow A(M)\,n-1MH + A^{\bullet}$$

I : initiator
M : monomer
AH: telogen

SCHEME 16.7 Mechanisms of telomerization.

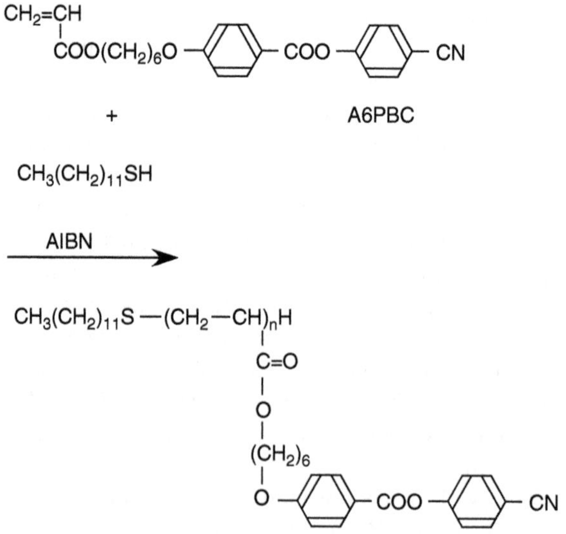
CH2=CH
COO(CH2)6O
COO
CN
+
A6PBC
CH3(CH2)11SH
AIBN
CH3(CH2)11S—(CH2—CH)nH
C=O
O
(CH2)6
O
COO
CN

SCHEME 16.8 Structures of telomers.

Although no in-plane reorientation was observed, the photochemical phase transition was induced by the photoisomerization of **BHAB** as can be seen in Figure 16.26. The changes in the birefringence of homopolymer/**BHAB** and Telomer

TABLE 16.3
Condition of Telomerization and Polymerization[a]

	Monomer A6PBC (g)	Telogen $C_{12}H_{25}SH$ (g)	Initiator AIBN (mg)
poly(A6PBC)	2.0	0	20
Telomer 1	1.9	0.1	20
Telomer 2	1.75	0.25	20
Telomer 3	1.65	0.35	20

[a] Polymerization was carried out in THF at 60°C for 6–24 h.

TABLE 16.4
Results of Telomerization and Polymerization

	T_{NI} (°C)	Degree of Polymerization	M_n NMR	M_n GPC	M_w	M_w/M_n
poly(A6PBC)	96	12.5	—	4400	5200	1.18
Telomer 1	64	6.8	2600	2600	3000	1.15
Telomer 2	41	2.6	1400	2000	2300	1.15
Telomer 3	40	2.0	1000	1400	1700	1.21

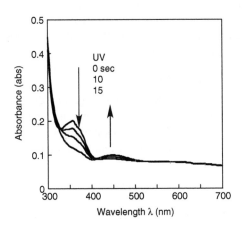

FIGURE 16.24 Change in absorption spectra of Telomer 2/BHAB (90:10 mol%) by ultraviolet irradiation.

2/BHAB films by UV and/or visible light irradiation are shown in Figure 16.26. Although the reversible photochemical phase transition between the nematic and the isotropic phases was induced for both films by irradiation at 22°C, the Telomer

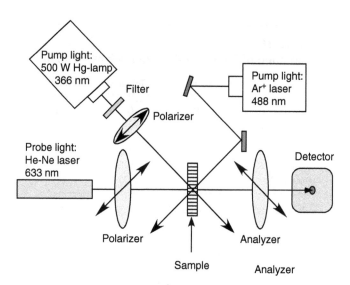

FIGURE 16.25 Experimental set-up for measurement of photochemical change in birefringence.

2/BHAB film was clearly seen to exhibit rapid change in birefringence in that the time required for the photochemical phase transition of the Telomer **2/BHAB** film was much shorter that that of the homopolymer/**BHAB** film.

The photochemical phase transition of the liquid crystalline systems doped with azobenzenes is related closely to irradiation temperature or isotropization temperature.[25] The isotropization temperature of the homopolymer is different from that of Telomer **2**. To diminish the influence of irradiation temperature, the response behavior was studied by irradiation at almost the same reduction temperature. Figure 16.27 shows the photochemical phase transition of the films composed of telomers and **BHAB** by UV and/or VIS irradiation at a T_{red} of 0.93 to 0.96. The time for the photochemical transition to the isotropic phase was reduced by the decrease in the molecular weights of telomers. The response was related to the facility of the molecular motion of the liquid crystalline side groups due to the disorganization effect of the photoisomerization of the azobenzene molecules in the systems. The increase in the facility of the molecular motion and fluidity of the telomers may be attributed to the effect of the molecular weight on photoresponse behavior.

SUMMARY

Properties of lightly crosslinked liquid crystalline networks and photoresponses of networks containing azo dyes were presented. Light crosslinking of liquid crystalline polymers provideds stability of the macroscopic molecular orientation and exhibited transition to the isotropic phase, indicating that the compounds possessed molecular motion and the ability to respond to external stimuli.

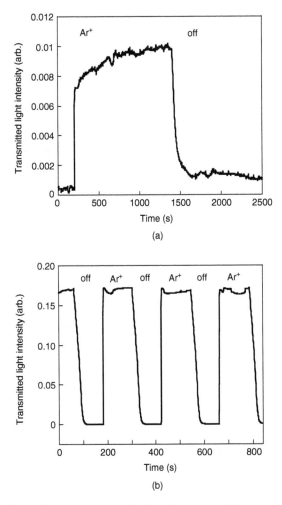

FIGURE 16.26 Photochemical changes in birefringence of homopolymer/BHAB and Telomer 2/BHAB films between crossed polarizers by irradiation of ultraviolet or VIS light at 22°C.

Optical switching was significantly affected by crosslinking density. Repetition rates ranged from a few microseconds to a few tens of microseconds; changes in birefringence ranged from 0.002 to 0.05. The applicability of liquid crystalline networks was demonstrated for real-time holographic data processing. Finally, the possible use of telomers for rapid responsive liquid crystalline systems was described briefly.

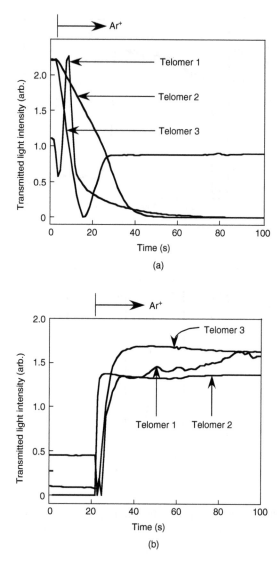

FIGURE 16.27 Photochemical changes in birefringence of telomer/BHAB films by irradiation of ultraviolet or VIS light.

REFERENCES

1. Cole, H.J. and Simon, R., High-resolution laser-addressed liquid crystal polymer storage display, *Polymer* 1985, 26, 1801.
2. Eich, M., Wendroff, J.H., Reck, B., and Ringsdorf, H., Reversible digital and holographic optical storage in polymeric liquid crystals, *Makromol. Chem. Rapid Commun.* 1987, 8, 59.

3. Ikeda, T., Horiuchi, S., Karanjit, D.B., Kurihara, S., and Tazuke, S., Photochemically induced isothermal phase transition in polymer liquid crystals with mesogenic phenyl benzoate side-chain. I. Calorimetric studies and order parameters, *Macromolecules* 1990, 23, 36.

4. Ikeda, T., Horiuchi, S., Karanjit, D.B., Kurihara, S., and Tazuke, S., Photochemically induced isothermal phase transition in polymer liquid crystals with mesogenic phenyl benzoate side-chain. II. Photochemically induced isothermal phase transition behaviors, *Macromolecules* 1990, 23, 42.

5. Ikeda, T., Kurihara, S., Karanjit, D.B., and Tazuke, S., Photochemically induced isothermal phase transition in polymer liquid crystals with mesogenic cyanobiphenyl side-chains, *Macromolecules* 1990, 23, 3938.

6. Sasaki, T., Ikeda, T., and Ichimura, K., Time-resolved observation of photochemical phase transition in polymer liquid crystals, *Macromolecules* 1992, 25, 3807.

7. Ikeda, T. and Tsutsumi, O., Optical switching and image storage by means of azobenzene liquid-crystal films, *Science* 1995, 268, 1873.

8. Ikeda, T., Sasaki, T., and Kim, H.-B., "Intrinsic" response of polymer liquid crystals in photochemical phase transition, *J. Phys. Chem.* 1991, 95, 509.

9. Tsutsumi, O., Shiono, T., Ikeda, T., and Galli, G., Photochemical phase transition behavior of nematic liquid crystals with azobenzene moieties as both mesogens and photosensitive chromophores, *J. Phys. Chem. B* 1997, 101, 1332.

10. Shishido, A., Tsutsumi, O., Kanazawa, A., Shiono, T., Ikeda, T., and Tamai, N., Distinct photochemical phase transition behavior of azobenzene liquid crystals evaluated by reflection-mode analysis, *J. Phys. Chem. B* 1997, 101, 2806

11. Hasegawa, M., Yamamoto, T., Kanazawa, A., Shiono, T., and Ikeda, T., Photochemically-induced dynamic grating by means of side-chain polymer liquid crystals, *Chem. Mater.* 1999, 11, 2764.

12. Bobrovsky, A.Y., Boiko, N.I., and Shibaev, V.P., Photosensitive cholesteric copolymers with spiropyran-containing side groups: novel materials for optical data recording, *Adv. Mater.* 1999, 11, 1025.

13. van de Witte, P., Brehmer, M., and Lub, J., LCD components obtained by patterning of chiral nematic polymer layers, *J. Mater. Chem.* 1999, 9, 2087.

14. Yamamoto, T., Hasegawa, M., Kanazawa, A., Shiono, T., and Ikeda, T., Holographic gratings and holographic image storage by photochemical phase transition of polymer azobenzene liquid-crystal films, *J. Mater. Chem.* 2000, 10, 337.

15. Kurihara, S., Masumoto, K., and Nonaka, T., Optical shutter driven photochemically from anisotropic polymer network containing liquid crystalline and azobenzene molecules, *App. Phys. Lett.* 1998, 73, 160.

16. Kurihara, S., Sakamoto, A., and Nonaka, T., Fast photochemical switching of liquid crystalline polymer network containing azobenzene molecules, *Macromolecules* 1998, 31, 4648.

17. Kurihara, S., Sakamoto, A., Yoneyama, D., and Nonaka, T., Photochemical switching behavior of liquid crystalline polymer networks containing azobenzene molecules, *Macromolecules* 1999, 32, 6493.

18. Sackmann, E., Photochemically induced reversible color changes in cholesteric liquid crystals, *J. Am. Chem. Soc.* 1971, 93, 7088.

19. Ichimura, K., Photoalignment of liquid-crystal systems, *Chem. Rev.*, 2000, 100, 1847.

20. Haas, W.E., Nelson, K.F., Adams, J.E., and Die, G.A., U.V. imaging with nematic chlorostilbenes, *J. Electrochem. Soc.* 1974, 121, 1667.

21. Kurihara, S., Ikeda, T., Tazuke, S., and Seto, J., Isothermal phase transition of liquid crystals induced by photoisomerization of doped spiropyrans, *J. Chem. Soc. Faraday Trans.* 1991, 87, 3251.

22. Irie, M., Darylethenes for memories and switches, *Chem. Rev.* 2000, 100, 1685.

23. Yokayama, Y., Fulgides for memories and switches, *Chem. Rev.* 2000, 100, 1717.

24. Dinescu, L. and Lemieux, R.P., Optical switching of a ferroelectric liquid crystal spatial light modulator by photoinduced polarization inversion, *Adv. Mater.* 1999, 11, 42.

25. Tazuke, S., Kurihara, S., and Ikeda, T., Amplified image recording in liquid crystal. Media by means of photochemically triggered phase transition, *Chem. Lett.* 1987, 911.

26. Clough, S.B., Blumstein, A., and Hsu, E.C., Structure and thermal expansion of some polymers with mesomorphic ordering, *Macromolecules* 1976, 9, 123.

27. Broer, D.J., Finkelmann, H., and Kondo, K., In-situ photopolymerization of an oriented liquid-crystalline acrylate, *Makromol. Chem.* 1988, 189, 185.

28. Broer, D.J. and Mol, G.N., In-situ photopolymerization of an oriented liquid-crystalline acrylate 2, *Makromol. Chem.* 1989, 190, 19.

29. Broer, D.J., Boven, J., and Mol, G.N., In-situ photopolymerization of an oriented liquid-crystalline acrylate 3, *Makromol. Chem.* 1989, 190, 2255.

30. Broer, D.J., Hikmet, R.A., and Challa, G., In-situ photopolymerization of an oriented liquid-crystalline acrylate 4, *Makromol. Chem.* 1989, 190, 3201.

31. Broer, D.J., Mol, G.N., and Challa, G., In-situ photopolymerization of an oriented liquid-crystalline acrylate 5, *Makromol. Chem.* 1991, 192, 59.

32. Broer, D.J. and Hynderickx, I., Three-dimensionally ordered polymer networks with a helicoidal structure, *Macromolecules* 1990, 23, 2474.

33. Hikmet, R.A., Lub, J., and Maassen Brink, P., Structure and mobility within anisotropic networks obtained by photopolymerization of liquid crystal molecules, *Macromolecules* 1992, 25, 4194.

34. Hikmet, R.A., Piezoelectric networks obtained by photopolymerization of liquid crystal molecules, *Macromolecules* 1992, 25, 5759.

35. Hikmet, R.A.M. and Lub, J., Anisotropic network gels obtained by photopolymerization in the liquid crystalline state: synthesis and application, *J. Prog. Pol. Sci.* 1996, 21, 1165.

36. Braun, D., Frick, G., Klimes, M., and Wendorf, J.H., Liquid crystal/liquid-crystalline network composite systems: structure formation and electrooptic properties, *Liq. Cryst.* 1992, 11, 929.

37. Hoyle, C.E., Watanabe, T., and Whitehead, J.B., Anisotropic network formation by photopolymerization of liquid crystal monomers in a low magnetic field, *Macromolecules* 1994, 27, 6581.

38. Kurihara, S., Ohta, H., and Nonaka, T., Synthesis and polymerization of liquid crystalline monomers having diene groups, *Polymer* 1995, 36, 849.

39. Kurihara, K., Iwamoto, K., and Nonaka, T., Preparation of thin films with well-defined molecular orientation of chromophores by polymerication of liquid crystalline monomers in an electric field, *J. Chem. Soc. Chem. Commun.* 1995, 2195.

40. Kurihara, S., Iwamoto, K., and Nonaka, T., Preparation and structure of polymer networks by polymerization of liquid crystalline monomers in DC electric field, *Polymer* 1998, 39, 3565.

41. Kurihara, S., Ishii, M., and Nonaka, T., Novel preparations of helical polymer and ionomer networks, *Macromolecules* 1997, 30, 313.

42. Portugall, M., Rigsdorf, H., and Zentel, R., Synthesis and phase behavior of liquid crystalline polyacrylate, *Makromol. Chem.* 1982, 183, 2311.

43. Kurihara, S., Sakamoto, A., and Nonaka, T., Optical switching of liquid crystalline polymer networks containing azobenzene molecules, *Macromolecules* 1999, 32, 6493.
44. Tsutsumi, O., Kitsunai, T., Kanazawa, A., Shiono, T., and Ikeda, T., Photochemical phase transition behavior of polymer azobenzene liquid crystals with electron-donating and accepting substituents at 4,4′-positions, *Macromolecules* 1998, 31, 355.
45. Ochi, M., Shimizu, Y., Nakanishi, Y., and Murata, Y., Effect of the network structure on thermal and mechanical properties of mesogenic epoxy resin cured with aromatic amine, *J. Polym. Sci.: Part B: Polym. Phys.* 1997, 35, 397.
46. Hikmet, R.A.M. and Broer, D.J., Dynamic mechanical properties of anisotropic networks formed by liquid crystalline acrylates, *Polymer* 1991, 32, 1627.
47. Kurihara, S., Yoneyama, D., and Nonaka, T., Photochemical switching behavior of liquid-crystalline networks; effect of molecular structure of azobenzene molecules, *Chem. Mater.* 2001, 13, 2807.
48. Andruzzi, L., Altomare, A., Ciardelli, F., Solaro, R., Hvilsted, S., and Ramanujam, P.S., Holographic gratings in azobenzene side-chain polymethacrylates, *Macromolecules* 1999, 32, 448.
49. Kumar, J., Li, L., Jiang, X.L., Kim, D.-Y., Lee, T.S., and Tripathy, S.K., Gradient force: the mechanism for surface relief grating formation in azobenzene functionalized polymers, *Appl. Phys. Lett.* 1998, 72, 2096.
50. Barrett, C.J., Nathansohn, A.L., and Rochon, P.L., Mechanism of optically inscribed high-efficiency diffraction gratings in azo polymer films, *J. Phys. Chem.* 1996, 100, 8836.
51. Sutherland, R.L., Natarajan, L.V., Tondiglia, V.P., and Bunning, T.J., Bragg gratings in an acrylate polymer consisting of periodic polymer-dispersed liquid-crystal planes, *Chem. Mater.* 1993, 5, 1533.
52. Tsutsumi, O., Demachi, Y., Kanazawa, A., Shiono, T., Ikeda, T., and Nagase, Y., Photochemical phase transition behavior of polymer liquid crystals induced by photochemical reaction of axobenzenes with strong donor-acceptor pairs, *J. Phys. Chem. B* 1998, 102, 2869.
53. Wildes, P.D., Pacifici, J.G., Irick, G., and Whitten, D.G., Solvent and substituent on the thermal isomerization of substituted azobenzenes. Flash spectroscopic study, *J. Am. Chem. Soc.* 1971, 93, 2004.
54. Stevens, H., Rehage, G., and Finkelmann, H., Phase transformations of liquid crystalling side-chain oligomers, *Macromolecules* 1984, 17, 851.
55. Zang, H., Yu, Z., Wan, X., Zhou, Q.-F., and Woo, E.M., Effects of molecular weight on liquid-crystalline behavior of a mesogen-jacketed liquid crystal polymer synthesized by atom transfer radical polymerization, *Polymer* 2002, 43, 2357.
56. Li, M.-H., Keler, P., Grelet, E., and Auroy, P., Liquid-crystalline polymethacrylates by atom-transfer radical polymerization at ambient temperature, *Macromol. Chem. Phys.* 2002, 203, 619.
57. Tain, Y., Watanabe, K., Kong, X., Abe, J., and Iyoda, T., Synthesis, nanostructures, and functionality of amphiphilic liquid crystalline flock copolymers with azobenzene moieties, *Macromolecules* 2002, 35, 3739.
58. Pragliola, S., Ober, C.K., Mather, P.T., and Joen, H.G., Mesogen-jacketed liquid crystalline polymers via stable free radical polymerization, *Macromol. Chem. Phys.* 1999, 200(10), 2338.
59. Yamada, K. and Koide, Y., Telomer type surfactants, *J. Jpn. Oil Chem. Soc.* 1981, 30, 2.

17 Engineering New Generation Drug Delivery Systems Based on Block Copolymer Micelles: Physicochemical Aspects

Eduardo Jule and Kazunori Kataoka

CONTENTS

INTRODUCTION

The concept of drug targeting as we know it appears as a necessity urged by some of the inherent complications and risks posed by the use of drugs. One of the major problems faced by pharmacology is the rapid metabolism of small molecules like therapeutic agents that are to be transported to infected sites and clearance (most particularly via urinary excretion, a phenomenon that occurs with particulates having molecular weights below ca. 40 kDa).

The purpose of a drug delivery system (DDS) is to ensure the transport of a therapeutic compound in a highly concentrated form from the circulation or other administration site to the site to be treated. The systemic distribution of a therapeutically active molecule generally results in its nonspecific distribution and subsequent accumulation at infected sites. However, a fraction of any dose is also distributed and accumulated at nontargeted sites, resulting in a not ineffective but nonoptimized treatment. Given the inherent toxicity of any therapeutic agent, accumulation at healthy sites generally results in undesired side effects that may complicate treatments. The second aim of a DDS can be described as ensuring the transport of therapeutically active molecules in a highly concentrated form and sparing sites not to be treated by means of passive or active targeting, as will be described in this chapter.

Drug carriers are generally of macromolecular or particulate nature and can be classified mainly as colloidal and noncolloidal. Although antibodies,[2] macromolecular prodrugs,[3-6] and many other systems have been extensively researched and have conveyed interesting results, only colloidal devices based on block copolymer micelles will be discussed here.

RETICULOENDOTHELIAL BARRIER

One of the major obstacles to the effective use of synthetic devices is the extremely rapid recognition and destruction of foreign particles by immunogenic responses that may prevent DDSs from reaching infected sites. These responses are mainly mediated by scavenger cells or what are commonly referred to as reticuloendothelial systems (RESs). These scavenger cells or mononuclear phagocyte systems (MPSs) are essentially present in the liver, spleen, and bone marrow[7] and ensure the permanent clearance of undesired species, whether they come from outside (e.g., bacteria) or inside (e.g., tumor or old red blood cells) the body.

Polystyrene particles, even of adequate size for nonspecific uptake (below 100 nm, as will be discussed later), will accumulate in the liver and spleen with half-lives as low as 50 s after administration.[8] Because MPSs are present in high amounts in the liver and spleen, these organs serve as filters for body fluids. This is an obvious advantage if targeted sites are within these organs but it can severely compromise the treatment of other organs.[9] The uptake of synthetic devices is essentially mediated by the adsorption of specific blood components called opsonins (immunoglobulin G, complement, and fibronectin) or by specific receptors on the surfaces of macrophages, so that special attention should be focused on the use of totally biocompatible materials capable of minimizing opsonization. As will be described in later sections, two parameters related to DDSs are defined as critical: surface and size.

WHY USE COLLOIDS?

Colloids have appeal because of the variety of physicochemical activities that can be achieved by particles displaying remarkable amounts of surface per unit of volume. Moreover, the use of appropriate surface coatings conveys steric stabilization of a noncoulombic nature and overcomes inherent colloidal instability[10] — a huge asset for a system to be to be administered into an organism. Many fundamental processes in nature occur on a colloidal scale and thus provide scientists with invaluable sources of inspiration for developing systems that may be of benefit to mankind.[11]

The fate of colloidal particles administered into the bloodstream will essentially be determined by two factors: their sizes and surfaces. When the particle size is relatively large (above 7 μm), lung capillaries rapidly clear colloids from circulation. Logically, this property can be exploited through what is defined as *passive targeting* and successful accumulation of drugs for chemotherapy can be achieved, as reported by Davis et al.[8] If the particle size is smaller than 7 μm, clearance from circulation is to be ensured by macrophages of the RES as previously described. Among the most studied systems are liposomes, polymeric micelles, and emulsions.[12] This discussion will center on recent advances in block copolymer micelle design, especially from a physicochemical view.

BLOCK COPOLYMER MICELLES

Block copolymers bearing blocks of dissimilar natures, i.e., a hydrophilic and a hydrophobic block, are known to associate in a spontaneous and facile way into colloidal particles called polymeric micelles. The resulting core–shell structure containing a compact inner core formed by the hydrophobic block surrounded by a palisade of hydrophilic chains is a unique architecture allowing the entrapment and transport of, say, drugs that are otherwise poorly soluble in water.[13,14]

Polyion complexes exploit electrostatic interactions between ionogenic block copolymers and oppositely charged polyions such as plasmid DNA, and have also produced core–shell structures[15,16] that have the required stability for prolonged circulation times. Moreover, complexes formed by a cationic block copolymer and negatively charged oligonucleotides with antisense activity have attracted much curiosity because of their capacity of delivering nucleic acids to targeted cells.[17,18] As if to complement these two kinds of driving forces, metal complexes have also been reported between polymers and platinous antitumor drugs.[19,20]

First proposed as drug carriers by Schmolka in the 1970s,[21] micelles have been the subject of intense research since then.[22] Micelles are characterized by small particle size (seldom exceeding 200 nm, a size comparable to certain viruses). They are generally characterized by a remarkable stability conferred by critical association concentrations (CACs) much lower than those of surfactant micelles.[23,24] As will be discussed later, a full understanding of this parameter is highly relevant. Under the strain of injection into the bloodstream, such self-assembled systems are prone to undergo dissociation into unimers. This reaction, of course, would bring their transport functions to a halt, while exposing the patient to unnecessary risk.

If the polymerization process is properly chosen, narrow size distributions can be achieved[25] — another great asset for DDSs. All these parameters are of fundamental importance as they ensure prolonged circulation times and thus accumulation at targeted sites. In order to be able to accumulate in, say, solid tumors, micelles or indeed any other DDSs must reach the proper sites and extravasate. In order to attain this, micelles must be able to circulate in the blood for extended periods and their particle size must allow exit from the bloodstream. Two types of targeting can be exploited to achieve accumulation of DDSs at desired sites and distinction will be made between passive and active targeting.

BENEFITS OF PASSIVE TARGETING: ENHANCED PERMEABILITY AND RETENTION (EPR) EFFECT

To satisfy their growing needs for oxygen and nutrients, tumors develop blood vessels excessively via a process called angiogenesis. This hypervascularization logically produces an abnormal hypertensive state. While normal tissues possess autoregulated blood flow rates even under induced high pressure, tumor tissues lack such homeostatic regulation.[26] As a result, endothelial intercellular gaps are passively widened at tumor sites.

Mediators such as vascular permeability factor (VPF), the vascular endothelial growth factor (VEGF) gene,[27,28] and many other substances, such as fibroblast growth factor (bFGF),[29] bradykinin, nitric oxide, peroxynitrate, matrix metalloproteinases (MMPs) and prostaglandins,[30,31] facilitate diffusion from vessels and are produced at high anomalous levels. The high levels of mediators in conjunction with the hypertensive state lead to "leaky" vessels through which diffusion is facilitated. As a result, large macromolecules or lipids undergo easy extravasation at tumor sites. Additionally, a defective lymphatic system conveys incomplete drainage of large species, resulting in high levels of retention of such species.

Such is the abhorrent structure of tumors. The combination of features described above generates what is commonly called the enhanced permeability and retention (EPR) effect elucidated by Maeda et al.,[32] on which much hope has been placed for selective treatment of an ever-growing number of patients suffering from carcinomas. Indeed, the EPR effect has more than once been described as the main path for tumor targeting and intracellular drug delivery.[33] It has been shown to enhance the accumulation of polymeric prodrugs and other systems such as polymeric micelles or liposomes for more than 100 hours.[34]

MDR phenomenon. Many difficulties remain to be overcome in order to achieve fully effective therapy. One is, of course, the multidrug resistance phenomenon. Most types of cancer cells possess the ability to mutate at an alarming rate, especially when subjected to the strain of selection. This naturally complicates cancer therapy in the sense that treatment with a specific drug can kill most neoplastic cells in a tumor, but not all of them, so that repeated administrations are required. Apart from the obvious concern about undesirable side toxicity, cells that survive chemotherapy will spread and generate more cells bearing resistance properties. Far more distressing is the fact that such cells can evolve and develop resistance to the original drug and to drugs to which they have not been exposed previously.[35,36]

Achieving effective cell death is a requirement for cancer chemotherapy. One of the main concepts underlying DDS is the transport of a therapeutically active agent in a highly concentrated form from the point of administration to the affected sites. Doses that would otherwise produce extreme toxicity if administered "naked" (directly) can produce the local action required for effective chemotherapy. Our group has consistently reported enhanced accumulations of polymeric micelles at tumors, mainly due to the EPR effect.[37–40] Poly(ethylene glycol)-poly(aspartic acid) (PEG-P(Asp)) micelles permitted the administration of doses of doxorubicin as high as 50 mg/kg, whereas doses of 20 mg/kg of free doxorubicin resulted in toxic deaths of mice.

BENEFITS OF ACTIVE TARGETING

Combining DDSs such as macromolecular prodrugs, liposomes, or micelles with biologically active molecules can produce a new array of bioconjugates and open new fields of applications otherwise unattainable with the separate components. Active targeting can be achieved through the use of a biomolecule that can be recognized by its corresponding receptors at desired sites, leading to enhanced accumulation where required.[41] Cells internalize macromolecular compounds through a specific mechanism called endocytosis. While some of its mechanisms are not fully understood, it is known that recognition of ligands by cell surface receptors can induce complex formation and subsequent internalization in a process called receptor-mediated endocytosis (RME).[42]

INSTALLATION OF TARGETING MOIETIES

Our group studied acetal-poly(ethylene glycol)-poly(D,L-lactide) (Ac-PEG-PDLLA) block copolymers as drug carriers since PEG-PDLLA micelles effectively encapsulated active molecules such as anticancer drugs,[43] DNA,[44] and others due to the outstanding biocompatibility of the hydrophobic group that degrades into D,L-lactide, a natural metabolite.

The most interesting features of this block copolymer are its end groups. Indeed, the acetal end yields an aldehyde group[45] after deprotection, through which further functionalization of the surface of micelles can be achieved. Thus, peptides[46] and carbohydrates[47] have been installed successfully on the surfaces of micelles and conveyed new ideas for designing DDSs.

Peptides

The biodistribution of particles is dictated by two essential factors: size and surface. The surface of a particle involves a number of factors, including charge. Negatively charged particles are uptaken preferentially by scavenger leukocytes, resulting in

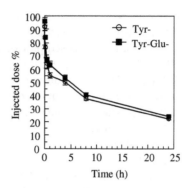

FIGURE 17.1 Blood clearance of Tyr-PEG-PDLLA micels and Tyr-Glu-PEG-PDLLA micelles in mice after intravenous injection (n = 4; average ± SEM). (From Yamamoto, Y. et al., *J. Control. Rel.*, 77, 27, 2001. With permission.)

rapid clearance from the body.[48,49] It is not unreasonable to assume that the biodistribution of micelles can be regulated through their surface charges.

Biodistribution of peptide-installed micelles. Yamamoto et al. prepared PEG-PDLLA micelles bearing neutral tyrosine (Tyr) and negatively charged tyrosylglutamic acid (Tyr-Glu) peptides.[46] The micelles bore very different zeta potentials: 1.3 and –10.6 mV, respectively. The difference is consistent with the properties of the individual ligands, proving that effective control of micelle surface charge can be achieved through the installation of peptides at the distal ends of the corona-forming PEG blocks. Studies on the biodistribution of the micelles in mice were conducted to assess the influence of surface charge on body distribution of the particles.[50] An impressive 25% of the initial dose was recovered from blood samples 24 hours after injection (Figure 17.1) — a prolonged time span when compared to those of systems reported previously.[51,52]

Blood clearance proceeded in two apparent steps: initial rapid clearance (half times ($t_{1/2}$) of 14.2 and 15.7 min for Tyr and Tyr-Glu micelles, respectively) followed by a slower phase ($t_{1/2}$ of 18.8 and 17.7 h, respectively). What is more striking about these clearance profiles is that they did not differ from one micelle type to another. The negative charges on the surfaces of Tyr-Glu micelles did not affect their distribution to leukocytes.

The tissue distribution of peptide-installed micelles appeared negligible at the kidneys and lungs (3% of the initial dose) while following a clearance profile similar to that of the bloodstream (see Reference 46). Liver and spleen uptakes were found to increase gradually over time although the number of micelles accumulating at these organs remained low (6 to 8% and 0.8 to 1% of the initial injected dose for the liver and spleen, respectively; data not shown). These results contrast dramatically with high accumulation values reported by other teams.[51,52] This feature may be explained by the low size distributions of PEG-PDLLA block copolymers and low micelle size, that is, low polymer size distributions result in low micelle size distributions and complete core–shell segregation. Smaller particle sizes might help PEG-PDLLA micelles to escape recognition and subsequent uptake by RES. Also, the tissue-to-blood concentration ratios (K_b) in the liver and spleen corresponded to the extracellular space volume after 24 and 8h, respectively (0.300),[53] indicating that micelles mainly accumulate at the extracellular space and undergo low intracellular uptake at these stages.

Micelles have remarkably long circulation times. Far more relevant is the fact that plasma samples recovered 24 h after injection were found to contain structures with apparent molecular weights that corresponded well to spherical structures such as micelles. PEG-PDLLA micelles can circulate in the bloodstream for extended times. This parameter is of utmost importance for achieving accumulation through the EPR effect. Micelle disintegration and PDLLA degradation led to considerable clearance from blood circulation, especially via urinary excretion (26% of the initial dose). Fecal excretion was relatively low (5%). The recovered fractions with molecular weights of 4,000 to 10,000 Da corresponded to the fast blood clearance observed during the first 15 min following injection, an occurrence certainly related to micelle disintegration under their CAC levels. This dynamic also urges us to better understand the physicochemical properties of these self-assembled systems.

Carbohydrates

Carbohydrates are some of the most abundant molecules in nature. Due to the extraordinary stereochemical encoding possibilities they offer, they play critical roles in biological processes, from energy storage to cellular recognition. Many such processes are regulated by carbohydrate–protein interactions[54] and this characteristic led to immense therapeutic interest, particularly related to specific recognition by cellular surface receptors.

The interactions of lactose-installed PEG-PDLLA micelles (lac-micelles) and natural lectins (*Ricinus communis* agglutinins or RCAs[55]) in simulating cellular surface receptors have been studied[56] and found to proceed in a highly specific manner, again providing evidence of the accessibility of ligands at the distal ends of micellar coronae.

SPR and CAC. Among the advantages of surface plasmon resonance (SPR) analysis is the possibility of assessing a wide variety of phenomena in real time without the need for cumbersome labeling.[57] SPR provides direct evidence on whether two species form complexes (be that through simple adsorption or through complex formation), or not. The sensitivity of the method allows detection of very low substrate concentrations. When lac-micelles were injected over surfaces bearing RCA lectins, complex formation was found to occur at very rapid rates, whereas complex dissociation occurred at extremely slow rates. The amount of complex formation was found to undergo dramatic enhancement in concentration range similar to CAC levels in micelles (Figure 17.2).[58] These observations conveyed valuable information as it became possible to recalculate CAC, resulting in values (6.4 ± 0.5 mg/L) in good agreement with those obtained based on the environment-dependent fluorescence of pyrene (7.7 ± 1.9 mg/L). It was also possible to speculate on the structure of the polymer in solution, based on the specific interactions of ligands installed on the surfaces of micelles and their corresponding receptors on SPR surfaces. At concentrations below CAC, unimers bound lectins at very low levels. Conversely, above CAC,

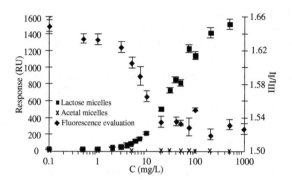

FIGURE 17.2 Binding of lac-micelles on a carboxymethyl (CM) resonance unit (RU) surface bearing 7000 RU of RCA-I lectins as a function of polymer concentration as evaluated by SPR (left axis). On the right axis, the I_I/I_{III} ratio of pyrene as evaluated by fluorescence evaluation. (From Jule, E. et al., *Langmuir*, 18, 10334, 2002. With permission from The American Chemical Society.)

micelle formation brought about the possibility of forming multivalent complexes because ligands at the surfaces of colloidal particles displayed high association numbers (>100, as established by static light scattering measurements; data not shown).

Why Is Multivalency So Interesting?

Efforts to achieve complex formation are often undermined by the intrinsic low affinities of carbohydrates toward lectins (10^{-3} to 10^{-4} M range[59]) — a situation of only limited interest for the design of drug delivery systems. Multivalency (binding of more than one ligand with one or many receptors) occurs widely in nature[60] and usually triggers a far different response from those from single interactions.

Cholera toxin intoxication is initiated when its five B subunits recognize and bind to the pentasaccharide moieties of GM1 ganglioside receptors. This process is usually followed by the injection of A subunits into the cytoplasm and subsequent activation of adenylate cyclase.[61] Analyses carried by microcalometry have shown that the five binding sites are not independent and that the final enthalpy can not be partitioned among the five B subchains.[62] The free energy of the system becomes cooperative because of the flexible structures of the B subunits. Based on the flexible structure of PEG,[63,64] we might expect that micelles will form multivalent complexes and enhanced complex formations with target receptors.

SPR and multivalency. To evaluate the impact of multivalency on the binding of lac-micelles to a surface simulating a cellular surface, micelles bearing different ligand functionalities (amounts of ligands per 100 copolymer chains) were prepared. Complex formation increased with an increase in the amounts of lactose on the surfaces of micelles. Above what seemed to be a critical value, the amount of complex formation increased nonlinearly, clearly indicating a cooperative effect among the various ligands present at the surfaces of lac-micelles (Figure 17.3). This specific accumulation at defined sites is certainly a property of interest in the design of drug delivery systems.

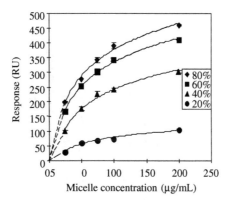

FIGURE 17.3 Recorded responses at equilibrium for micelles bearing different ligand densities at different concentrations. Numbers next to symbols correspond to ligand density. Dotted fragments indicate transition phase between unimers and micelles. (From Jule, E. et al., *Bioconjugate Chem.*, 14, 117, 2003. With permission from The American Chemical Society.)

Ligand densities and kinetic constants. Lac-micelles were found to associate with lectins at very high association rates, an evaluation also carried out with SPR. Far more remarkable were dissociation rates. The systems were found to form strong stable complexes with equilibrium dissociation rates in the nanomolar range,[65] similar to the ranges of certain viruses.[66]

We also evaluated the influence of ligand densities on kinetic constants to determine how the densities influence parameters such as stoichiometry, rate of complex formation and inter-receptor distance.[67] Kinetic association constants were found to increase with increasing ligand density. This is not illogical since higher amounts of ligands allow binding to the lectin beds at a faster pace. An increase in ligand density seemed to cause a tremendous decrease in kinetic dissociation constants, not an increase in kinetic association constants (Figure 17.4) as pointed out by Whitesides' group.[60]

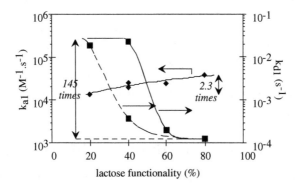

FIGURE 17.4 Driving kinetic constants ka1 (u) and kd1 (n) as a function of lactose functionality. Diamonds (♦) represent kinetic constants for lac-micelles 40% fitted with the trivalent model. (From Jule, E. et al., *Bioconjugate Chem.*, 14, 177, 2003. With permission from The American Chemical Society.)

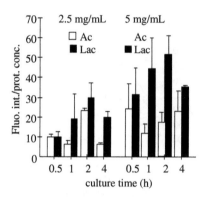

FIGURE 17.5 Cellular uptake of Ac-PEG-PDLLA and lac-PEG-PDLLA micelles by human hepatoblastoma (HepG$_2$). Fluorescence intensity related to protein concentration (ng/mL) is plotted against culture time for two micelle concentrations (n = 3; average ± SEM).

It is also possible to gain insight into the influence of ligand density on other properties such as the binding ability of a system. While micelles bearing high ligand densities were found to form trivalent complexes with lectins, micelles bearing much lower densities were still found to form bivalent complexes.[65] Lac-micelles tended to form multivalent complexes, a feature that might be explained by the flexible structure of PEG. While higher ligand densities led to enhanced kinetic and equilibrium constants, lower ligand densities were more effective if pursued on a molecular basis, as reported by the Kiessling group.[68]

All these simulations produced encouraging results and allow us to propose that lac-micelles form strong multivalent complexes in the presence of asialoglycoprotein receptors on the surfaces of hepatocytes. *In vitro* assays in our laboratory revealed how the uptake of PEG-PDLLA micelles is time- and concentration-dependent. They also demonstrated how uptake by human hepatoblastoma (HepG$_2$) is ligand-dependent since lac-micelles are endocytosed almost four times more than their unmodified counterparts (acetal-PEG-PDLLA micelles; see Figure 17.5). These assays are promising, particularly when combined with our biodistribution studies that showed that the installation of ligands did not affect micellar blood disposition. Because tumor masses are located outside the microvasculature, extravasation is a fundamental prerequisite for the interaction of ligand-installed micelles and tumor cell surfaces. Lac-micelles may escape recognition by RES, extravasate, and thus interact with cellular surfaces at intercellular spaces, leading to enhanced intracellular accumulation following RME.

THERMAL CHARACTERIZATION OF MICELLES

Micelles showed great promise for ensuring the transport of a wide variety of molecules such as anticancer agents, genes, and even enzymes.[69,70] It seemed encouraging to proceed with *in vitro* and *in vivo* assays although we should remember that micelles are macromolecular dynamic systems and that a fundamental understanding of their properties is of the utmost importance.

As noted earlier, PDLLA has been used as a hydrophobic block for micelle preparation because of its biodegradability and facility of accommodating various types of drugs. PLLA has a slow degradation profile and is incompatible with some drugs.[71] While PDLLA is a candidate for the design of micelles, special care should be taken in understanding its fundamental properties. Similarly, fundamental studies of dynamic macromolecular assemblies such as polymeric micelles should be pursued.

PDLLA underwent a glass transition in a temperature range similar to that of physiological conditions.[72] It is logical then to contemplate the possibility that PEG-PDLLA micelles show critical changes in important properties such as CAC, size, association number, and chain exchange rate.

T_g of PDLLA. We first investigated the thermal properties of PEG-PDLLA micelles using ^{1}H nuclear magnetic resonance (NMR) measurement. ^{1}H NMR is a powerful tool for assessing the mobility of polymer strands on supramolecular assemblies such as micelles.[73] While peaks corresponding to methine (δ = 5.2 ppm) and methyl (δ = 2.4 ppm) protons of the PDLLA block were not observed at 25°C, an increase in temperature above 40°C clearly rendered these peaks observable (data not shown). This temperature is slightly higher than that of the wet glass transition [T_g (wet)] of the DLLA segments of micelles as aqueous entities (38°C) determined by differential scanning calorimetry (DSC). This urges us to obtain further insight into other micellar properties at this temperature range.[74]

The CAC is an important parameter directly related to the stability of micelles. Block copolymer micelles such as PEG-PDLLA were stabilized by a combination of intermolecular forces.[75] Under the strain of dilution following injection into the bloodstream, these structures were prone to premature disruption accompanied by the release of the encapsulated drug, bringing their transport function to a halt while exposing the patient to unnecessary risk. These studies evaluated the CAC levels of micelles using the environment-dependent fluorescence of pyrene. The intensities of pyrene vibronic bands exhibited strong dependence on solvent environment.[76] The intensity of the 0,0 band (I_1) underwent a remarkable increase in polar environments whereas the intensity of the 0,2 band (I_3) exhibited maximum variations when related to I_1. Their ratio has been long used to assess changes in the polarities of microenvironments surrounding pyrene, particularly in micellar solutions.[77] The CAC values of micelles increased with increases of temperature above 40°C, clearly pointing to a decrease in the stability of PEG-PDLLA micelles as the mobility of the PDLLA segment increased.

When plotting CAC in an Arrhenius plot against 1/T, the resulting figure clearly separated into two regions, with a break point at 40°C (Figure 17.6). Above 40°C, the logarithm of the CAC decreased with an increase in 1/T in a linear manner. It was then possible to calculate the changes in standard enthalpy, free energy, and entropy (ΔH^0, ΔG^0, and ΔS^0, respectively) according to the following equations describing the relationship of CAC and temperature:[78]

$$\Delta H^0 \sim R \, d \ln(CAC)/dT^{-1}$$

$$\Delta G^0 \sim RT \ln(CAC)$$

$$\Delta S^0 = (\Delta H^0 - \Delta G^0)/T$$

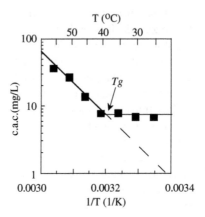

FIGURE 17.6 Arrhenius plots of CAC (mg/L) of PEG-PDLLA micelles. (From Yamamoto, Y. et al., *J. Control. Rel.*, 82, 359, 2002. With permission.)

The resulting values were -89.3 kJ mol^{-1}, -79.9 kJ mol^{-1}, and -29.1 J mol^{-1} K^{-1}, respectively. Note the remarkable change in standard enthalpy at this temperature range.

Micelle structure. Our evaluation also allowed us to speculate about micelle structures in this often controversial concentration range. As shown in Figure 17.6, micelle disintegration occurs at a concentration higher than the value expected from a simple linear extrapolation for temperatures below 40°C. This phenomenon was further confirmed by a decrease in scattering intensity as established by light scattering measurements.[74]

Excimer formation. To deepen our understanding of micelle dynamics and the glass transition of PDLLA, we further studied the behavior of the core using pyrene as a fluorescent probe and drug model. A pyrene derivative was chemically bound to the PDLLA end in a facile and quantitative way using a carbonyl cyanide derivative (Py).[74] Micelles prepared using this PEG-PDLLA-Py displayed fluorescence spectra corresponding to those of excited-state Py dimers at room temperature.[79] This result was consistent with that for the compact glassy core at this temperature.

Excimer formation was then used to obtain valuable information on the behavior of micellar cores, especially under the influence of temperature. A temperature increase, particularly when approaching the glass transition of PDLLA, entailed a decrease of excimer formation as the polymer chain mobility increased.[80] The core appeared to remain stable in physiological thermal conditions. Even at temperatures higher than the glass transition temperature of PDLLA, this stability was ensured over periods that overlapped the duration of blood circulation of these micelles.[50]

Chain exchange reactions. Despite their remarkable stability, block copolymer micelles should not be assumed to be immutable systems like polystyrene beads. Intermicellar chain exchange can be evidenced using lac-PEG-PDLLA and PEG-PDLLA micelles.[74] Further proof was yielded when the fluorescence spectra of excimer-displaying micelles became time-dependent upon mixture with "empty" micelles.[80] This exchange was accelerated with an increase in temperature, especially beyond the T_g of PDLLA. Again, fundamental studies on the dynamic character of polymeric micelles provided insight into the dynamic properties of the compact core and about micellar systems as a whole. These inherent properties are certainly to be exploited as micelles bearing different ligands can be prepared readily.

Micelles are indeed fit candidates for entrapment and transport of a wide variety of compounds. Special care must be taken to understand fundamental properties such as their uptake by RME and their biodistribution.

CONCLUSION

Tremendous progress has been made in the field of drug delivery systems, especially regarding polymeric micelles. In 2003, a doxorubicin block copolymer micelle formulation was undergoing a Phase II clinical trial for pancreatic cancer at the National Cancer Center of Japan. Another paclitaxel formulation is expected to begin a Phase I clinical study soon. Polymeric micelle formulations are certainly highly promising candidates in the treatment of cancers.

While many limitations such as those posed by size or surface properties have been overcome, more difficult problems remain, including improving micelle stability under the strain of dilution and better formulation of polymers to further decrease CAC values. *In vitro* and *in vivo* trials have yielded encouraging results and should be expanded to provide further insight into micelle tissue distribution and intracellular distribution.

Physicochemical simulations and studies should accompany such assays. Properties such as CAC, apparent molecular weight, association number, and even kinetic constants are interesting from a fundamental point of view, but they also exert certain repercussions on macromolecular properties. These factors will play roles in the designs of new generations of drug delivery systems.

REFERENCES

1. Seymour, L., Duncan, R., Strohalm, J., Ulbrich, K., and Kopecek, J., Effect of molecular weight (M_w) of N-(2-hydroxypropyl)methacrylamide copolymers on body distribution and rate of excretion after subcutaneous, intraperitoneal, and intravenous administration to rats, *J. Biomed. Mat. Res.*, 21, 1341, 1987.
2. Tietze, L., Feuerstein, T., Fecher, A., Haunert, F., Panknin, O., Borchers, U., Schuberth, I., and Aleves, F., Proof of principle in the selective treatment of cancer by antibody-directed enzyme prodrug therapy: the development of a highly potent prodrug, *Ang. Chem. Int. Ed.*, 41, 759, 2002.
3. Shiah, J., Dvorak, M., Kopeckova, P., Sun, Y., Peterson, C., and Kopecek, J., Biodistribution and antitumor efficacy of long-circulating N-(2-hydroxypropyl) methacrylamide copolymer–doxorubicin conjugates in nude mice, *Eur. J. Cancer*, 37, 131, 2001.
4. Minko, T., Kopeckova, P., Pozharov, V., and Kopecek, J., HPMA copolymer-bound adriamycin overcomes *MDR1* gene-encoded resistance in a human ovarian carcinoma cell line, *J. Control. Rel.*, 54, 223, 1998.

5. Loadman, P., Bibby, M., Double, J., Al-Shakhaa, W., and Duncan, R., Pharmaco-kinetics of PK1 and doxorubicin in experimental colon tumor models with differing responses to PK1, *Clin. Cancer Res.*, 5, 3682, 1999.

6. Maeda, H., Wu, J., Sawa, T., Matsumura, Y., and Hori, K., Tumor vascular perme-ability and the EPR effect in macromolecular therapeutics: a review, *J. Control. Rel.*, 65, 271, 2000.

7. Kawai, Y., Smedsrod, B., Elvevold, K., and Wake, K., Uptake of lithium carmine by sinusoidal enodthelial and Kupffer cells of the rat liver: new insights into the classical vital staining and the reticulo-endothelial system, *Cell Tissue Res.*, 292, 395, 1998.

8. Illum, L. and Davis, S., Organ uptake of intravenously administrated colloidal parti-cles can be altered using a non-ionic surfactant (Poloxamer 388), *FEBS Lett.*, 167, 79, 1983.

9. Davis, S. and Illum, L., Colloidal delivery systems: opportunities and challenges, in *Site-Specific Drug Delivery*, John Wiley & Sons, New York, 93, 1986.

10. Napper, D. and Netschey, A., Studies of the steric stabilization of colloidal particles, *J. Colloidal Interface Sci.*, 37, 528, 1971.

11. Hemsley, A. and Griffiths, P., Architecture in the microcosm: biocolloids, self-assem-bly and pattern formation, *Philos. Trans. R. Soc. London*, 358, 547, 2000.

12. Muller, R., *Colloidal Carriers for Controlled Drug Delivery and Targeting: Modifi-cation, Characterization and* in Vivo *Distribution*, CRC Press, Boca Raton, FL, 1991.

13. Kwon, G. and Kataoka, K., Block copolymer micelles as long-circulating drug vehi-cles, *Adv. Drug Delivery Rev.*, 16, 295, 1995.

14. Cammas, S., Suzuki, K., Sone, C., Sakurai, Y., Kataoka, K., and Okano, T., Thermo-responsive polymer nanoparticles with a core-shell micelle structure as site-specific drug carriers, *J. Control. Rel.*, 48, 157, 1997.

15. Harada, A. and Kataoka, K., Formation of polyion complex micelles in aqueous milieu from a pair of oppositely-charged block copolymers with poly(ethylene glycol) segments, *Macromolecules*, 28, 5294, 1995.

16. Kabanov, A., Vinogradov, S., Suzdaletseva, Y., and Alakhov, V., Water-soluble block polycations as carriers for oligonucleotide delivery, *Bioconjugate Chem.*, 6, 639, 1995.

17. Kataoka, K., Togawa, H., Harada, A., Yasugi, K., Matsumoto, T., and Katayose, S., Spontaneous formation of polyion complex micelles with narrow distribution from antisense oligonucleotide and cationic block copolymer in physiological saline, *Mac-romolecules*, 29, 8556, 1996.

18. Kabanov, A., Bronich, T., Kabanov, V., Yu, K., and Eisenberg, A., Soluble stoichio-metric complexes from poly(N-ethyl-4-vinylpyridinium) cations and poly(ethylene oxide) block-polymethacrylate anions, *Macromolecules*, 29, 6797, 1996.

19. Nishiyama, N., Yokoyama, M., Aoyagi, T., Okano, T., Sakurai, Y., and Kataoka, K., Preparation and characterization of self-assembled polymer-metal complex micelles from *cis*-dichlorodiamineplatinum (II) and poly(ethylene glycol)-poly(α, β-aspartic acid) block copolymer in an aqueous medium, *Langmuir*, 15, 377, 1999.

20. Nishiyama, N. and Kataoka, K., Preparation and characterization of size-controlled polymeric micelles with time-modulated decaying property as a novel drug delivery system, *J. Control. Rel.*, 74, 83, 2001.

21. Schmolka, I., A review of block copolymer surfactants, *J. Am. Oil Chem. Soc.*, 54, 110, 1977.

22. Jones, M. and Leroux, J., Polymeric micelles: a new generation of colloidal drug carriers, *Eur. J. Pharm. Biopharm.*, 48, 101, 1999.

23. Wilhelm, M., Zhao, C., Wang, Y., Xu, R., Winnik, M., Mura, J., Riess, G., and Croucher, M., Poly(styrene-ethylene oxide) block copolymer micelle formation in water: a fluorescence probe study, *Macromolecules*, 24, 1033, 1991.

24. Astafieva, I., Zhong, X., and Eisenberg, A., Critical micellization phenomena in block polyelectrolyte solutions, *Macromolecules*, 26, 7339, 1993.

25. Yasugi, K., Nagasaki, Y., Kato, M., and Kataoka, K., Preparation and characterization of polymer micelles from poly(ethylene glycol)-poly(D,L-lactide) block copolymers as potential drug carriers, *J. Control. Rel.*, 62, 89, 1999.

26. Maeda, H. and Matsumura, Y., Tumorotropic and lymphotropic principles of macromolecular drugs, *Crit. Rev. Therap. Drug Carrier Syst.*, 6, 193, 1989.

27. Dvorak, H., Brown, L., Detmar, M., and Dvorak, A., Vascular permeability factor/vascular endothelial growth factor: microvascular hyperpermeability, and angiogenesis, *Am. J., Pathol.*, 146, 1029, 1995.

28. Hobbs, S., Monsky, W., Yuan, F., Roberts, W., Griffith, L., Torchlin, V., and Jain, R., Regulation of transport pathways in tumor vessels: role of tumor type and microenvironment, *Proc. Natl. Acad. Sci. USA*, 95, 4607, 1998.

29. Jain, R., Delivery of molecular and cellular medicine to solid tumors, *Adv. Drug Deliv. Rev.*, 46, 149, 2001.

30. Maeda, H., The enhanced permeability and retention (EPR) effect in tumor vasculature: the key role of tumor-selective macromolecular drug targeting, *Adv. Enzyme Regul.*, 41, 189, 2001.

31. Wu, J., Akaike, T., and Maeda, H., Modulation of enhanced vascular permeability in tumors by a bradykinin antagonist, a cyclooxygenase inhibitor, and a nitric oxide scavenger, *Cancer Res.*, 58, 159, 1998.

32. Matsumura, Y. and Maeda, H., A new concept for macromolecular therapeutics in cancer chemotherapy: mechanism of tumoritropic accumulation of proteins and the antitumor agent Smancs, *Cancer Res.*, 46, 6387, 1986.

33. Baban, D. and Seymour, L., Control of tumour vascular permeability, *Adv. Drug Delivery Rev.*, 34, 109, 1998.

34. Duncan, R., Polymer conjugates for tumour targeting and intracytoplasmic delivery: the EPR effect as a common gateway? *Pharm. Sci. Technol. Today*, 2, 441, 1999.

35. Simon, S. and Schindler, M., Cell biological mechanisms of multidrug resistance in tumors, *Proc. Natl. Acad. Sci. USA*, 91, 3497, 1994.

36. Van Bambeke, F., Balzi, E., and Tulkens, P., Antibiotic efflux pumps, *Biochem. Pharmacol.*, 60, 457, 2000.

37. Yokoyama, M., Miyauchi, M., Yamada, N., Okano, T., Sakurai, Y., Kataoka, K., and Inoue, S., Polymeric micelles as novel drug carrier: adriamycin-conjugated poly(ethylene glycol)-poly(aspartic acid) block copolymers, *J. Control. Rel.*, 11, 269, 1990.

38. Yokoyama, M., Okano, T., Sakurai, Y., Ekimoto, H., Shibazaki, C., and Kataoka, K., Toxicity and antitumor activity against solid tumors of micelle-forming polymeric anticancer drug and its extremely long circulation in blood, *Cancer Res.*, 51, 3229, 1991.

39. Kataoka, K., Kwon, S., Yokoyama, M., Okano, T., and Sakurai, Y., Block copolymer micelles as vehicles for drug delivery, *J. Control. Rel.*, 24, 119, 1993.

40. Kwon, G., Suwa, S., Yokoyama, M., Okano, T., Sakurai, Y., and Kataoka, K., Enhanced tumor accumulation and prolonged circulation times of micelle-forming poly (ethylene oxide-aspartate) block copolymer-adriamycin conjugates, *J. Control. Rel.*, 29, 17, 1994.

41. Kullberg, E., Bergstrand, N., Carlsson, J., Edwards, K., Johnsson, M., Sjöberg, S., and Gedda, L., Development of EGF-conjugated liposomes for targeted delivery of DNA-binding agents, *Bioconjugate Chem.*, 13, 737, 2002.

42. Ashwell, G. and Harford, J. Carbohydrate-specific receptors of the liver, *Ann. Rev. Biochem.*, 51, 531, 1982.
43. Govender, T., Riley, T., Ehtezazi, T., Garnett, M., Stolnik, S., Illum, L., and Davis, S., Defining the drug incorporation properties of PLA-PEG nanoparticles, *Int. J. Pharm.*, 19, 95, 2000.
44. Perez, C., Sanchez, A., Putnam, D., Ting, D., Langer, R., and Alonso, M., Poly(lactic acid)-poly(ethylene glycol) nanoparticles as new carriers for the delivery of plasmid DNA, *J. Control. Rel.*, 75, 211, 2001.
45. Scholz, C., Iijima, M., Nagasaki Y., and Kataoka, K., A novel reactive polymeric micelle with aldehyde groups on its surface, *Macromolecules*, 28, 7295, 1995.
46. Yamamoto, Y., Nagasaki, Y., Kato, M., and Kataoka, K., Surface charge modulation of poly(ethylene glycol)-poly(D,L-lactide) block copolymer micelles: conjugation of charged peptides, *Colloids Surfaces B Biointerfaces*, 16, 135, 1999.
47. Yasugi, K., Nakamura, T., Nagasaki, Y., Kato, M., and Kataoka, K., Sugar-installed polymer micelles: synthesis and micellization of poly(ethylene glycol)-poly(D,L-lactide) block copolymers having sugar groups at the PEG chain end, *Macromolecules*, 32, 8024, 1999.
48. Takakura, Y., Fujita, T., Hashida, M., and Sezaki, H., Disposition characteristics of macromolecules in tumor-bearing mice, *Pharm. Res.*, 7, 339, 1990.
49. Takakura, Y. and Hashida, M., Macromolecular carrier systems for targeted drug delivery: pharmacokinetic considerations on biodistribution, *Pharm. Res.*, 13, 820, 1996.
50. Yamamoto, Y., Nagasaki, Y., Kato, Y., Sugiyama, Y., and Kataoka, K., Long circulating poly(ethylene glycol)-poly(D,L-lactide) block copolymer micelles with modulated surface charge, *J. Control. Rel.*, 77, 27, 2001.
51. Bazile, D., Prudhomme, C., Bassoullet, M., Marlard, M., Spenlehauer, G., and Veillard, M., Stealth Me-PEG-PLA nanoparticles avoid uptake by the mononuclear phagocytes system, *J. Pharm. Sci.*, 84, 493, 1995.
52. Burt, H., Zhang, X., Toleikis, P., Embree, L. and Hunter, W., Development of copolymers of poly(D,L-lactide) and methoxypolythylene glycol as micellar carriers for Paclitaxel, *Colloids Surfaces B Biointerfaces*, 16, 161, 1999.
53. Allen, T. and Hansen, C., Pharmacokinetics of stealth versus conventional liposomes: effect of dose, *Biochim. Biophys. Acta*, 1068, 133, 1991.
54. Dwek, R., Glycobiology: toward understanding the function of sugars, *Chem. Rev.*, 96, 683, 1996.
55. Lis, H. and Sharon, N., Lectins: carbohydrate-specific proteins that mediate cellular recognition, *Chem. Rev.*, 98, 637, 1998.
56. Nagasaki, Y., Yasugi, K., Yamamoto, Y., Harada, A., and Kataoka, K., Sugar-installed block copolymer micelles: their preparation and specific interaction with lectin molecules, *Biomacromolecules*, 2, 1067, 2001.
57. Karlsson, R. and Fält, A., Experimental design for kinetic analysis of protein–protein interactions with surface plasmon resonance biosensors, *J. Immunol. Methods*, 200, 121, 1997.
58. Jule, E., Nagasaki, Y., and Kataoka, K., Surface plasmon resonance study on the interaction between lactose-installed poly(ethylene glycol)-poly(D,L-lactide) block copolymer micelles and lectins immobilized on a gold surface, *Langmuir*, 18, 10334, 2002.
59. Solís, D., Fernández, P., Díaz-Mauriño, T., Jiménez-Barbero, J., and Martín-Lomas, M., Hydrogen-bonding pattern of methyl β-lactoside binding to the *Ricinus communis* lectins, *Eur. J. Biochem.*, 214, 677, 1993.

60. Mammen, M. and Choi, S., and Whitesides, G., Polyvalent interactions in biological systems: implications for design and use of multivalent ligands and inhibitors, *Ang. Chem. Int. Ed.*, 37, 2754, 1998.

61. Kuziemko, G., Stroth, M., and Stevens, R., Cholera toxin binding affinity and specificity for gangliosides determined by surface plasmon resonance, *Biochemistry*, 35, 6375, 1996.

62. Schön, A. and Freire, E., Thermodynamics of intersubunit interactions in cholera toxin upon binding to the oligosaccharide portion of its cell surface receptor, ganglioside G_{MI}, *Biochemistry*, 28, 5019, 1989.

63. Milton, H.J., *Poly(ethylene glycol) Chemistry*, Plenum Press, New York, 1992.

64. Otsuka, H., Nagasaki, Y., and Kataoka, K., Surface characterization of functionalized polylactide through the coating with heterobifunctional poly(ethylene glycol)/polylactide block copolymers, *Biomacromolecules*, 1, 39, 2000.

65. Jule, E., Nagasaki, Y., and Kataoka, K., Lactose-installed poly(ethylene glycol)-poly(D,L-lactide) block copolymer micelles exhibit fast-rate binding and high affinity toward a protein bed simulating a cell surface, *Bioconjugate Chem.*, 14, 177, 2003.

66. Lortat-Jacob, H., Chouin, E., Cusack, S., and van Raaij, M., Kinetic analysis of adenovirus fiber binding to its receptor reveals an avidity mechanism for trimeric receptor–ligand interactions, *J. Biol. Chem.*, 276, 9009, 2000.

67. MacKenzie, C., Hirama, T., Deng, S., Bundle, D., Narang, S., and Young, N., Analysis by surface plasmon resonance of the influence of valence on the ligand binding affinity and kinetics of anti-carbohydrate antibody, *J. Biol. Chem.*, 271, 1527, 1996.

68. Cairo, C., Gestwicki, J., Kanai, M., and Kiessling, L., Control of multivalent interactions by binding epitope density, *J. Am. Chem. Soc.*, 124, 1615, 2002.

69. Harada, A. and Kataoka, K., Novel polyion complex micelles entrapping enzyme molecules in the core: preparation of narrowly distributed micelles from lysozyme and poly(ethyleneglycol)-poly(aspartic acid) block copolymer in aqueous medium, *Macromolecules*, 31, 288, 1998.

70. Harada, A. and Kataoka, K., Novel polyion complex micelles entrapping enzyme molecules in the core. [II]: characterization of the micelles prepared at non-stoichiometric mixing ratios, *Langmuir*, 15, 4208, 1999.

71. Zhang, X., Goosen, M., Wyss, U., and Pichora, D., Biodegradable polymers for orthopedic applications, *Rev. Macromol. Chem. Phys.*, C33, 81, 1993.

72. Steendam, R., van Steenbergen, M., Hennink, W., Frijlink, H., and Lerk, C., Effect of molecular weight and glass transition on relaxation and release behaviour of poly(D,L-lactic acid) tablets, *J. Control. Rel.*, 70, 71, 2001.

73. Riley, T., Stonik, S., Heald, C., Xiong, C., Garnett, M., Illum, L., and Davis, S., Physicochemical evaluation of nanoparticles assembled from poly(lactic acid)-poly(ethylene glycol) (PLA-PEG) block copolymers as drug delivery vehicles, *Langmuir*, 17, 3168, 2001.

74. Yamamoto, Y., Yasugi, K., Harada, A., Nagasaki, Y., and Kataoka, K., Temperature related change in the property of poly(ethylene glycol)-poly(D,L-lactide) block copolymer micelles in aqueous milieu relevant to drug delivery systems, *J. Control. Rel.*, 82, 359, 2002.

75. Kataoka, K., Harada, A., and Nagasaki, Y., Block copolymer micelles for drug delivery: design, characterization and biological significance, *Adv. Drug Delivery Rev.*, 47, 113, 2001.

76. Nakajima, A., Solvent effect on the vibrational structures of the fluorescence and absorption spectra of pyrene, *Bull. Chem. Soc. Jpn.*, 44, 3272, 1971.

77. Kalyanasundaram, K. and Thomas, J., Environmental effects on vibronic band inten-
    sities in pyrene monomer fluorescence and their application in studies of micellar
    systems, *J. Am. Chem. Soc.*, 99, 2039, 1977.
78. Shen, H., Zhang, L., and Eisenberg, A., Thermodynamics of crew-cut micelle for-
    mation of polystyrene-b-poly(acrylic acid) diblock copolymers in DMF/H_2O mixture,
    J. Phys. Chem. B, 101, 4697, 1997.
79. Winnik, F., Photophysics of preassociated pyrenes in aqueous polymer solutions and
    in other organized media, *Chem. Rev.*, 93, 587, 1993.
80. Jule, E., Yamamoto, Y., Thouvenin, M., Nagasaki, Y., and Kataoka, K., Thermal
    characterization of poly(ethylene glycol)-poly(D,L-lactide) block copolymer micelles
    based on pyrene excimer formation, in preparation.

18 Fast Responsive Nanoparticles of Hydrophobically Modified Poly(Amino Acid)s and Proteinoids

Jong-Duk Kim, Seung Rim Yang, Yong Woo Cho, and Kinam Park

CONTENTS

INTRODUCTION

Efficient delivery of poorly soluble drugs and macromolecular drugs such as peptides, proteins, and deoxyribonucleic acids (DNAs), is one of the major issues in drug delivery. Among the useful carriers are biocompatible amino acid-based copolymers that self-assemble into nano-sized micelle-like aggregates of various morphologies in aqueous solutions. Their diverse properties and nanosized dimensions can enhance accessibility to target sites with rapid responses to environmental changes.

Proteinoids are usually synthesized by anhydrous thermal condensation of amino acids,[1,2] dissolve in neutral or basic aqueous solutions, and form microspheres when the solutions are acidified.[3] Drug molecules can be encapsulated in the inner chambers of proteinoid microspheres.[4-7] Because more than 20 different amino acids exist, the diverse composition and properties of proteinoids are attractive for drug delivery.[4-6] Poly(amino acid)s grafted with side chains form water-soluble self-aggregates with hydrophobic cores[8] or hydrophilic shells,[9] depending on the hydrophilicity of the side chains. A hydrophobic core can incorporate lipophilic drugs, while a hydrophilic corona or outer shell exerts steric repulsion against uptake by the reticuloendothelial system. These nano-sized aggregates also have fairly narrow size distribution, low critical aggregation concentration, slow rate of dissociation, and high drug-loading capacity for pharmaceutical applications.

This chapter describes the synthesis of amphiphilic poly(amino acid)s and proteinoids, the properties of self-aggregates and nanoparticles, and their responses to external stimuli. Due to their nano-sized dimensions, their responses to changes in environmental stimuli are extremely fast, and this property can be useful in various applications.

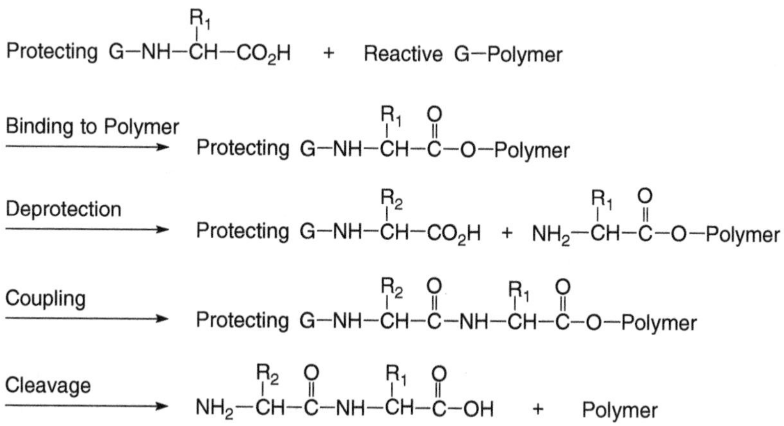

Protecting G—NH—CH(R_1)—CO$_2$H + Reactive G—Polymer

Binding to Polymer
$\longrightarrow$ Protecting G—NH—CH(R_1)—C(O)—O—Polymer

Deprotection
$\longrightarrow$ Protecting G—NH—CH(R_2)—CO$_2$H + NH$_2$—CH(R_1)—C(O)—O—Polymer

Coupling
$\longrightarrow$ Protecting G—NH—CH(R_2)—C(O)—NH—CH(R_1)—C(O)—O—Polymer

Cleavage
$\longrightarrow$ NH$_2$—CH(R_2)—C(O)—NH—CH(R_1)—C(O)—OH + Polymer

FIGURE 18.1 Solid phase peptide synthesis.

SYNTHESIS AND SELF-ASSEMBLY

Amphiphilic poly(amino acid)s or proteinoids form hydrophobic cores covered with hydrophilic surfaces to avoid contact with water. This organization process of nano-sized self-assemblies is thermodynamically driven and spontaneous.[9–12]

POLYPEPTIDES AND POLY(AMINO ACID)S

Solid Phase Peptide Synthesis

Hydrophilic and hydrophobic segments of poly(amino acid)s can be synthesized by a solid phase peptide synthetic route.[13] Amino acids can be assembled into a peptide of any desired sequence while the other end of the chain is anchored to an insoluble support. After the desired sequence of amino acids has been linked together on the support, a reagent can be applied to cleave the chain from the support and liberate the finished peptide into solution. All the reactions involved in the synthesis are commercially available and homogeneous products can be obtained.[14] This basic idea of synthesis is illustrated in Figure 18.1. Many naturally occurring peptides have been synthesized by the solid phase method and modified for the study of structure–activity correlations.

Polymerization of α-Amino Acid-N-Carboxyanhydrides (NCAs)

Solid phase peptide synthesis is neither useful nor practical for direct preparation of large polypeptides because of unavoidable deletions and truncations resulting from incomplete deprotection and coupling steps. The most economical and expeditious process for synthesis of long polypeptide chains is polymerization of α-amino acid-N-carboxyanhydrides (NCAs).[15,16] Considerable variety of NCAs allows exceptional diversity in the types of polypeptides. NCA polymerization has been initiated using many different nucleophiles and bases; the most common are primary amines

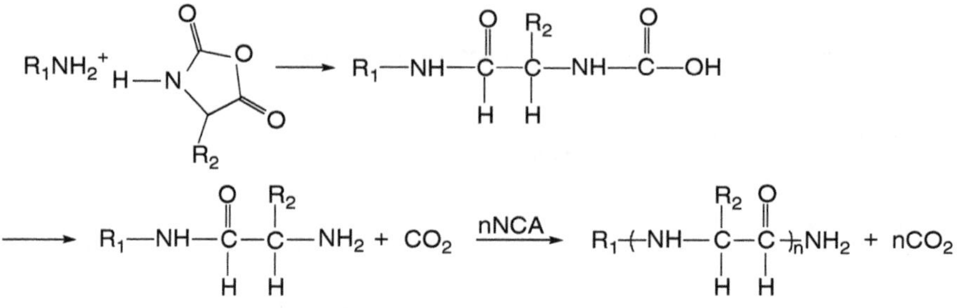

FIGURE 18.2 Amine mechanism of NCA polymerization.

and alkoxide anions.[15,16] Optimal polymerization conditions have often been determined empirically for individual NCAs, and no universal initiators or conditions that can be used for all monomers have yet been found.

The most likely pathway of NCA polymerization is the amine mechanism shown in Figure 18.2. Conventional NCA polymerization, however, has an inherent problem: lack of control over the reactivity of the growing polymer chain end during the course of polymerization. Use of transition metal complexes as end groups may control the addition of each NCA monomer to the polymer chain ends. Highly effective zero-valent nickel and cobalt initiators allowed living polymerization of NCAs into high molecular weight polypeptides via an unprecedented activation of NCAs into covalent propagating species. The additions of different NCA monomers allowed formation of block copolypeptides of defined sequence and composition.[15–19]

PROTEINOIDS

A peptide bond is formed when water is produced from the $-COOH$ and $-NH_2$ groups present in two different amino acids or peptides. The Gibbs free energy ($\Delta G°$) of bond formation is in the range of 2 to 4 Kcal/mole[20] as shown by the following equation:

$$^+H_3NCHRCOO^- + {}^+H_3NCHR'COO^- \rightarrow {}^+H_3NCHRCONHCHR'COO^- + H_2O$$

$$\Delta G° = 2 \sim 4 \text{ Kcal/mole}$$

The supply of energy equivalent to 4 Kcal/mole will lead to a reaction to produce a peptide bond and water. If the system is closed, it soon reaches equilibrium with water, and amino acids will be dissolved in an aqueous solution instead of formation of a peptide bond. For this reason, peptide bond formation required removal of water either by evaporation or by chemical reaction with polyphosphoric acid,[21] cyanamide, or dicyanamide.[22] Aspartic acid (or glutamic acid) polymerized to polyaspartylimide and underwent internal ring opening in aqueous solution of high pH to form poly(aspartic acid).[23]

If glutamic acid is heated above 100°C in a dry state, it cyclizes to form hot liquid pyroglutamic acid.[24] Pyroglutamic acid was found at the N terminals of thermal copoly(amino acids).[25] Aspartic acid and glutamic acid thermally copolymerized together to form poly(aspartylglutamic acid).[21]

Ground mixtures of dry amino acids containing at least small proportions of charged amino acids were heated to temperatures in the range of 120 to 200°C. Different amino acids in the mixture may have produced different degrees of acidity (or basicity) and hydrophilicity (or hydrophobicity). Certain amino acids preferred in condensation to occupy higher percentages. Thus, the residue sequence may have exhibited nonrandomness and limited heterogeneity in proteinoids.

An example of proteinoid synthesis starts with heating glutamic acid (5 g) to a molten state in a nitrogen atmosphere. The molten mass was kept stirred at 170°C, and to it was added 5 g of aspartic acid and 2.5 g of an equimolar mixture of the other 17 basic and neutral amino acids. The mixture was kept heated at 170°C under stirring in a nitrogen atmosphere for 6 h. The highly viscous brown paste formed was cooled to room temperature to solidify into a hard, glassy mass. The product was then dissolved in 100 ml of 10% aqueous solution of sodium bicarbonate. The solution was filtered, neutralized with dilute acetic acid, and dialyzed through a cellulose membrane against distilled water for 48 h (water changed every 6 h). The molecular weight cut-off (MWCO) of the membrane was 3500. The contents of the dialysis tube were dried at 45°C under vacuum.[26,27]

POLY(AMINO ACID)-BASED AMPHIPHILIC COPOLYMERS

Block Copolymers

Block copolymers can be synthesized by copolymerization of a water-soluble monomer with a hydrophobic comonomer[28] or by block copolymerization of reactive polymer end groups.[29-31] Regarding poly(amino acid)-based block copolymers, emphasis has been placed on micelles made of poly(ethylene oxide) (PEO), e.g., PEO-b-poly(L-amino acid).[32] Kataoka et al. prepared PEO-b-poly(β-benzyl-L-aspartate) and engineered the chemical structures of core-forming blocks through partial replacement of the benzyl group by an aliphatic chain and cetyl ester residue.[33,34]

They also synthesized PEO-b-poly(L-lysine) and prepared a polyion complex with genes, oligonucleotides, and enzymes.[35-37] Di- and tri-block copolymers of PEO-b-poly(γ-benzyl-L-glutamate) were also prepared.[38,39] PEO-b-poly(L-amino acid) was synthesized by the ring opening polymerization of amino acid NCAs initiated by the terminal primary amino group of α-methoxy-ω-aminopoly(ethylene glycol) as shown in Figure 18.3.[40]

Diblock copoly(α-amino acid)s were synthesized to form nanoparticles. Constandis et al. presented a new family of copoly(α-amino acids) including poly(leucine-b-sodium glutamate). These compounds self-assemble to form nontoxic and biodegradable nanoparticles for controlled release of insulin[41] (see Figure 18.4). Deming et al. synthesized several diblock copolypetide amphiphiles with charged and hydrophobic segments to prepare hydrogels with different copolymer chain lengths, compositions, and chain conformations.[42]

Graft Copolymers

Graft copolymers can be synthesized by attaching hydrophobic moieties such as long alkyl chains or bulky cholesterol derivatives to water-soluble polymer backbones.[43-45]

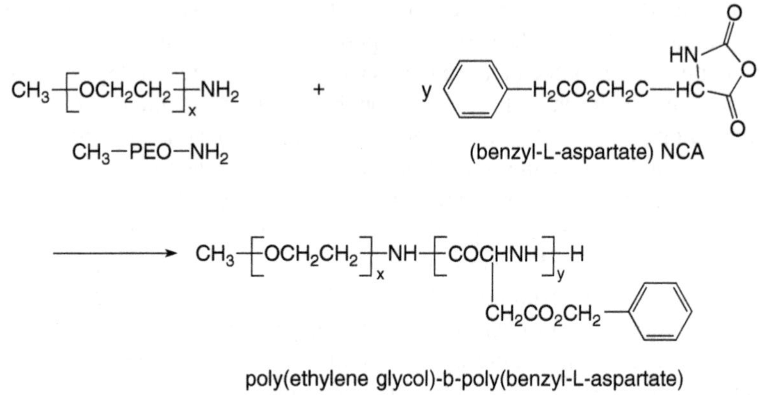

poly(ethylene glycol)-b-poly(benzyl-L-aspartate)

FIGURE 18.3 Synthesis of poly(ethylene oxide)-b-poly(β-benzyl-L-aspartate).

L-methyl glutamate NCA

Poly(sodium glutamate-b-leucine)

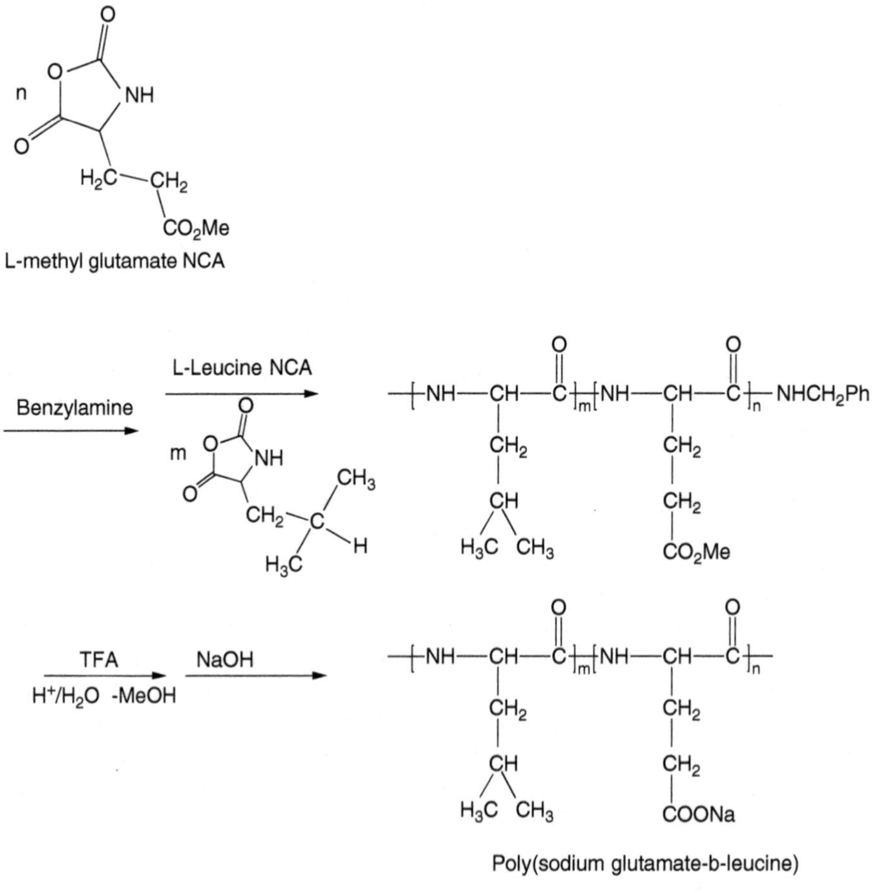

FIGURE 18.4 Synthesis of poly(sodium glutamate-block-leucine).

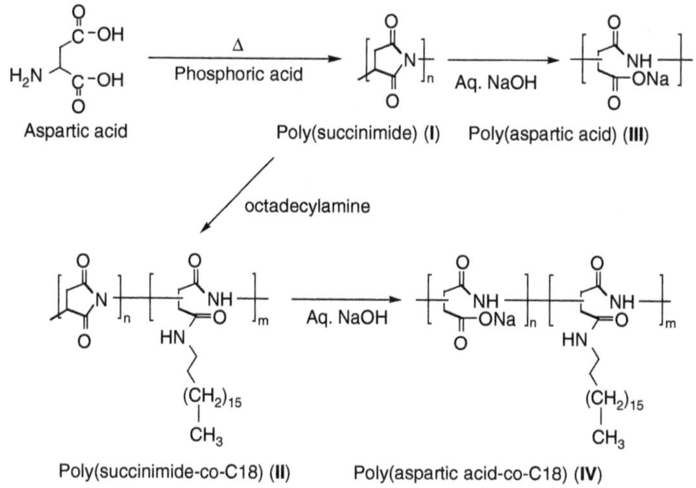

FIGURE 18.5 Synthesis of PSI and poly(aspartic acid) with long alkyl groups. (From Kang, H.S. et al., *Langmuir*, 17, 7501, 2001. With permission.)

An example of a graft poly(amino acid)-based copolymer is shown in Figure 18.5.[9] Polysuccinimide (PSI) was synthesized by thermal condensation of aspartic acid with phosphoric acid, and then an alkyl chain was conjugated by aminolysis of PSI with alkylamine. The remaining succinimide units were hydrolyzed with NaOH, which converted to poly(sodium aspartate). The degree of substitution (DS) is the mole percent of the attached unit of alkyl group per total succinimide unit. The DS was determined by both [1]H-nuclear magnetic resonance (NMR) and elemental analysis.

Poly(2-hydroxyethyl aspartamide) (PHEA) was synthesized by aminolysis of PSI with ethanolamine and dehydrocholic acid-conjugated PHEA was prepared by esterification in the presence of carbodiimide as a coupling reagent.[46] Polycaprolactone (PCL)-grafted polyasparagine was carried with amine-terminated PCL and PSI, and followed by aminolysis to polyasparagine.[47] Poly(L-lysine) was often modified with several moieties because of primary ε-amine groups in poly(L-lysine) as shown in Figure 18.6.

Poly(L-lysine)-g-PLGA micelles were used to produce compact nanoparticle complexes with plasmid DNA that could efficiently protect the complexed DNA.[48] Biodegradable PLGA chains were grafted to a cationic poly(L-lysine) backbone by reacting a carboxylic terminal end group of PLGA with primary ε-amine groups in poly(L-lysine). A cholesterol-bearing poly(L-lysine) was synthesized by a condensation reaction of cholesteryl N-(6-isocyanatehexyl) carbamate with poly(L-lysine).[49] Graft copolymers composed of the poly(L-lactic acid-co-L-lysine) (PLAL) backbone, and poly(L-lysine), poly(D,L-alanine), or poly(L-aspartic acid) side chains were synthesized with various sequences and graft densities.[50] Amphiphilic block or graft copolymers form self-assemblies, nano-sized micelle-like aggregates of various morphologies in aqueous solution.

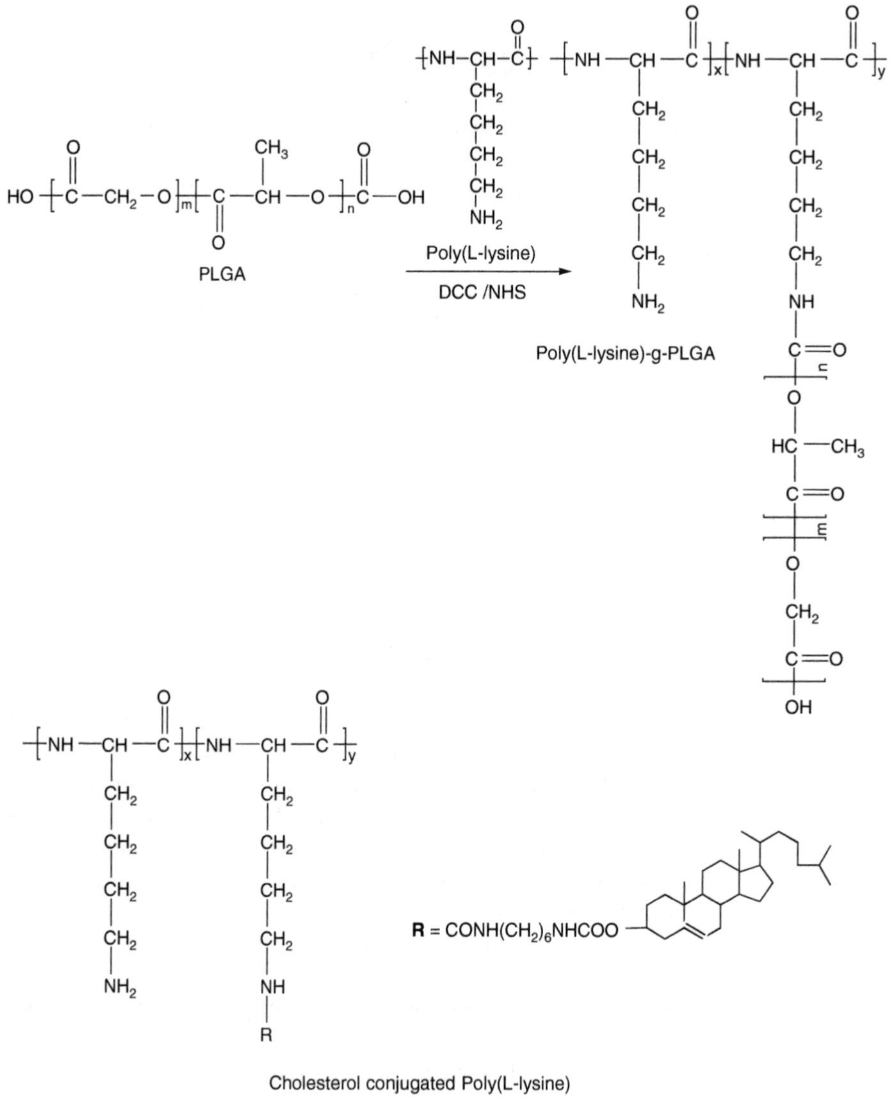

FIGURE 18.6 Poly(L-lysine) graft copolymer.

STRUCTURES AND FUNCTIONS

MICELLE AGGREGATES

Amphiphilic block or graft copolymers have been found to form self-assembled, nano-sized micelle-like aggregates in aqueous solutions and have been studied for possible applications as drug carriers.[29,51] The hydrophobic microdomains of self-aggregates can act as hosts for many hydrophobic molecules. The drug delivery potential of polysaccharides with steroids[9,52–55] and poly(amino acid)s with side chains[9,46,47] has also received attention.

Critical Association Concentration

Micelle-like aggregates start to form at critical association concentration (CAC), a parameter similar to the critical micellization concentrations (CMCs) of surfactant micelles. The most common method to determine the CACs of polymeric micelles is using a hydrophobic fluorescence probe sensitive to changes in environmental polarities.[56,57]

Self-aggregates are thermodynamically stable if the total copolymer concentration is above CAC.[11] A drug delivery system is subject to a "sink condition" or severe dilution upon intravenous injection. The total blood volume of an average individual is approximately 5 l. Thus, intravenous injection of 100 ml of a 2% (w/w) PCL_{21}-b-PEO_{44} micelle solution results in a copolymer concentration of 400 μg/ml in the blood. Therefore it is important to know the CAC levels of copolymers. The CMC values for PBLA-b-PEO are known to be 5 to 18 μg/ml,[58,59] while the CMC for a PLA-b-PEO system was found to be 35 μg/ml.[53] Figure 18.7 shows the CACs of three polyaminoacid graft copolymers of PAsp-g-alkyl,[9] PHEA-g-DHA,[46] and PAsn-g-PCL.[47] In fact, the CACs of PAsn-g-PCL are as small as a tenth of the sizes of the others. Since the PCL side chain forms a crystalline phase, it is expected that the graft copolymer may have a small CAC.

The CAC decreased as the grafting density of hydrophobic groups increased, as seen in the CMCs of surfactants. For most of the low molecular weight surfactants

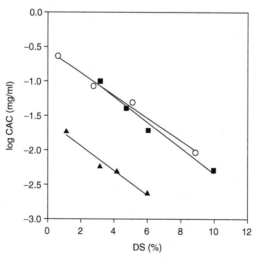

▲   CAC of PAsn-g-PCL as a function of DS

■   CAC of PHEA-g-DHA as a function of DS

○   CAC of PAsp-g-alkyl as a function of DS

FIGURE 18.7 Critical aggregation concentration (CAC) of poly(amino acid)s grafted with hydrophobic moieties determined by emission fluorescence spectra of pyrene.

in aqueous solutions, the free energy of micellization was proportional to the length of the alkyl, DHA, and PCL chains as described in this equation:[60]

$$\Delta G^\circ = RT \log cmc \qquad (18.1)$$

For a homologous straight-chain ionic surfactant in an aqueous solution, a relation between CMC and the number of carbon atoms N in the alkyl chain was found via the following equation:[61]

$$\log CMC = A - BN \qquad (18.2)$$

where A and B depend on the specific ion type and temperature. However, the relation can be modified into Equation (18.3) in the case of an anionic copolymer grafted with an alkyl chain:

$$\log CAC = A - B[DS] \qquad (18.3)$$

The CACs of PAsp-C18 series and other systems showed linear relationships according to Equation (18.3), as shown in Figure 18.7. The degree of substitution (DS) of the PAsp-C18 series can be correlated with the lengths of the alkyl groups in the above relation.

Size Distribution

The sizes of colloidal particles influence circulation time and organ distribution *in vivo*. Particles smaller than 200 nm are known to be less susceptible to clearance by the reticuloendothelial system and those smaller than 5 μm have access to small capillaries.[62] Most theories of micelle formation are based on the equilibrium thermodynamic approach. However, aggregates of poly(amino acid)-g-hydrophobic groups such as PAsp-alkyl[9] are not formed under equilibrium conditions due to the rigidities of grafted alkyl chains at room temperature.

Therefore, the aggregation property of a graft copolymer in aqueous solution should be regarded as kinetically controlled. In bimodal distribution, the primary aggregate can be considered thermodynamically stable and associated by both intramolecular and intermolecular interactions of grafted alkyl chains. The large secondary aggregate can be formed mainly by intermolecular interactions because the aggregate formation is kinetically controlled. After the incubation of aggregate solution at 60°C, the size of primary aggregate was maintained and the intensity increased, while the scattering intensity of secondary aggregate was remarkably reduced by melting of octadecyl chains and reconstitution of PAsp-C18 into primary aggregates as shown in Figure 18.8.

Micelle size is controlled by several factors, among which are the lengths of the hydrophobic groups and the lengths of the hydrophilic groups.[63] Several different studies led to the development of scaling relations.[52,64] The graft copolymers with poly(amino acid) backbones also form self-aggregates in aqueous solutions. Interestingly, the hydrodynamic diameters of self-aggregates were reduced as DS

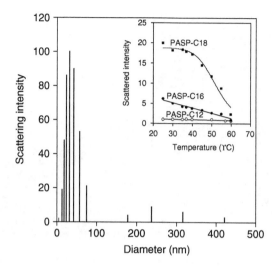

FIGURE 18.8 Size distiribution of C18-D10 after reconstitution by melting of octadecyl chain. Inset (b) represents the dependence of light scattering intensity on heating, indicating disorganization of secondary aggregate by breaking hydrophobic domains of intermolecular interaction. (From Kang, H.S. et al., *Langmuir,* 17, 7501, 2001. With permission.)

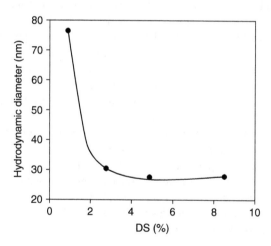

FIGURE 18.9 Plot of number–average mean diameter of PAsn-g-alkyl vs. DS of octadecyl group. (From Kang, H.S. et al., *Langmuir,* 17, 7501, 2001. With permission.)

increased as shown Figure 18.9. This size reduction may be attributed to the large curvature K created by both chain stiffness and strong hydrophobic interactions of neighboring hydrophobic groups. It is believed that the graft copolymer (having a higher DS) forms smaller aggregates due to stronger hydrophobic interactions of grafted hydrophobic groups with increases in the packing density of hydrophobic groups in self-aggregates. Such a reduction in size was observed when alkyl, DHA, or PCL was grafted into a poly(amino acid) backbone.

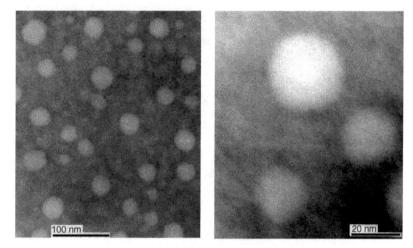

FIGURE 18.10 Transmission electron microscopy photographs of PAsn-g-PCL. (From Jeong, J.H. et al., *Polymer*, 44, 583, 2003. With permission.)

Morphologies

Amphiphilic molecules self-assemble in aqueous media, and the morphologies of these self-assemblies were examined by transmission electron microscopy (TEM). The spherical shape was the most common. However, if the length of the core-forming block was much greater than that of the corona-forming block, the morphologies were shaped like rods, vesicles, lamellae, large compound micelles, tubules, and hexagonally packed hollow hoops.[52,64,65] Formation of various morphologies of aggregates may be explained by a force balance effect involving the degree of stretching of the core-forming blocks, the interfacial energy between the micelle core and the solvent, and intercorona chain interactions.[52,66]

Figure 18.10 consists of two transmission electron micrographs of poly(asparagine)-g-poly(caprolactone) with negative staining that clearly show spherical shapes of self-aggregates as light parts surrounded by negative staining. The hydrophobic moieties conjugated to one poly(amino acid) backbone chain were sufficient to gather and form hydrophobic domains. In this case, a micelle was formed by a single polymer chain. Such unimeric micelles were designated *self-aggregates* and *flower-type aggregates* as shown in Figure 18.10.

PROTEINOIDS

Proteinoids are random copolymers formed from amino acids. The inorganic poly-condensation of amino acids into peptide bonds occurs at temperatures over $140°C$ or can form protein-like chains from a mixture of 20 common amino acids at only $70°C$ in the presence of phosphoric acid or amidinium carbodiimide in aqueous solution.[1,2] Formation of proteinoids is due to the hydrophobic interaction of protonated carboxyl groups present in the glutamic and aspartic acid residues of proteinoid chains. The synthesis of proteinoids requires excessive amounts of glutamic acid and aspartic acid; they provide the reaction-initiating materials, pyroglutamic acid and polyaspartic acid, in the condensation reactions of amino acids.[2]

Molecular Weights of Proteinoids

The mean molecular weights of proteinoids were determined by end-group assay and sedimentation velocity analyses in an ultracentrifuge.[1] The average molecular weights ranged from 4000 to 10,000, and increased with higher reaction temperatures and longer heating times. Also, the acidic or basic characteristics affected molecular weights. Proteinoids with higher acidic amino acid portions tended to have low molecular weights, and those with higher basic amino acid portions had high molecular weights. Some thermal polylysines had mean molecular weights above 10,000 as measured by sedimentation equilibrium analysis.[67] The mean molecular weights observed for proteinoids fell within the lower end of the molecular-weight ranges of natural proteins.[2]

Solubility and Precipitability of Proteinoids

Solubility of proteinoids is a function of composition. Depending on which amino acids are used in the reactant mixture, proteinoids show different solubility properties. Proteinoids rich in hydrophobic amino acids such as valine and leucine are less soluble in water. Therefore, solubility and other physical properties are controllable through a choice of reaction conditions and selection of amino acids. It is also possible to obtain proteinoids corresponding to each of the various classes of proteins, such as albumins, globulins, and histones.[1]

Proteinoids can be precipitated from aqueous solution by trichloroacetic acid, picric acid, phosphotungstic acid, sulfosalicylic acid, zinc hydroxide, nitric acid, phosphomolybdic acid, mercury sublimate, and hot methanol.[68] Some of these reagents are conventionally used for precipitating proteins. Salting-in by dilute concentrations of salt and salting-out by high concentrations of ammonium sulfate are also applicable to proteinoids since proteins respond to salt concentrations.[2]

Proteinoid Microspheres

Proteinoids can form microspheres through changes in temperature or the pH of the dispersion medium.[69] The compositions and properties of proteinoids can be varied easily using different combinations of more than 20 available amino acids.[70,71] Proteinoids dissolve in neutral and basic aqueous solutions and form microspheres when the solutions are acidified and drug or peptide molecules can be encapsulated in the inner chambers of the formed microspheres. This process of microsphere formation is caused by the hydrophobic interaction of protonated carboxyl groups present in the glutamic and aspartic acid residues in proteinoid chains. Fox and Dose proposed that proteinoid microspheres played a major role in the origin of life.[2]

Conformations and Structures

α-Helices and β-sheets are the major secondary structural motifs that organize the three-dimensional geometries of proteins.[69] Amino acids have been extensively studied for their ability to form helical and sheet structures.[5,6] Several block copolymers with identical compositions and different sequences, e.g., (Val–Lys)n, Ala_{20}–Glu_{20}–Phe_8, Glu_{20}–Ala_{20}–Phe_8, and others form very different helical structures in the same environment.[70]

NANOCAPSULES

Hydrophobic drugs have been delivered via polymeric micelles made of biodegradable hydrophobic and hydrophilic polymer blocks. The hydrophobic drug is entrapped in the hydrophobic core and the hydrophilic corona serves as a stabilizing interface between the hydrophobic core and the external aqueous medium. Poly(amino acid)s are promising alternatives for delivery of hydrophobic drugs because they are easy to make and their amino acid side chains offer sites for crosslinking, drug conjugation, or pendent group modification for improved physicochemical properties.[71,72]

Drug Entrapment

In general, the amount of drug loaded into polymer aggregates by physical means is dependent on several factors including the molecular volume of solubilizate, interfacial tension of solubilizate against water, length of the core and shell-forming block of the copolymer, polymer and solubilizate concentrations,[73] and the Flory–Huggins interaction parameter.[74,75] Bader et al. reported the first application of proteinoids in drug delivery in 1984.[76] A sulfide derivative of cyclophosphamide (an anticancer drug analogue) was conjugated to lysine residues of a PEO-poly(L-lysine) block copolymer. Since then, various types of drug delivery systems based on poly(amino acid) copolymers have been investigated (Table 18.1).

For example, the primary hydroxyl group of poly(2-hydroxyethyl aspartamide) (PHEA) composed of an amino acid derivative based on aspartic acid can offer a conjugation site for attaching a drug. Methotrexate (MTX) was easily loaded into the hydrophobic cores of PHEA-C18 aggregates by sonication.[77] The amount of entrapped MTX in 1 g of copolymer was calculated to be 3.39 mg/DS. MTX is soluble in distilled water to an extent due to the presence of carboxylic and free amine groups despite overall hydrophobic nature. MTX, however, was highly

TABLE 18.1
Nanocapsules Based on Poly(Amino Acid)s Used for Drug Delivery

Nanocapsule System	Entrapped Molecule	Loading Method	Ref.
PEO-b-poly(L-lysine)	Cyclophosphamide	Chemical and physical	82
PHEA-g-C18	Methotrexate	Chemical and physical	77
PEO-g-P(Asp)	Doxorubicin	Chemical complex	62,73
Poly(L-lysine)-g-PLGA	Plasmid DNA	Adsorption	48
Poly(L-leucine-b-L-glutamate)	Insulin	Physical	41
PEO-PBLA	Indomethacin	Physical	80
PEO-PHSA	Amphotericin B		79

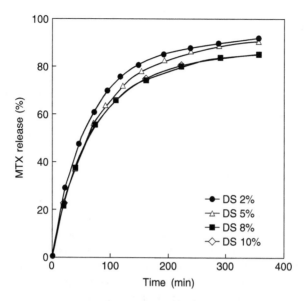

FIGURE 18.11 MTX release profile from PHEA-C18 in pH 7.0 buffer at 37°C. (From Kang, H.S. et al., *J. Control. Rel.*, 81, 135, 2002. With permission.)

partitioned in the hydrophobic domains of the proteinoids and the partitioning constant increased with the DS of the octadecyl group.

Release Kinetics

The release of drug from an aggregate depends upon the rate of diffusion of the entrapped drug, aggregate stability, and the rate of biodegradation of the copolymer.[11] Figure 18.11 shows the MTX release profile from PHEA-C18 at pH 7.0. Its solubility at pH 7.0 increased abruptly due to the transformation of the carboxylic group into salt form. The release rate from aggregates was rapid due to direct contact with the aqueous media even though MTX was incorporated in the hydrophobic core. The same results were also found when nanoparticles released a hydrophobic drug containing a carboxylic group.[31] La et al. found that indomethacin was maintained within micelles for a long time at pH 1.2 and released rapidly at pH 6.5.[78] The cores of aggregates formed from the more hydrophilic polymers may contain appreciable amounts of water, and the release of drugs from such cores has been found to proceed rapidly.[79,80]

INTERACTION AND TRANSITION

STIMULUS SENSITIVITY

pH Sensitivity

Proteinoids and poly(amino acid)s can form polyelectrolyte complexes by electrostatic interactions with biological molecules that can be reversible by changing the

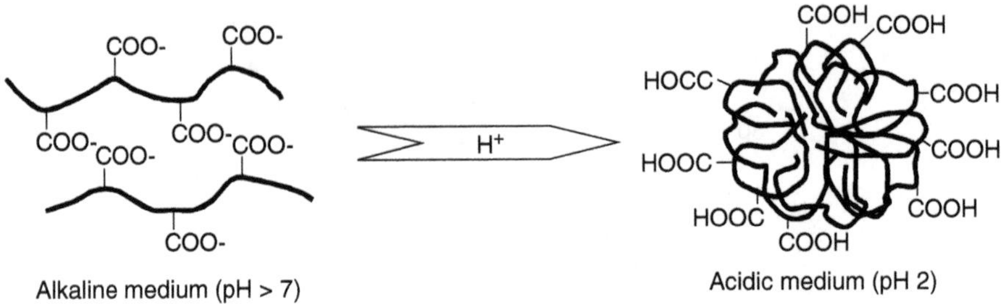

FIGURE 18.12 Self-assembly of a proteinoid to a microsphere in acidic aqueous medium.

pH.[81] Incorporated drugs can be released easily when the complexes dissolve. The pH-sensitive dissolution of nanoparticles formed by complexation of polyaminoacids with dodecanoic acid (C12) was adjusted by choosing proper amino acids. The particle stability against basic conditions increased with increasing pK_a values of poly(amino acid)s.[82] Proteinoids of all naturally occurring amino acids were insoluble in acidic media and dissolved in neutral and alkaline media[64,83] as shown in Figure 18.12. Thus, a drug can be loaded into proteinoids by changing the pH of the medium.[84–86]

Thermosensitivity

Thermoresponsive hydrogels based on crosslinked copolymers of N-isopropylacrylamide (NIPAM) and poly(amino acid)s were prepared[87] using two kinds of reactive NIPAM-based copolymers containing poly(amino acid)s as side-chain groups and activated ester groups. The polymer chains were easily crosslinked by simply mixing in aqueous solution. The swelling ratio measurements of hydrogels showed large volume changes dependent on temperature changes. Such temperature-dependent large volume changes can be used for development of injectable or implantable drug delivery systems.

A block copolymer consisting of biodegradable poly(lactic acid) and nonbiodegradable PEO was developed as an injectable thermoresponsive polymer.[88] Precise control over the molecular architecture was required for control of the thermoresponsive properties. The reaction of polysuccinimide with a mixture of 5-aminopentanol and 6-aminohexanol produced a new thermoresponsive polymer based on a biodegradable poly(amino acid), poly(N-substituted alpha/beta-asparagine), showing a clear lower critical solution temperature (LCST) in water as shown in Figure 18.13.[89] This thermoresponsive poly(amino acid) had a hydroxy group in the side chain and functional molecules such as drugs and probes could be easily introduced. Proteinoid aggregation occurred upon a temperature increase above the LCST of the chain.[90,91]

Environment Sensitivity

The thiol groups of cysteines can be utilized for making stabilized nanoparticles by crosslinking of cysteine-containing blocks by disulfide bonds.[92,93] The thiol groups

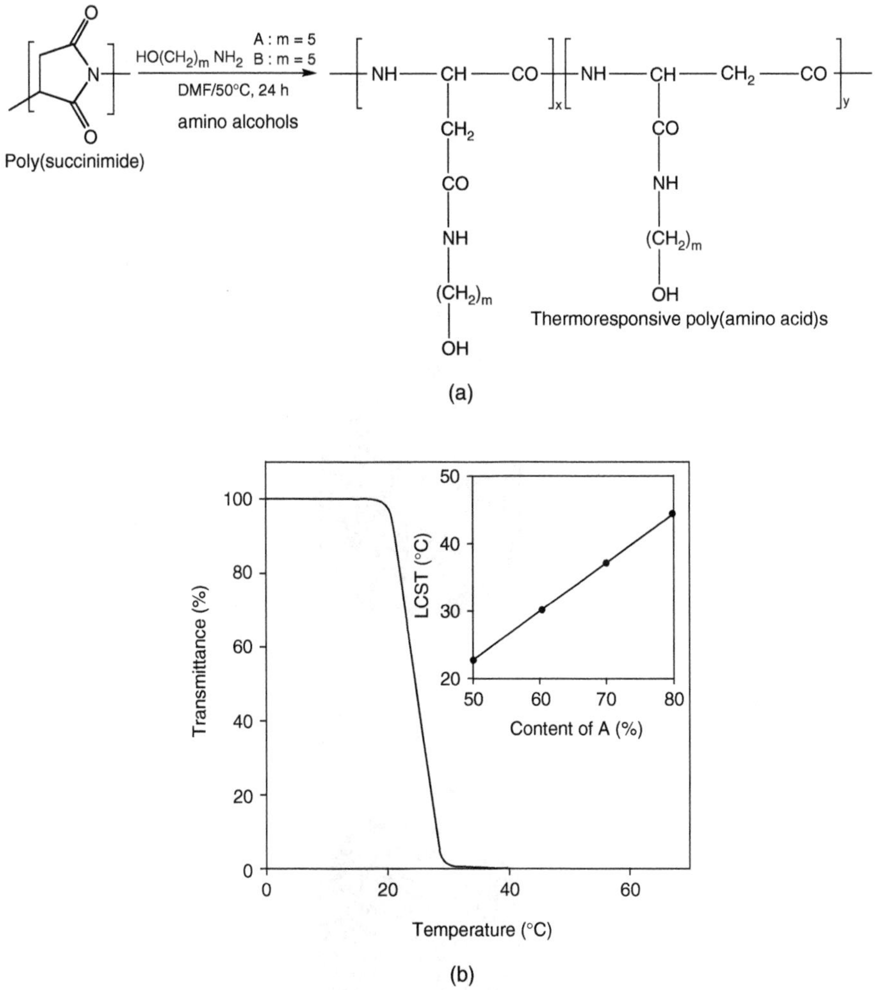

FIGURE 18.13 The structure (a) and LCST behavior (b) of biodegradable thermosensitive poly(amino acid)s. (From Yoich, T. et al., *Chem. Commun.,* 106, 107, 2003. With permission.)

on a small fraction of the lysine repeating units of PEO-b-poly(L-lysine) diblock copolymers formed micelles with reversible crosslinking as shown in Figure 18.14. The advantage of micelles with disulfide crosslinkages in drug delivery is that the cleavage of disulfide bonds would occur within cells because intracellular compartments have stronger reducing environments than extracellular fluids do. Such micelles are useful in the delivery of oligonucleotides into cells.

Photosensitivity

Poly(amino acid)s with photochromic side chains can respond to light with reversible variations between disordered and regularly folded chains such as α-helices and β-structures. Such changes are accompanied by changes in physicochemical properties.

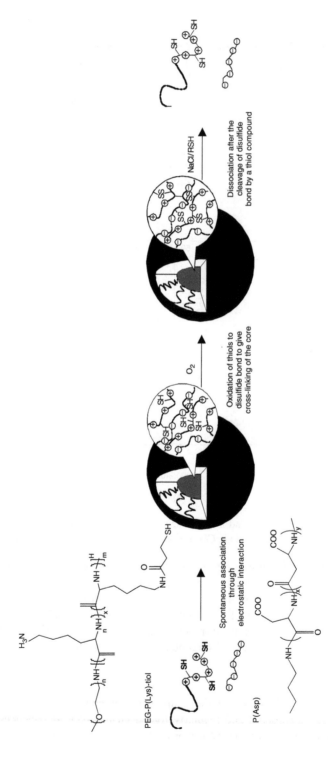

FIGURE 18.14 Reversibly crosslinked micelles from thiol-modified PEG-PLL block copolymers. (From Kakizawa, Y. et al., *J. Am. Chem. Soc.*, 121, 11247, 1999. With permission.)

Poly(α-amino acid)s containing azobenzene and spiropyran groups in the side chains showed the most significant photoresponse effects.[94] The molecular and supramolecular structures of these polypeptides can be photomodulated using the photosensitive side chains as effectors. The extents and types of photoresponses include photo-induced transitions between coil and alpha-helix, photostimulated aggregation and disaggregation processes, and reversible changes of viscosity and solubility. Photochromic poly(α-amino acid) systems actually behave as amplifiers and transducers of primary photochemical events occurring in side chains.

INTERACTIONS WITH BIOMOLECULES

Hydrophobically modified poly(amino acid)s can interact with biomolecules such as genes, proteins, liposomes, and cell membranes by hydrophobic and electrostatic interactions. Oppositely charged macromolecules can form polyion complexes with poly(amino acid) segments. The incorporation of DNA, peptides, and proteins in poly(amino acid)-based nanoparticles may also lead to stabilization against digestive enzymes such as nuclease and facilitate uptake into cells.[95]

Binding of Proteins to Proteinoids

Bovine serum albumin (BSA) has a high affinity for hydrophobic molecules.[96] Lysozyme, which is deactivated by surfactants, fatty acids, and steroids, shows binding to hydrophobically modified proteinoids.[97] When a proteinoid dispersion and lysozyme solution were mixed, precipitates were formed immediately.

Interactions of Hydrophobically Modified Proteinoids with Liposomal Membranes

The surfaces of liposomes were modified with water-soluble polymers to increase the circulation time in blood, specific targeting, and responsiveness to external stimuli.[98] The anchoring of the polymer onto liposomes was done by using hydrophobically modified water-soluble polymers.[99,100] The liposome with hydrophobically modified proteinoids showed surfaces protected from surfactants as shown in Figure 18.15. The hydrophobically modified proteinoids on liposomal membranes resulted in liposome stabilization and liposome-sized alterations and they can be used as surface modifiers of liposomes with specific properties.

Interactions with Cell Membranes and Cell-Penetrating Peptides

Membrane interactions with amphiphatic polypeptides result from a delicate balance of hydrophobic and electrostatic interactions. These interactions and self-assembling tendencies may result in the formation of pore-like structures or other membrane-disruptive assemblies. Hydrophobically modified poly(amino acid)s interact with cell membranes and show properties similar to those of amphipathic polypeptides.

Some poly(amino acid)s can bind to short, highly basic peptides such as TAT (basic sequence from the HIV-1 TAT protein), antennapedia, and transportan for rapid translocation into cells.[101] A novel transport peptide that was rich in arginine

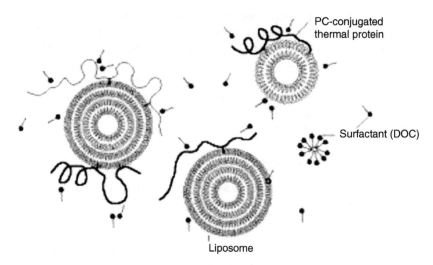

FIGURE 18.15 Putative morphology of liposomes associated with hydrophobically modified proteinoids.

and proline permitted its cargo to translocate across membranes into cytoplasm.[102] A 10-residue proline-rich peptide with two arginine residues was capable of delivering a noncovalently linked protein into cells. Thus, proline-rich peptides represent a potentially new class of cell-permeating peptides for intracellular delivery of protein cargos.[103,104]

Many arginine-rich peptides including those having branched chain structures show efficient intracellular delivery. For that reason, the presence of a ubiquitous internalization mechanism for arginine-rich peptides has been suggested.[105,106] The transfection efficiency in gene delivery depends on the number and positioning of histidine residues in the peptide.[107] Histidine-rich molecules allow the transfer of plasmid and oligonucleotides in cultured cells. The biological activity of antisense oligodeoxynucleotides was increased more than 20-fold when they were complexed with highly histidylated oligolysine into small cationic spherical particles of 35 nm. We have evidence that imidazole protonation mediates the effects of these molecules in endosomes.[108] It appears that the systematic designs of poly(amino acid)s can increase or alter interactions with cell membranes and subsequent transport across cell membranes.

POLY(AMINO ACID) AS A MULTIFUNCTIONAL CARRIER

POLY(AMINO ACID) CONJUGATES

A primary advantage of poly(amino acid)-based nanoparticles is that they allow attachment of drugs, drug compatible moieties, genes or intelligent vectors through free functional groups (e.g., amine and carboxylic acid) of amino acid chains. Ringsdorf et al. attached a cytotoxic agent to the poly(L-lysine) block of a PEO-b-poly(L-lysine) copolymer to form micelles.[109] Yokoyama et al. attached doxorubicin onto the poly(aspartic acid) backbone through an amide bond.[34,110] To overcome the excessive stability of an amide linkage between a drug and core forming block, an ester bond was used to form a hydrolyzable micelle-forming conjugate.[9,111]

Protein or peptide conjugation can also be synthesized using methods based on the formation of disulfide bridges.[112,113] Poly(amino acid)s contain primary amino groups that can be used to introduce thiol groups on polymer backbones. These thiol groups can then be used to couple a variety of compounds such as proteins and peptides by disulfide bonds or thioether linkages. Poly(L-lysine) was substituted with small ligands such as lectin and sugar receptorm that acted as recognition signals.[114–116] Another new methodology was synthesizing glycopeptides by the ring opening polymerization of sugar-substituted α-amino acid N-carboyanhydrides (NCAs).[117,118]

Bioavailability

Drug delivery vehicles must meet several requirements such as water solubility, nontoxicity, nonimmunogenicity, biodegradability, *in vivo* stability, and selective delivery to target sites. Poly(amino acid)-based carriers are of interest because they can undergo hydrolysis and/or enzymatic degradation and produce biocompatible monomers. Biodegradability and immunogenicity depend on the chemical structures and/or physcochemical properties of the poly(amino acid) chains.[119–122] The degree of immune response is dependent on the number of different amino acids in a molecule.[123] A study of adriamycin-conjugated poly(glutamic acid) showed that an antibody was formed.[124,125] Poly(L-lysine) appears to be a good macromolecular carrier due to its unique properties such as ease of attachment of drug molecules, biodegradability, and stimulation of endocytosis.

A high cationic electrostatic charge can lead to cytotoxicity because it is not specific to target cells. Concerns about toxicity led to the development of new approaches such as conjugation of sugar-targeting moieties in which any free lysine ε-amines were acylated with δ-gluconolactone. The polymer remained degradable but was electrically neutral and had high water solubility.[123,126] The inclusion of other amino acids onto a poly(L-lysine) backbone can reduce toxicity to cell cultures.

Hudecz et al. investigated branched polypeptides based on poly(L-lysine)s as carriers.[127] Branched polypeptides were used as synthetic antigens since the antigenicity of amino acid polymers increased in polymers with many different components.[122] Before branched polypeptides can be used as carriers, nonimmunogenic structures must be found. Although all poly(L-amino acid)s are not perfect candidates as drug carriers owing to their potential nonspecific toxicity, structural modifications could lead to nontoxic carriers. Poly(amino acid)s can serve as highly promising biodegradable drug delivery vehicles that can respond quickly to environmental stimuli.[128]

ACKNOWLEDGMENT

The authors acknowledge financial support from and thank the BK Project and the Ministry of Science and Technology of Korea.

REFERENCES

1. Fox, S.W. and Harada, K., The thermal copolymerization of amino acids common to protein, *J. Am. Chem. Soc.*, 82, 3745, 1960.
2. Fox, S.W. and Dose, K., *Molecular Evolution and the Origin of Life*, W.H. Freeman, San Francisco, 1972.
3. Madhan-Kumar, A.B., Jayakumar, R., and Panduranga Rao, K., Synthesis and aggregational behavior of acidic proteinoid, *J. Poly. Sci. A Poly. Chem.*, 34, 2915, 1996.
4. Steiner, S.S. and Rosen, R., Delivery systems for pharmacological agents encapsulated with proteinoids, U.S. Patent 4,925,673, 1990.
5. Steiner, S.S. and Clinical Technologies Associates, Inc., Orally administerable ANF, U.S. Patent 4,983,402, 1991.
6. Milstein, S.J. and Kantor, M.L., Proteinoid carriers and methods for preparation and use thereof, U.S. Patent 5,578,323, 1996.
7. Santiago, N., Milstein, S., Rivera, T., Garcia, E., Zaidi, T., Hong, H., and Bucher, D., Oral immunization of rats with proteinoid micospheres encalsulating influenza virus antigens, *Pharm. Res.*, 10, 1243, 1993.
8. Ottsuka, H., Nakasaki, Y., and Kataoka, K., Self-assembly of poly(ethylene glycol)-based block copolymers for biomedical applications, *Curr. Opin. Colloid Interf. Sci.*, 6, 3, 2001.
9. Kang, H.S., Yang, S.R., Kim, J.D., Han, S.H., and Chang, I.S., Effects of grafted alkyl groups on aggregation behavior of amphiphilic poly(aspartic acid), *Langmuir*, 17, 7501, 2001.
10. Nagarajan, R. and Ganesh, C., Block copolymer self-assembly in selective solvents: theory of solubilization in spherical micelles, *Macromolecules*, 22, 4312, 1989.
11. Allen, C., Maysinger, D., and Eisenberg, A., Nano-engineering block copolymer aggregates for drug delivery, *Colloid Surface B*, 16, 3, 1999.
12. Deming, T.J., Facile synthesis of block copolypeptides of defined architecture, *Nature*, 390, 386, 1997.
13. Merrifield, R.B., Solid phase peptide synthesis. II. The synthesis of bradykinin, *J. Am. Chem. Soc.*, 86, 304, 1964.
14. Stewart, J.M. and Young, J.D., *Solid Phase Peptide Synthesis*, Freeman, San Francisco, 1969.
15. Kricheldorf, H.R., *α-Amino Acid-N-Carboxyanhydrides and Related Materials*, Springer, New York, 1987.
16. Kricheldorf, H.R. and Penczek, S., *Models of Biopolymers by Ring-Opening Polymerization*, CRC Press, Boca Raton, FL, 1990.
17. Deming, T.J., Amino acid-derived nickel cycles: intermediates in nickel-mediated polypeptide synthesis, *J. Am. Chem. Soc.*, 120, 4240, 1998.
18. Deming, T.J., Living polymerization of α-amino acid-N-carboxyanhydrides, *J. Polym. Sci. Polym. Chem.*, 38, 3011, 2000.
19. Deming, T.J., Methodologies for preparation of synthetic clock copolyepeptides: materials with future promise in drug delivery, *Adv. Drug Delivery Rev.*, 54, 1145, 2002.
20. Borsook, H. and Huffman, H.M., *Chemistry of the Amino acids and Proteins*, Charles C Thomas, Springfield, IL, 1944, p. 822.
21. Harada, K. and Fox, S.W., Characterization of thermal polymers of neutral α-amino acids with dicarboxylic amino acids or lysine, *Arch. Biochem.Biophys.*, 109, 49, 1965.
22. Steinman, G., Lemman, R.M., and Clavin, M., Cyanamide: a possible compound in chemical evolution, *Proc. Natl. Acad. Sci. USA*, 52, 27, 1964.

23. Vegotsky, A., Harada, K., and Fox, S.W., The thermal copolymerization of amino acids common to protein, *J. Am. Chem. Soc.*, 80, 3361, 1958.
24. Fox, S.W., Harada, K., Woods, K.R., and Windsor, C.R., Amino acid compositions of proteinoids, *Arch. Biochem. Biophys.*, 102, 439, 1963.
25. Fox, S.W., Syren, R.M., and Windsor, C.R., Thermal copoly(amino acids) as inhibitors of glyoxalase I, in *Cuba Foundation Symposium*, 67, 175, 1978.
26. Bae, S.K. and Kim, J.D., Aggregation behaviors and their pH sensitivity of cholestrol-conjugated proteinoids composed of glutamic acid and aspartic acid matrix, *J. Biomed. Mat. Res.*, 64A, 282, 2003.
27. Bae, S.K., Association Properties of Proteinoids and Lipid-Conjugated Proteinoids and Their Applications as Biopolymers, Ph.D. thesis, Korea Advanced Institute of Science and Technology, 2000.
28. Ezzell, S.A., Hoyle, C.E., Greed, D., and McCormick, C.L., Water-soluble copolymers. 40. Photophysical studies of the solution behavior of associative pyrenesulfonamide-labeled polyacrylamides, *Macromolecules*, 25, 1887, 1992.
29. Yokoyama, M., Fukushima, S., Uehara, R., Okamoto, K., Kataoka, K., Sakurai, Y., and Okano, T., Characterization of physical entrapment and chemical conjugation of adriamycin in polymeric micelles and their design for *in vivo* delivery to a solid tumor, *J. Control. Rel.*, 50, 79, 1998.
30. Harada, A. and Kataoka, K., Formation of polyion complex micelles in an aqueous milieu from a pair of oppositely charged block copolymers with poly(ethylene glycol) segments, *Macromolecules*, 28, 5294, 1995.
31. Nah, J.W., Jeong, Y.I., and Cho, C.S., Clonazepam release from core-shell type nanoparticles composed of poly(gamma-benzyl L-glutamate) as the hydrophobic part and poly(ethylene oxide) as the hydrophilic part, *J. Polym. Sci. Polym. Phys.*, 36, 415, 1998.
32. Lavasanifar, A., Samuel, J., and Kwon, G.S., Poly(ethylene oxide)-*block*-poly(L-amino acid) micelles for drug delivery, *Adv. Drug Delivery Rev.*, 54, 169, 2002.
33. Tokoyama, M., Satoh, A., Sakurai, Y., Okano, T., Matsumura, Y., Kakizoe, T., and Kataoka, K., Incorporation of water-insoluble anticancer drug into polymeric micelles and control of their particle size, *J. Control. Rel.*, 55, 219, 1998.
34. Yokoyama, M., Kwon, G.S., Okano, T., Sakurai, Y., Sato, T., and Kataoka, K., Preparation of micelle-forming polymer-drug conjugates, *Bioconjugate Chem.*, 3, 295, 1992.
35. Harada, A., Cammas, S., and Kataoka, K., Stabilized α helix structure of poly(L-lysine)-block-poly(ethylene glycol) in aqueous medium through supramolecular assembly, *Macromolecules*, 29, 6183, 1996.
36. Kataoka, K., Ishihara, A., Harada, A., and Miyazaki, H., Effect of the secondary structure of poly(L-lysine) segments on the micellization in aqueous milieu of poly(ethylene glycol)-poly(L-lysine) block copolymer partially substituted with a hydrocinnamoyl group at the N-position, *Macomolecules*, 31, 6071, 1998.
37. Harada, A., Togawa, H., and Kataoka, H., Physicochemical properties and nuclease resistance of antisense oligodeoxynucleotides entrapped in the core of polyion complex micelles composed of poly(ethylene glycol)–poly(L-Lysine) block copolymers, *Europ. J. Pharm. Sci.*, 13, 35, 2001.
38. Jeong, Y.I., Cheon, J.B., Kim, S.H., Nah, J.W., Lee, Y.M., Sung, Y.K., Akaike, T., and Cho, C.S., Enhanced transdermal delivery of AZT (Zidovudine) using iontophoresis and penetration enhancer, *J. Control. Rel.*, 51, 169, 1998.
39. Nah, J.W., Jeong, Y.I., and Cho, C.S., Norfloxacin release from polymeric micelle of poly(gamma-benzyl L-glutamate) poly(ethylene oxide) poly(gamma-benzyl L-glutamate) block copolymer, *Bull. Korean Chem. Soc.*, 19, 962, 1998.

40. Harada, A. and Kataoka, K., Novel polyion complex micelles entrapping enzyme molecules in the core: preparation of narrowly distributed micelles from lysozyme and poly(ethylene glycol)-poly(aspartic acid) block copolymer in aqueous medium, *Macromolecules*, 31, 288, 1998.

41. Constancis, A., Meyreix, R., Bryson, N., Huille, S., Grosselin, J.M., Gulik-Krzywicki, T., and Soula, G., Macromolecular colloids of diblock poly(amino acids) that bind insulin, *J. Colloid Interface Sci.*, 217, 357, 1999.

42. Nowak, A.P., Breedveld, V., Pakstis, L., Ozbas, B., Pine, D.J., Pochan, D., and Deming, T.J., Rapidly recovering hydrogel scaffolds from self-assembling diblock copolypeptide amphiphilics, *Nature*, 417, 424, 2002.

43. Akiyoshi, K., Yamaguchi, S., and Sunamoto, J., Self-aggregates of hydrophobic polysaccharide derivatives, *J. Chem. Lett.*, 1263, 1991.

44. Nichfor, M., Lopes, A., Carpov, A., and Melo, E., Aggregation in water of dextran hydrophobically modified with bile acids, *Macromolecules*, 32, 7078, 1999.

45. Lee, K.Y., Jo, W.H., Kwon, I.C., Kim, Y.H., and Jeong, S.Y., Structural determination and interior polarity of self-aggregates prepared from deoxycholic acid-modified chitosan in water, *Macromolecules*, 31, 378, 1998.

46. Yang, S.R., Jeong, J.H., Park, K., and Kim, J.D., Self-aggregates of hydrophobically modified poly(2-hydroxyethyl aspartamide) in aqueous solution, *Colloid Poly. Sci.*, 281, 852, 2003.

47. Jeong, J.H., Kang, H.S., Yang, S.R., and Kim, J.D., Polymer micelle-like aggregates of novel amphiphilic biodegradable poly(asparagine) grafted with poly(caprolactone), *Polymer*, 44, 583, 2003.

48. Jeong, J.H. and Park, T.G., Poly(L-lysine)-g-poly(D,L-lactic-co-glycolic acid) micelles for low cytotoxic biodegradable gene delivery carriers, *J. Control. Rel.*, 82, 159, 2002.

49. Akiyoshi, K., Ueminami, A., Kurumada, S., and Nomura, Y., Self-association of cholesteryl-bearing poly(L-lysine) in water and control of its secondary structure by host–guest interaction with cyclodextrin, *Macromolecules*, 33, 6752, 2000.

50. Caponetti, G., Hrkach, J.S., Kriwet, B., Poh, M., Lotan, N., Colombo, P., and Langer, R., Microparticles of novel branched copolymers of lactic acid and amino acids: preparation and characterization, *J. Pharm. Sci.*, 88, 136, 1999.

51. Kataoka, K., Harada, A., and Katasaki, Y., Block copolymer micelles for drug delivery: design, characterization and biological significance, *Adv. Drug Delivery Rev.*, 47, 113, 2001.

52. Zhang, L., Yu, K., and Eisenberg, A., Ion-induced morphological changes in "crew-cut" aggregates of amphiphilic block copolymers, *Science*, 268, 1728, 1995.

53. Hagan, S.A., Coombes, A.G.A., Garnett, M.C., Dunn, S.E., Davies, M.C., Illum, L., and Davis, S.S., Polylactide-poly(ethylene glycol) copolymers as drug delivery systems. 1. Characterization of water dispersible micelle-forming systems, *Langmuir*, 12, 2153, 1996.

54. Cammas, S., Suzuki, K., Sone, C., Sakurai, Y., Kataoka, K., and Okano, T., Thermo-responsive polymer nanoparticles with a core-shell micelle structure as site-specific drug carriers, *J. Control. Rel.*, 48, 157, 1997.

55. Kim, S.Y., Shin, I.G., Lee, Y.M., Cho, C.S., and Sung, Y.K., Methoxy poly(ethylene glycol) and ε-caprolactone amphiphilic block copolymeric micelle containing indomethacin. II. Micelle formation and drug release behaviours, *J. Control. Rel.*, 51, 13, 1998.

56. Kenneth, C., Dowling, J.K., and Thomas, A., Novel micellar synthesis and photo-physical characterization of water-soluble acrylamide-styrene block copolymers, *Macromolecules*, 23, 1059, 1990.

57. Wilhelm, M., Zhao, C.L., Wang, Y., Xu, R., and Winnik, M.A., Poly(styrene-ethylene oxide) block copolymer micelle formation in water: a fluorescence probe study, *Macromolecules,* 24, 1033, 1991.

58. La, S.B. and Okano, T., Polymeric micelles as new drug carriers, *Adv. Drug Delivery Rev.*, 21, 107, 1996.

59. Kwon, G., Naito, M., Yokoyama, M., Okano, T., Sakurai, Y., and Kataoka, K., Micelles based on AB block copolymers of poly(ethylene oxide) and poly(beta-benzyl L-aspartate), *Langmuir*, 9, 945, 1993.

60. Mayers, D., *Surfactant Science and Technology,* VCH, New York, 1988, chap. 3.

61. Rosen, M.J., *Surfactants and Interfacial Phenomena*, 1st ed., John Wiley & Sons, New York, 1978, chap. 3.

62. Yokoyama, M., Okano, T., Sakurai, Y., Fukushima, S., Okamoto, K., and Kataoka, K., Selective delivery of adriamycin to a solid tumor using a polymeric micelle carrier system, *J. Drug Target.*, 7, 171, 1999.

63. Nagarajan, R. and Ganesh, K., Block copolymer self-assembly in selective solvents: spherical micelles with segregated cores, *J. Chem. Phys.*, 90, 5843, 1989.

64. Zhang, L. and Eisenberg, A., Formation of crew-cut aggregates of various morphologies from amphiphilic block copolymers in solution, *Polym. Adv. Technol.*, 9, 677, 1998.

65. Zhang, L., Barlow, J., and Eisenberg, A., Scaling relations and coronal dimensions in aqueous block polyelectrolyte micelles, *Macromolecules*, 28, 6055, 1995.

66. Zhang, L. and Eisenberg, A., Multiple morphologies and characteristics of "crew-cut" micelle-like aggregates of polystyrene-*b*-poly(acrylic acid) diblock copolymers in aqueous solutions, *J. Am. Chem. Soc.*, 118, 3168, 1996.

67. Hennon, G., Plaquet, R., Dantrevaux, M., and Biserte, G., Synthesis of amino acid polymers by thermal polycondensation and study of certain physiochemical properties, *Biochimie*, 53, 215, 1971.

68. Krampitz, G., Amino acid copolymerizates, *Naturwissenschaften*, 46, 558, 1959.

69. Madhan-Kumar, A.B., Jayakumar, R., and Panduranga, R.K., Synthesis and aggregational behavior of acidic proteinoid, *J. Poly. Sci. A Poly. Chem.*, 34, 2915, 1996.

70. Madhan-Kumar, A.B. and Panduranga, R.K., Preparation and characterization of pH-sensitive proteinoid microspheres for the oral delivery of methotrexate, *Biomaterials*, 19, 725, 1998.

71. Campbell, P., Glover, G.I., and Gunn, J.M., Inhibition of intracellular protein degradation by pepstatin, poly(L-lysine), and pepstatinyl-poly(L-lysine), *Biochem. Biophys.*, 203, 676, 1980.

72. Van Heeswijk, W.A.R. et al., The synthesis and characterization of polypeptide-adriamycin conjugates and its complexes with adriamycin, *J. Control. Rel.*, 1, 301, 1985.

73. Yokoyama, M., Okano, T., Sakurai, Y., and Kataoka, K., Improved synthesis of adriamycin-conjugated poly(ethylene oxide)-poly(aspartic acid) block copolymer and formation of unimodal micellar structure with controlled amount of physically entrapped adriamycin, *J. Control. Rel.*, 32, 269, 1994.

74. Gadelle, F., Koros, W.J., and Schechter, R.S., Solubilization of aromatic solutes in block copolymers, *Macromolecules*, 28, 4883, 1995.

75. Kabanov, A.V., Chekhonin, V.P., Alakhov, V.Y., Batrakova E.V., Lebedev, A.S., Meliknubarov, N.S., Arzhakov, S.A., Levashov, A.V., Morozov, G.V., Severin, E.S., and Kabanov, V.A., The neuroleptic activity of haloperidol increases after its solubilization in surfactant micelles: micelles as microcontainers for drug targeting, *FEBS Lett.*, 258, 343, 1989.

76. Bader, H., Ringsdorf, H., and Schmidt, B., Watersoluble polymers in medicine, *Angew. Chem.*, 123/124, 457, 1984.

77. Kang, H.S., Kim, J.D., Han, S.H., and Chang, I.S., Self-aggregates of poly(2-hydroxyethylaspartamide) copolymers loaded with methotrexate by physical and chemical entrapments, *J. Control. Rel.*, 81, 135, 2002.

78. La, S.B., Okano, T., and Kataoka, K., Preparation and characterization of the micelle-forming polymeric drug indomethacin-incorporated poly(ethylene oxide)-poly(β-benzyl L-aspartate) block copolymer micelles, *J. Pharm. Sci.*, 85, 85, 1996.

79. Lavasanifar, A., Samuel, J., and Kwon, G.S., Micelles of poly(ethylene oxide)-*block*-poly(*N*-alkyl stearate L-aspartamide): synthetic analogues of lipoproteins for drug delivery, *J. Biomed. Mater. Res.*, 52, 831, 2000.

80. Teng, Y., Morrison, M.E., Munk, P., Webber, S.E., and Prochazka, K., Release kinetics studies of aromatic molecules into water from block polymer micelles, *Macromolecules*, 31, 3578, 1998.

81. Tirrell, D.A. and Linhardt, J.G., pH-Induced fusion and lysis of phosphatidylcholine vesicles by the hydrophobic polyelectrolyte poly(2-ethylacrylic acid), *Langmuir*, 16, 122, 2000.

82. Sascha, A.F. and Hunemann, F., pH-sensitive nanoparticles of poly(amino acid) dodecanoate complexes, *Int. J. Pharm.*, 230, 11, 2001.

83. Fox, S.W., How did life begin? Recent experiments suggest an integrated origin of anabolism, protein, and cell boundaries, *Science*, 132, 200, 1960.

84. Santiago, N. et al., Oral immunization of rats with proteinoid microspheres encapsulating influenza virus antigens, *Pharm. Res.*, 10, 1243, 1993.

85. Haratake, M., Zhao, R., and Ottenbrite, R.M., A study of aggregation behavior of oligopeptides. I. Aggregation characteristics and effects of drugs, *Poly. Preprints*, 37, 131, 1996.

86. Yang, Y.Z., Antoun, S., Ottenbrite, R.M., and Milstein, S., Amino acid oligomer microspheres as drug delivery systems. 1. Synthesis of oligo(amino acids) via NCAs and their microsphere formation, *J. Bioact. Compat. Poly.*, 11, 219, 1996.

87. Yoshida, T., Aoyagi, T., Kokufuta, E., and Okano, T., Newly designed hydrogel with both sensitive thermoresponse and biodegradability, *J. Poly. Sci. A Poly. Chem.*, 41, 779, 2003.

88. Jeong, B., Bae, Y.H., Lee, D.S., and Kim, S.W., Biodegradable block copolymers as injectable drug-delivery systems, *Nature*, 388, 860, 1997.

89. Yoichi, T., Motoichi, K., Hiroshi, U., Toyoji, K., and Shiro, K., Biodegradable thermoresponsive poly(amino acid)s, *Chem. Commun.*, 106, 2003.

90. Heskins, M. and Guillet, J.E., Solution properties of poly(*N*-isopropylacrylamide), *J. Macromol. Sci. Chem.*, A2, 1441, 1968.

91. Chun, S.W. and Kim, J.D., A novel hydrogel-dispersed composite membrane of poly(N-isopropylacrylamide) in a gelatin matrix and its thermally actuated permeation of 4-acetamidophen, *J. Control. Rel.*, 38, 39, 1996.

92. Kakizawa, Y., Harada, A., and Kataoka, K., Environment-sensitive stabilization of core-shell structured polyion complex micelle by reversible cross-linking of the core through disulfide bond, *J. Am. Chem. Soc.*, 121, 11247, 1999.

93. Kakizawa, Y., Harada, A., and Kataoka, K., Glutathione-sensitive stabilization of block copolymer micelles composed of antisense DNA and thiolated poly(ethylene glycol)-block-poly(L-lysine): a potential carrier for systemic delivery of antisense DNA, *Biomacromolecules*, 2, 491, 2001.

94. Osvald, P., Adriano, F., and Francesco, C., Photochromic poly(α-amino acid)s: photomodulation of molecular and supramolecular structure, *React. Funct. Poly.*, 26, 185, 1995.

95. Lucas, P., Milroy, D.A., Thomas, B.J., Moss, S.H., and Pouton, C.W., Pharmaceutical and biological properties of poly(amino acid)/DNA polyplexes, *J. Drug Target.*, 7, 143, 1999.

96. Andersson, L.O., *Plasma Proteins*, John Wiley & Sons, New York, 1979, p. 43.

97. Imoto, T. and Johnson, L.N., *The Enzymes,* 3rd ed., vol. 7, Academic Press, New York, 1972, p. 666.

98. Largic, D.D. and Needham, D., The "stealth" liposome: a prototypical biomaterial, *Chem. Rev.*, 95, 2601, 1995.

99. Ringsdorf, H., Sackmann, E., Simon, J., and Winnik, F.M., Interactions of liposomes and hydrophobically modified poly-(N-isopropylacrylamides): an attempt to model the cytoskeleton, *Biochem. Biophys. Acta* 1153, 335, 1993.

100. Ringsdorf, H., Venzmer, J., and Winnik, F.M., Interaction of hydrophobically modified poly-n-isopropylacrylamides with model membranes or playing a molecular accordion, *Angew. Chem. Int. Ed. Engl.,* 30, 315, 1991.

101. Lindsay, M.A., Peptide-mediated cell delivery: application in protein target validation, *Curr. Opin. Pharm.*, 2, 587, 2002.

102. Eom, K.D., Miao, Z.W., Yang, J.L., and Tam, J.P., Tandem ligation of multipartite peptides with cell-permeable activity, *J. Am. Chem. Soc.,* 125, 73, 2003.

103. Sadler, K., Eom, K.D., Yang, J.L., Dimitrova, Y., and Tam, J.P., Translocating proline-rich peptides from the antimicrobial peptide bactenecin 7, *Biochemistry*, 41, 14150, 2002.

104. Chen, B.X. and Erlanger, B.F., Intracellular delivery of monoclonal antibodies, *Immunol. Lett.*, 84, 63, 2002.

105. Futaki, S., Arginine-rich peptides: potential for intracellular delivery of macromolecules and the mystery of the translocation mechanisms, *Int. J. Pharm.*, 245, 1, 2002.

106. Futaki, S., Nakase, I., Suzuki, T., Zhang, Y.J., and Sugiura, Y., Translocation of branched-chain arginine peptides through cell membranes: flexibility in the spatial disposition of positive charges in membrane-permeable peptides, *Biochemistry*, 41, 7925, 2002.

107. Kichler, A., Leborgne, C., Marz, J., Danos, O., and Bechinger, B., Histidine-rich amphipathic peptide antibiotics promote efficient delivery of DNA into mammalian cells, *Proc. Natl. Acad. Sci. USA.*, 100, 1564, 2003.

108. Pichon, C., Goncalves, C., and Midoux, P., Histidine-rich peptides and polymers for nucleic acids delivery, *Adv. Drug Delivery Rev.*, 53, 75, 2001.

109. Pattern, M.K., Lloyd, J.B., Horpel, G., and Ringsdorf, H., Micelle-forming block copolymers: pinocytosis by macrophages and interaction with model membranes, *Macromol. Chem. Phys.*, 186, 725, 1985.

110. Yokoyama, M., Inoue, S., Kataoka, K., Yui, N., and Sakurai, Y., Preparation of adriamycin-conjugated poly(ethylene glycol)-poly(aspartic acid) block copolymer: a new type of polymeric anticancer agent, *Macromol. Chem. Rapid Commun.*, 8, 431, 1987.

111. Li, Y. and Kwon, G.S., Methotrexate Esters of Poly(ethylene oxide)-block-poly(2-hydroxyethyl-L-aspartamide). I. Effects of the level of methotrexate conjugation on the stability of micelles and on drug release, *Pharm. Res.*, 17, 607, 2000.

112. Carlsson, J., Drevin, H., and Axen, R., Protein thiolation and reversible protein-protein conjugation. N-Succinimidyl 3-(2-pyridyldithio)propionate: a new heterobifunctional reagent, *Biochem. J.*, 173, 723, 1978.

113. Wanger, E., Cotton, M., Mechtler, K., Kirlappos, H., and Birnsteil, M., DNA-binding transferrin conjugates as functional gene-delivery agents: synthesis by linkage of polylysine or ethidium homodimer to the transferrin carbohydrate moiety, *Bioconjugate Chem.*, 2, 226, 1991.

114. Monsigny, M., Roche, A.C., Midous, P., and Mayer, R., Glycoconjugates as carriers for specific delivery of therapeutic drugs and genes, *Adv. Drug Delivery Rev.*, 14, 1, 1994.

115. Shoichiro, A., Masayuki, N., Yoxhiyuki, T., Toshihiro, A., and Atsushi, M., Synthesis of novel polyampholyte comb-type copolymers consisting of a poly(L-lysine) backbone and hyaluronic acid side chains for a DNA carrier, *Bioconjugate Chem.*, 9, 476, 1998.

116. Kunz, H., Synthesis of glycopeptides, partial structures of biological recognition components, *Angew. Chem. Int. Ed. Engl.*, 26, 294, 1987.

117. Rude, E., Westphal, O., Hurwits, E., Fuchs, S., and Sela, M., Synthesis and antigenic properties of sugar-polypeptide conjugates, *Immunochemistry*, 3, 137, 1966.

118. Keigo, A., Kaname, T., and Masahiko, O., Glycopeptide synthesis by an α-amino acid N-carboxyanhydride (NCA) method: ring opening polymerization of a sugar-substituted NCA, *Macromolecules*, 27, 875, 1994.

119. Chiu, H.C., Kopeckova, P., Deshmane, S.S., and Kopecek, J., Lysosomal degradability of poly(alpha-amino acids), *J. Biomed. Mater. Res.*, 34, 381, 1997.

120. McCormick-Thomson, L.A., Sgouras, D., and Duncan, R., Poly(amino acid) copolymers as potential soluble drug delivery system. 2. Body distribution and preliminary biocompatibility testing *in vitro* and *in vivo*, *J. Bioact. Compt. Polym.*, 4, 252, 1989.

121. Shen, W.C. and Ryser, H.J., Poly(L-lysine) and poly(D-lysine) conjugates of methotrexate: different inhibitory effect on drug resistant cells, *Mol. Pharmacol.*, 16, 614, 1979.

122. Rihova, B. and Riha, I., Immunological problems of polymer-bound dugs, *Crit. Rev. Ther. Drug Carrier Syst.*, 1, 311, 1985.

123. Midoux, P., Negre, E., Roche, A.C., Mayer, R., Monsigny, M., Balzarini, J., De Clercq, E., Mayer, E., Ghaffer, A., and Gangemi, J.D., Drug-targeting-anti-HSV-1 activity of mannosylated polymer-bound 9-(2-phosphonylmethoxyethyl)adenine, *Biochem. Biophys. Res. Commun.*, 167, 1044, 1990.

124. Marre, A.D., Seymour, L.W., and Schacht, E., Evaluation of the hydrolytic and enzymatic stability of macromolecular mitomycin C derivatives, *J. Control. Rel.*, 31, 89, 1994.

125. Hoes, C.J.T., Potman, W., van Heeswijk, W.A.R., Mud, J., de Grooth, B.G., Greve, J., and Feijen, J., Optimization of macromolecular prodrugs of the antitumor antibiotic adriamycin, *J. Control. Rel.*, 2, 205, 1985.

126. Negre, E., Chance, M.L., Hanboula, S.Y., Monsigny, M., Roche, A.C., Mayer, R.M., and Hommel, M., Antileishmanial drug targeting through glycosylated polymers specifically internalized by macrophage membrane lectins, *Antimicrob. Agents Chemother.*, 36, 2228, 1992.

127. Hudecz, F., Gaal, D., Kurucz, I., Lanyi, A., Kovacs, A.L., Mezo, G., Rajnavolgyi, E., and Szekerke, M., Carrier design: cytotoxicity and immunogenicity of synthetic branched polypeptides with poly(L-lysine) backbone, *J. Control. Rel.*, 19, 231, 1992.

128. Drobnik, J., Biodegradable soluble macromolecules as drug carriers, *Adv. Drug Delivery Rev.*, 3, 229, 1989.

19 Fast Biodegradable Polymers

Wim E. Hennink, Jan Hein van Steenis, and Cornelus F. van Nostrum

CONTENTS

INTRODUCTION

Biodegradable polymers have found widespread application in many technological areas. They are used as biomaterials for drug delivery purposes, for example, as degradable sutures, orthopedic implants, and as scaffolds for tissue engineering applications.[1-8] These materials are not only of academic interest, but they have found commercial applications in a great number of clinical products.[9] In addition to their utility in the biomedical and pharmaceutical fields, biodegradable polymers are also used in environmentally friendly packaging materials.[10-12]

In principle polymers can be degraded via a variety of routes, including heat (pyrolysis), radiation (ultraviolet, gamma), oxidative agents (ozone, peroxides), strong acids and bases, and "simply" by water. This chapter focuses on biodegradable polymers used for biomedical and pharmaceutical applications. These polymers degrade under physiological conditions almost exclusively by chemical or enzymatic hydrolysis of labile bonds present in the main chains, crosslinks, or in side groups. Responsive synthetic systems that react in relatively short times (seconds to minutes; see other chapters in this book) to an external stimulus (temperature, heat, pH) are well known. In contrast, degradation of polymers at 37°C triggered, for example, by pH, takes hours or days to months. Therefore, *rapid* biodegradability as used in this chapter should be interpreted as a relative value.

The advantages of biodegradability of polymers used for the applications mentioned above are obvious. One major benefit is the fact that a biodegradable system or implant does not have to be removed when it has fulfilled its intended task. Of course, care should be taken to ensure that nontoxic degradation products are formed. In principle, this can be guaranteed by using polymers composed of endogenous compounds and this explains the popularity of the poly(lactic acid) and poly(glycolic acid) families of polymers.

Biodegradability can be used to modulate the properties of systems, e.g., to control the releases of biologically active substances (drugs, pharmaceutically active proteins, antigens, vaccines) from polymers. This chapter presents an overview of some important classes of biodegradable polymers. Their properties, particularly their degradation characteristics, are described and strategies to modulate their biodegradability levels are discussed. Three main classes of biodegradable polymeric systems are discussed, namely hydrophobic materials, insoluble but swellable systems (hydrogels), and fully soluble polymers.

BIODEGRADABLE HYDROPHOBIC POLYMERS

POLYMER DEGRADATION: GENERAL CONSIDERATIONS

A great variety of biodegradable polymers (also called bioerodible polymers) have been developed. These polymers degrade due to hydrolytically sensitive groups by which the monomers that form the polymer are connected with each other. During degradation, low molecular weight water-soluble degradation products (monomers and oligomers) are formed and leave the remaining solid material by diffusion. The degradation products are excreted via the kidneys, further degraded as oligomers, or metabolized as in the case of lactic acid into water and CO_2. Table 19.1 presents an overview of the factors that affect the degradation of polymeric materials.

Table 19.1 shows that the biodegradation rate of a material depends on several factors among which are the geometry and porosity of the degradable device.[13] The biodegradation rate also depends on typical polymer characteristics such as the type, presence of comonomers, and molecular weight.

Hydrophobic polymers with hydrolyzable bonds mainly degrade via chemical hydrolysis; enzymatic catalysis does not play a role. Since water is necessary for the degradation process, the degradation time (the time required to fully dissolve a solid material made of a biodegradable polymer) depends on the water-absorbing capacity of the material and the chemical nature of the hydrolyzable bonds. Although the materials discussed in this section are hydrophobic and therefore do not dissolve

TABLE 19.1
Factors Affecting Hydrolytic Degradation Behavior
of Biodegradable Polyesters

Water permeability and solubility (hydrophilicity and hydrophobicity)
Chemical composition
Mechanism of hydrolysis (noncatalytic, autocatalytic, enzymatic)
Additives (acids, bases, monomers, solvents, drugs)
Morphology (crystalline, amorphous)
Device dimensions (size, shape, surface-to-volume ratio)
Porosity
Glass transition temperature (glassy, rubbery)
Molecular weight and molecular weight distribution
Physicochemical factors (ion exchange, ionic strength, pH)
Sterilization
Site of implantation

Source: Anderson, J.M., in *Biomedical Applications of Synthetic Biodegradable Polymers,* Hollinger, J.O., Ed., CRC Press, Boca Raton, FL,
1995, chap. 10.

in water, they still are able to absorb some water when placed in an aqueous environment. Generally speaking, for a certain class of related polymers (the poly(lactic acid) family) the higher the water-absorbing capacity of a material, the faster the degradation.

An important factor governing the degradation rates of polymers is the chemical nature of the bonds by which the monomers are covalently linked. As a rule, rate increases in the order of amide ← ester ← carbonate ← anhydride.[2]

Another important factor that affects biodegradation time and other characteristics of polymeric materials is the morphology of the matrix. Many degradable polymers (poly(L-lactic acid) [PLLA] and poly-ε-caprolactone) with regular structures can crystallize. In addition to a crystalline phase, these materials also have amorphous (noncrystalline) phases. The presence of a crystalline phase has large consequences for the biodegradation of materials made from these polymers. First, because crystallites are well-ordered structures with low free volumes, the water-absorbing capacity of a polymeric material decreases with increasing crystallinity. Because water is necessary for the biodegradation of polymeric materials, decreasing water absorbing capacity increases biodegradation time.

Second, the hydrolytically sensitive groups in the crystalline phase are far less susceptible to hydrolysis than the same bonds in the amorphous phase because the crystallites are essentially impermeable to water molecules. This means that in semicrystalline materials, the degradation starts in the amorphous phase. As a consequence, the crystallinity in the remaining system increases during degradation. In later stages, the crystalline regions degrade, mainly via surface erosion. The biodegradability of poly(lactic acid) and related polymers has been extensively studied especially by Vert's research group.[14–17] The lessons learned from this polymer are

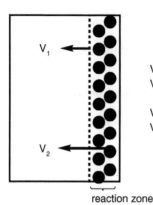

V_1 = rate of water permeation
V_2 = rate of polymer hydrolysis

$V_1 > V_2$: reaction zone increases with time → bulk hydrolysis
$V_1 < V_2$: reaction zone at surface → surface erosion

reaction zone

FIGURE 19.1 Bulk hydrolysis versus surface erosion. (From Anderson, J.M., in *Biomedical Applications of Synthetic Biodegradable Polymers,* Hollinger, J.O., Ed., CRC Press, Boca Raton, FL, 1995, chap. 10.)

also applicable to other systems as will be discussed in more detail in the following sections.

DEGRADATION: SURFACE EROSION VS. BULK HYDROLYSIS

Degradable polymers can be subdivided into different categories according to their chemical compositions. Another way to categorize them is according to their degradation behavior, namely degradation by surface erosion or bulk hydrolysis (Figure 19.1).

For the biodegradation of polymeric materials, water is necessary to hydrolyze the chemical bonds present in polymer chains. Even hydrophobic polymers absorb water when placed in an aqueous environment. Two extreme situations can be distinguished. Once the chemical hydrolysis of the labile bonds present in the degradable material is faster than the in-diffusion of water from the surrounding, surface degradation (frequently called surface erosion) occurs.[18] This degradation process is characterized by a continuous mass loss of the material over time. Moreover, the molecular weight of the polymer in the nondegraded part of the matrix does not undergo a change.

Members of the poly(anhydride) family of polymers (Figure 19.2) as developed by Langer et al.[19–21] essentially degrade via the surface erosion process. The biodegradation times of poly(anhydrides) depend on the polymer structures between the anhydride bonds. Aliphatic poly(anhydrides) degrade within days whereas aromatic systems degrade over months to years.

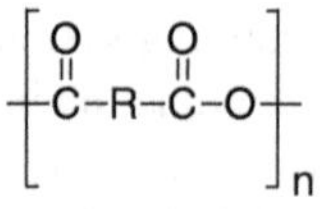

$$\left[\begin{array}{c} \overset{O}{\underset{\|}{C}}-R-\overset{O}{\underset{\|}{C}}-O \end{array}\right]_n$$

FIGURE 19.2 General structure of polyanhydride.

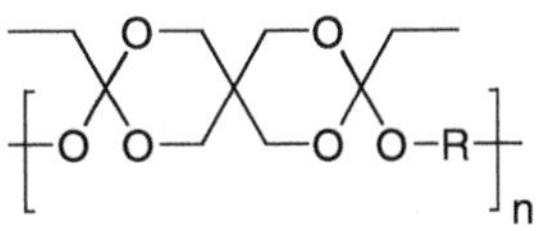

FIGURE 19.3 General structure of poly(ortho ester).

Another category of well studied materials that degrade by surface erosion are the polyorthoester systems (Figure 19.3) as designed by Heller and coworkers.[22,23]

The biodegradation time of a poly(orthoester) can be controlled by polymer composition and can range from a couple days to months. The introduction of α-hydroxyacid segments is an effective method for shortening the degradation times of poly(orthoesters).[24]

Surface erodible systems are attractive for the design of controlled release systems. When a drug is homogeneously distributed over the matrix of a surface erodible system, the release of the drug essentially follows the polymer mass loss, resulting in a more or less zero order release of a drug for the duration of the degradation process.[24]

The other category of degradable materials degrades via bulk hydrolysis processes, not by surface erosion. The main group representative of such bulk degrading materials is the well-known and well-studied poly(lactic acid) family. For these materials, water penetration into the material is faster than the hydrolysis of their labile bonds (Figure 19.1). This means that when placed in an aqueous environment, these systems are saturated with water and hydrolysis consequently occurs through the homogeneous matrix. Initially, the degradation of these materials can only be determined through a decrease in molecular weight of the polymer caused by random hydrolytic cleavages of ester bonds.[25] In later stages of the degradation process, when the molecular weight has dropped to a certain level, soluble degradation products are formed which in turn are associated with mass loss.

Three points should be made regarding biomaterials that degrade via surface erosion or bulk hydrolysis. First, polymers that exclusively degrade via only one of the mechanisms do not exist in practice. In fact, polymers degrade predominantly via the surface erosion route (with some contribution of bulk degradation) and vice versa. Second, although polymeric materials initially degrade by the bulk hydrolysis mechanism, heterogeneous degradation occurs in later stages of the process, as demonstrated by Vert and coworkers for poly(lactic acid) and related polymers. The core of the material degrades faster than the shell due to accumulation of low molecular weight acidic degradation products [lactic acid (oligomers)] in the material that catalyze the hydrolysis of remaining intact ester bonds.[26] Third, PLLA is degraded by surface erosion after incubation in an aqueous solution of high pH.[27] The implication of this finding is that the degradation mechanism may change once the pH of the surroundings changes.

BIODEGRADABLE ALIPHATIC POLYESTERS

In principle, linear aliphatic polyesters can be obtained by polycondensation of aliphatic compounds having both hydroxyl groups and carboxylic acid groups or by

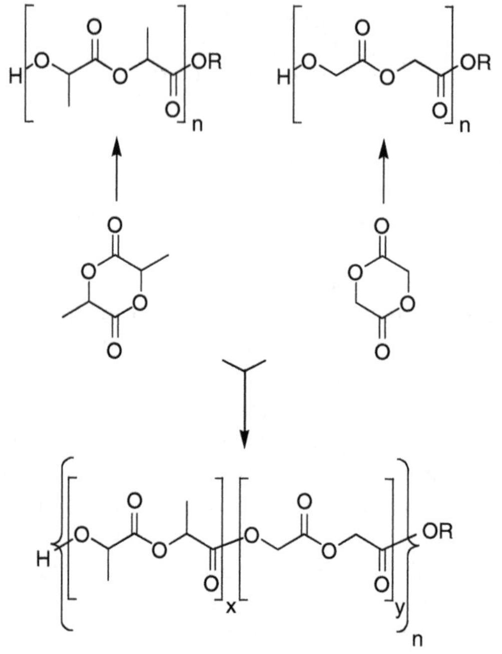

FIGURE 19.4 Synthesis of poly(lactic acid) and poly(glycolic acid) and their copolymers from cyclic precursors.

reaction of compounds having two hydroxyl groups with compounds having two carboxylic acid groups. Branched and crosslinked structures can be obtained by using trifunctional and higher functional monomers. Indeed, a great variety of linear aliphatic polyesters have been synthesized chemically.[28–30] Natural polyesters are also known. Certain microorganisms can convert glucose or other sugars into aliphatic polyesters under certain conditions, then use them as carbon and energy sources. A well-known example of these materials is poly(hydroxybutyrate or PHB).[31,32]

An important class of hydrophobic biodegradable polyesters is the poly(lactic acid) family of polymers. Poly(lactic acid) and its copolymers with glycolic acid have very good biocompatibility and yield nontoxic endogenous compounds as degradation products.[33–35] These polymers have been studied for a variety of biomedical, biotechnological, and pharmaceutical applications.

Poly(lactic acid) can be synthesized by a polycondensation reaction of lactic acid at high temperature.[36] This route, however, yields relatively low molecular weight polymers. High molecular weight poly(lactic acid) and poly(glycolic acid) and their copolymers can be synthesized routinely by ring opening polymerization of the dilactone of lactic acid or glycolic acid using stannous 2-ethyl hexanoate or zinc powder as a catalyst (Figure 19.4).[17,37] Moreover, by synthesizing poly(α-hydroxy) acids via controlled ring opening polymerization, polymers with low polydispersities and block copolymers with well-defined structures can be produced.[38] Because poly(lactic acid) and poly(glycolic acid) are most commonly synthesized

TABLE 19.2
Biodegradation Times of Lactic Acid/Glycolic Acid Polymers

Polymer	Biodegradation Time (Months)
Poly(L-lactide)	18–24
Poly(D,L-lactide)	12–16
Poly (glycolide)	2–4
50:50 Poly(DL-lactide-co-glycolide)	2
85:15 Poly(DL-lactide-co-glycolide)	5
90:10 Poly(DL-lactide-co-caprolactone)	2

Source: From Lewis, D.H., in *Biodegradable Polymers as Drug Delivery Systems,* Chasin, M. and Langer, R., Eds., Marcel Dekker, New York, 1990. With permission.

from lactide and glycolide, respectively, their polymers are also known as polylactide and polyglycolide.

Table 19.2 summarizes the degradation times of lactic acid and glycolic acid copolymers. Since lactic acid is a chiral compound, both L and D (or S and R) forms can be distinguished. Poly(L-lactic acid) (PLLA) and poly(D-lactic acid) are rather hydrophobic semicrystalline polymers that show relatively slow biodegradation behaviors (around 18 to 24 mo).[40] The crystallinity in these polymers can be eliminated by copolymerization of L-lactide and D-lactide (or meso-lactide), yielding poly(D,L-lactic acid) — a hydrophobic amorphous material with a faster degradation time (12 to 16 mo) than PLLA. The biodegradability of poly(D,L-lactic acid) can further be modulated by copolymerization with glycolide; poly(lactic acid)-co-glycolic acid 50:50 (PL(G)A) has a degradation time of 2 mo.

This increased degradation time as compared to poly(D,L-lactic acid) arises for a number of reasons. First, the copolymer has no crystallinity, and as noted earlier, amorphous polymers degrade faster than their crystalline counterparts. Second, glycolic acid is more hydrophilic than lactic acid. This implies that the water-absorbing capacity of PL(G)A is slightly higher than that of PLLA. Higher water content results in faster hydrolytic degradation because water is the reactive species. Moreover, a higher water content leads to a higher dielectric constant in the degrading matrix. Ester hydrolysis proceeds faster with increasing dielectric constant of the medium.[40] Third, the ester bond between glycolic acid and glycolic acid or lactic acid is more susceptible to degradation than an ester bond between two lactic acid molecules.[1] The rapidly degrading PL(G)A 50:50 polymer is presently under investigation for the controlled release of certain pharmaceutically active peptides and proteins.[41–43]

The degradation kinetics of PL(G)A are further affected by additives such as metal salts,[44] monomers,[45] basic compounds such as corals,[46] acidic drugs,[47] superoxide ions,[48] and catalysts such as $SnOct_2$ and zinc metal.[49] To stabilize proteins in PL(G)A microspheres, additives such as $Mg(OH)_2$ have been used.[42] These additives however, may also affect the biodegradation times of PL(G)A microspheres.

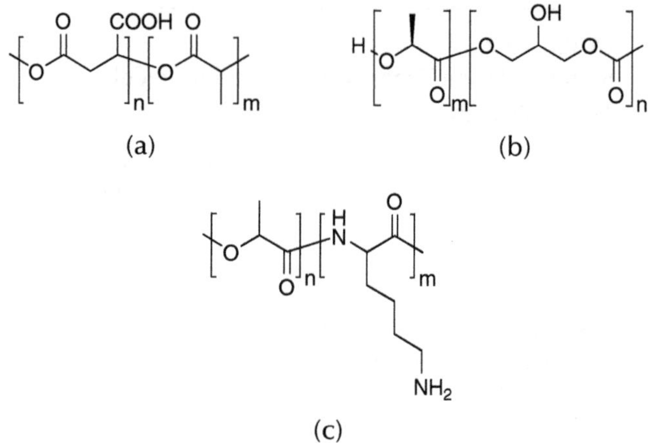

FIGURE 19.5 Biodegradable polyesters with pendant functional groups. (a) Poly(L-lactide-co-*RS*-β-malic acid). (From He, B. et al., *Polymer*, 44, 989, 2003. With permission.) (b) Poly(carbonate ester) of glycerol and lactic acid. (From Ray, W.C. and Grinstaff, M.W., *Macromolecules*, 36, 3557, 2003. With permission.) (c) Poly(lactic acid-co-lysine). (From Liu, Y. et al., *Eur. Polym. J.*, 39, 977, 2003. With permission.)

An important and obvious strategy to modulate (shorten) the biodegradation times of aliphatic polyesters is to hydrophilize these polymer systems via the introduction of functional (e.g., OH, COOH, or NH$_2$) side groups in the polymer chains, the introduction of hydrophilic blocks in the polymer chains, or blending with hydrophilic polymers. Functionalized polyesters have been synthesized recently[50-55] and Figure 19.5 shows some representative structures.

The properties, particularly biodegradability, of these newly synthesized polymers have not been studied in full detail yet. However, it is likely that these functionalized polyesters degrade more rapidly than their nonfunctionalized counterparts. Two reasons can be given to substantiate this hypothesis. First, functional groups increase the hydrophilicity of a polymer. Since water is necessary for hydrolytic degradation, a higher water content of polymeric material will increase degradation rate. Additionally, a higher water content in the material will result in a higher dielectric constant in the homogeneous material. In a study published recently, a higher dielectric constant of the medium caused a higher susceptibility of ester bonds for hydrolysis.[49]

Second, these hydrophilic functional groups may also act as catalysts in the degradation of ester bonds present in the polymer chains. When the content of the hydrophilic monomer exceeds a certain limit, the polymers can become fully water-soluble. These functionalized water-soluble polyesters can be used for the delivery of DNA when cationic groups are introduced or for the design of macromolecular prodrugs when carboxylic acid or hydroxyl groups present in side chains are used for the covalent attachments of drug molecules.[56]

Aliphatic polyesters can also be hydrophilized by synthesizing block or graft copolymers of PL(G)A and poly(ethylene glycol) (PEG) or dextran. In fact, the materials formed (hydrogels) have high water-absorbing capacities; their properties will be discussed in the next section.

Finally, blending is an important method of tailoring material properties to mask unfavorable characteristics and strengthen desired qualities such as improved degradability. PLLA has been blended with PEG[57] and poly(vinylpyrrolidone) (PVP).[58] PLLA is partially miscible with both PEG and PVP, resulting in increased water absorbing capacity and decreased crystallinity of the PLLA. Both factors are favorable for increasing the degradation rate of PLLA, as was observed for the PLLA and PEG blends.[57]

BIODEGRADABLE HYDROGELS

Hydrogels are polymeric networks that absorb and retain large amounts of water. In a polymeric network, the hydrophilic groups or domains present are hydrated in an aqueous environment, thereby creating a hydrogel structure. Crosslinks of a chemical or physical nature are present to prevent dissolution of the gel.[59,60] Because of their water-absorbing capacity, hydrogels are currently used for contact lenses and protein separation. To be effective in such applications, the gels must remain stable and not degrade under conditions in which they are used.

Biodegradability is advantageous for certain applications such as drug delivery.[59,60] Degradable hydrogels are often used as drug delivery materials because they are generally biocompatible and their aqueous compositions make them suitable depots for sensitive compounds such as pharmaceutically active proteins. If the size of the protein is smaller than the meshes in the hydrogel matrix, the release of the protein is governed by Fickian diffusion. In contrast, when the protein is larger than the average pores of the gel, the release is dependent on the degradation of the hydrogel.[61] The control of the degradation rate is therefore very important for adjusting the release rates of the incorporated drugs.

Long-lasting delivery systems require slow biodegradation of the hydrogel, while other applications may require a relatively fast release of drugs through rapid degradation. It is beyond the scope of this chapter to summarize the extensive literature on degradable hydrogels. We will summarize recent developments to illustrate the potentials of biodegradable hydrogels and possibilities of modulating their properties, in particular their biodegradability. The next section will cover dextran hydrogels and PEG-PL(G)A-based systems.

HYDROGEL DEGRADATION: SURFACE EROSION VS. BULK HYDROLYSIS?

As noted earlier, the degradation of relatively hydrophobic polymers proceeds via surface erosion or bulk hydrolysis. When systems are used in their wetted forms, such as by injection or implantation of a previously hydrated gel, it is unlikely that the gels will degrade chemically via surface erosion because the network already contains a large amount of water and low molecular weight ions (e.g., hydroxyl ions) that catalyze the hydrolysis of labile bonds present in the gel can diffuse almost freely through the gel. Conversely, when a dried gel is put into an aqueous environment, in principle these materials can degrade via surface erosion. However, the dried gel will rapidly absorb water because of its hydrophilic character. Thus, in practice, hydrogels chemically degrade via a bulk hydrolysis process.

Hydrogels can also degrade by enzymatic action. Examples of such systems are gelatins, starches, and dextran hydrogels that can be degraded by trypsin, amylase, and dextranase, respectively.[59] When an enzyme is added to a preformed hydrogel, surface erosion occurs. In general, the degradation time increases with increasing concentration of enzyme and decreases with increasing crosslinking density of the gel, as noted in the literature concerning the degradation of crosslinked dextran gels by dextranase.[62]

Enzymes can also degrade hydrogels by bulk degradation. For these systems a matching enzyme is added to a hydrogel formulation before the crosslinking reaction is carried out. Again, the time to dissolve the gels is dependent on the amount of enzyme present in the gel and the crosslink density of the gel, as demonstrated for dextran hydrogels with entrapped dextranase.[63] When the crosslink density is too high, the enzyme is not capable of cleaving bonds in the polymer network and the gel remains stable over time.[64]

CHEMICALLY CROSSLINKED DEXTRAN HYDROGELS

Dextran is a naturally occurring water-soluble polysaccharide with excellent biocompatibility, used as a blood plasma expander. For that reason it is a good candidate for hydrogel preparation. One way to prepare hydrogels from water-soluble polymers is through network formation by chemical crosslinking. The method we used was aqueous free radical polymerization of dextrans modified with methacrylate groups. Dextran derivatized with methacrylate esters (dex-MA, Figure 19.6a) was obtained by reaction of the polysaccharide with glycidyl methacrylate.[65,66] In the corresponding crosslinked

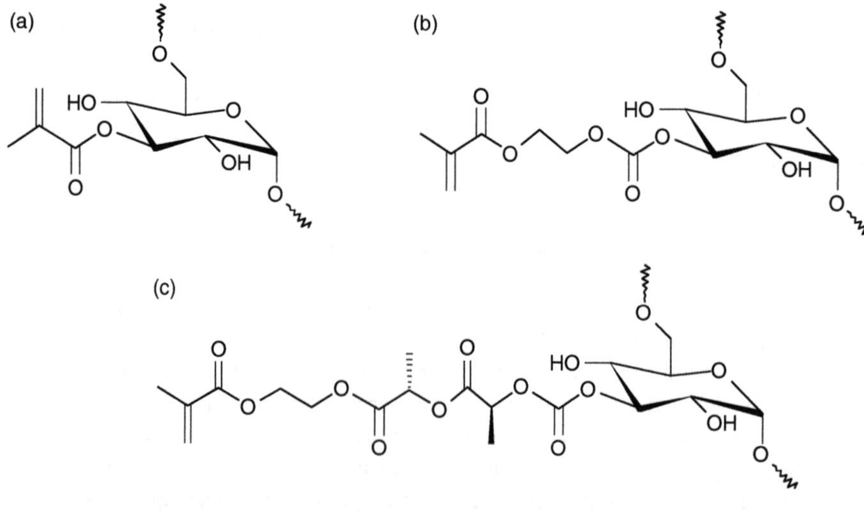

FIGURE 19.6 Polymerizable dextran derivatives used for the preparation of hydrogels. (From Van Dijk-Wolthuis, W.N.E. et al., *Macromolecules*, 30, 3411, 1997 and Van Dijk-Wolthuis, W.N.E. et al., *Macromolecules*, 30, 4639, 1997. With permission.)

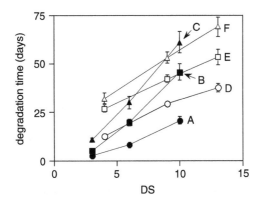

FIGURE 19.7 Degradation times of dex-HEMA (open symbols) and dex-lactate-HEMA hydrogels (closed symbols) as a function of degree of substitution (number of methacrylate groups/100 glucopyranose residues) at various initial water contents. A: dex-lactate-HEMA 90%; B: 80%; C: 70%; D: dex-HEMA 90%; E: 80%; F: 70%. (From Van Dijk-Wolthuis, W.N.E. et al., *Macromolecules*, 30, 4639, 1997. With permission.)

networks, the ester bonds appeared very stable. Under physiological conditions, dex-MA hydrogels showed few signs of degradation over a 5-month period.[67] On the other hand, when hydrolytically sensitive spacers were introduced between the methacrylate groups and the dextran backbone, degradation was significantly enhanced.

Hydrogels prepared from dextran to which 2-hydroxyethyl methacrylate units were coupled via a carbonate bond (dex-HEMA, Figure 19.6b) degraded under physiological conditions, probably due to the hydrolytical instability of the carbonate bonds. Further increase of the degradation rate was achieved by introducing additional oligolactate spacers between the HEMA units and the backbone (dex-lactate-HEMA, Figure 19.6c). As shown in Figure 19.7, the degradation time of dex-lactate-HEMA can be fine-tuned by the degree of substitution of dextran and the initial water content of the hydrogels from 2 days to 2 months.[67] As a consequence, the release rates of encapsulated proteins can be tailored to a similar extent.

PHYSICALLY CROSSLINKED DEXTRAN HYDROGELS

Crosslinking of polymers to form hydrogels by chemical means has the disadvantage that the required conditions may affect the encapsulated drugs. This is especially the case when highly sensitive biomolecules such as proteins and genes are the therapeutic compounds. Network formation by physical interactions between groups or segments of polymers is favored.[60] We applied the concept of stereocomplex formation to create physical crosslinks in biodegradable dextran hydrogels. Dextran was substituted with oligolactic acid side chains containing L-lactic acid (dex-L-OLA) or D-lactic acid enantiomers (dex-D-OLA; Figure 19.8).

These graft copolymers are soluble in water when short OLA grafts are attached to the dextran backbone. Interestingly, when aqueous solutions of dex-L-OLA and dex-D-OLA with minimum chain lengths of 11 lactic acid units are mixed, the L-OLA and D-OLA grafts associate to form so-called stereocomplex crystallites

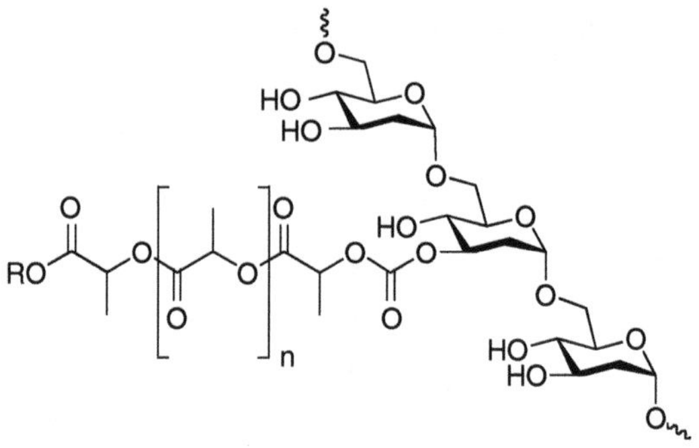

FIGURE 19.8 Dextran grafted with oligolactate chains. (From De Jong, S.J. et al., *Macromolecules*, 33, 3680, 2000. With permission.)

and viscoelastic gels. These hydrogels are thermoreversible; they can be dissolved and reconstructed upon heating and cooling, respectively.[68] Degradation of the dex-OLA gels occurs through hydrolysis of the OLA grafts. After an initial swelling phase, the gels fully degraded in 1 to 7 d, depending on the degree of substitution of dextran and the initial water contents of the gels.[69]

A more detailed investigation of the degradation of one of the single enantiomers (dex-L-OLA) revealed that the amount of lactic acid still grafted to the backbone decreased with a half-life of about 2 days (physiological conditions). Mass spectrometry analysis of the degradation products suggested that the carbonate bond connecting the dextran with the lactic acid oligomer was hydrolyzed first. This may be attributed to the neighboring dextran hydroxy groups that stabilize the transition state during hydrolysis. This phenomenon results in the removal of a complete side chain that then further degrades to smaller oligomers.[69] HPLC analysis showed that the degradation of the latter oligomers proceeded stepwise from their hydroxy termini with half-lives of a couple hours at pH 7. One lactic acid dimer was split off in each step by a process called backbiting.[40]

DEGRADABLE HYDROGELS BASED ON AMPHIPHILIC COPOLYMERS OF PL(G)A AND PEG

Blockcopolymers of PEG and PL(G)LA (Figure 19.9 shows a representative structure) were synthesized with the aim of using the polymers for the delivery of certain pharmaceutically active proteins.[70–72]

PEG was introduced to increase the water-absorbing capacity of PL(G)A systems. By controlling the water content, the intention was to simultaneously control the compatibility with entrapped proteins, their release rates, and the degradation

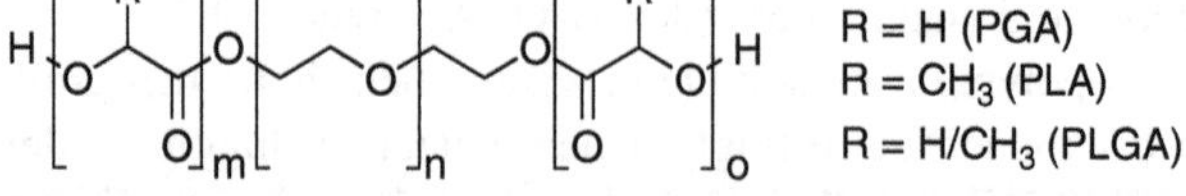

R = H (PGA)
R = CH₃ (PLA)
R = H/CH₃ (PLGA)

FIGURE 19.9 A-B-A triblock copolymer of PEG and poly(α-hydroxy acids).

behavior of the PEG-PL(G)A hydrogels. Other hydrophilic polymers such as poly(vinyl alcohol)[73] were combined with PL(G)A; PEG was combined with other aliphatic polyesters such as poly(ε-caprolactone)[74] and poly(R-3-hydroxy butyrate)[75] with the same goal in mind. ABA block copolymers (Figure 19.9) of PLA (A block) and PEG (B block) were soluble in water when the degree of polymerization (DP) $DP_{PEO}/DP_{PLA} > 4$.[76] When this ratio was <4, turbid aqueous solutions were obtained, likely due to the formation of micelles.[76]

ABA block copolymers of PL(G)A (A block) and PEG (B block) with long PL(G)A blocks were soluble in typical solvents for PL(G)A-like dichloromethane and chloroform. Drug-loaded systems based on these triblock copolymers were prepared essentially using the same methods (e.g., solvent evaporation) developed for the preparation of PL(G)A microspheres.[71,77–79] The research on the degradation behavior of hydrogels based on PL(G)A-PEG-PL(G)A blockcopolymers has been summarized by Kissel et al.[72] The degradation of these polymers was unpredictable because the degradation behavior of PL(G)A is complex and because of the complicated phase behavior of these systems. No general rules on the degradation of PL(G)A-PEG-PL(G)A have been devised yet.

PLA-PEG-PLA and PGA-PEG-PGA are soluble in water and consequently do not form hydrogels when the degree of polymerization of the polyester chains is <5 and the molecular weight of the PEG block is 1 to 20 kDa.[76] Hydrogels based on these blockcopolymers were obtained by the reaction of the hydroxyl termini with acryloyl chloride followed by a radical polymerization of the acrylated PLLA-PEG-PLLA polymers.[80] The degradation times of the gels obtained under physiological conditions were dependent on composition and varied from 1 to 120 d. Generally speaking, the longer the PEG chains, the less dense the network and the shorter the degradation time. Further, systems with PGA segments degraded faster than comparable systems with PLA. The degradation behaviors of these gels were modeled by Martens and Metters et al. and the developed models clearly describe the observed degradation and mass loss profiles.[81,82]

A major breakthrough was realized after it was found that PEG-PL(G)A-PEG block copolymers were soluble in water at room temperature and solidified when brought to 37°C.[83,84] This sol–gel behavior depended on the molecular weights of the PEG and PL(G)A blocks and the polymer concentration in water.[84,85] This behavior makes these systems very attractive for biodegradable injectable *in situ* drug delivery systems.[84,86] No detailed degradation studies have been reported yet. The PEG-PL(G)A-PEG copolymers are, as expected, degradable and have half-lives around 30 days *in vivo*.[86] No structure–biodegradability relationships have been reported.

BIODEGRADABLE SOLUBLE POLYMERS

WATER SOLUBLE POLYMERS FOR TUMOR TARGETING

Water-soluble polymers can be degraded enzymatically [polymers based on natural poly(α-amino acids)][87,88] or chemically. Water-soluble, nondegradable polymers can be removed from the circulation by excretion via the kidneys if the molecular weight is not too high (e.g., <40 kDa for dextran).[89] Soluble polymers are presently under investigation as targeted delivery systems, for example, for cytostatic drugs. The drugs are covalently linked to polymers via degradable linkers.

Worth mentioning is the important work done by Kopecek, Ulbrich, and Duncan on poly(N-(2-hydroxypropyl)methacrylamide)–doxorubicin conjugates.[56,90–92] The polymers are designed in such a way that they are stable in the general circulation and degraded in the endosomal and lysosomal compartments of tumor cells. This process liberates (releases) the polymer-bound drug by interpolating a peptide spacer between the polymer backbone and doxorubicin that is specifically cleaved by proteases present in the cell organelles. As a result, a high concentration of the cytostatic drug is delivered intracellularly, but not outside the cells. Thus, the side effects of the toxic drug are minimized. Tumor cell recognition and uptake of the polymeric prodrug are promoted by the coupling of a targeting ligand [monoclonal antibodies (fragments), galactose] to the polymer–drug conjugate.[56]

In a more recent approach, doxorubicin was coupled to the polymer backbone via a hydrazone bond that was stable under physiological conditions (pH 7.4) and hydrolytically degraded in a mild acidic environment.[92] This means that the drug was released once the polymer–drug conjugate entered the endosomal and lysosomal compartments of cells. The advantage of this chemically degrading system over an enzymatically degrading polymeric prodrug is that release of the drug is independent of proteolytic activity in the endosomes.[89]

DEGRADABLE POLYMERS FOR GENE DELIVERY

Gene therapy has been proposed to treat diseases such as cystic fibrosis that originate from inherited genetic deficiencies and also to treat acquired genetic disorders such as cancer, cardiovascular disease, and rheumatoid arthritis.[93,94] In order to express the exogenous gene, the DNA must be delivered into the nucleus of the target cell. Since DNA is a large hydrophilic molecule with an overall negative charge, it does not easily pass through cellular membranes. Furthermore, DNA must be protected from degradation by deoxyribonucleases (DNases).

To obtain acceptable gene expression levels, the use of a carrier, e.g., a cationic polymer, is required to bring the plasmid into the target cell.[95] Known polymeric carriers such as polyethylenimine (pEI), poly(2-dimethylaminoethyl methacrylate) (pDMAEMA), and poly-L-lysine (pLL), are nonbiodegradable (pEI and pDMAEMA) or show low transfection activity (pLL).[96,97]

Considerable efforts have been made in recent years to design biodegradable polycations that can be used as synthetic DNA carriers. The use of degradable carriers would allow controlled release of encapsulated DNA after it is taken up by target tissues or cells, followed by subsequent metabolism and excretion of the carrier. A sufficiently long lifetime of the carrier, i.e., a few hours, is required in order to allow the polymer–DNA complexes to reach the target sites unaffected after intravenous or other administration. However, to deliver and release DNA efficiently into cells, a carrier should preferably be degraded within a few days.

The use of degradable polyesters as gene delivery systems has some advantages, since they form nontoxic degradation products. For example, PL(G)A microspheres

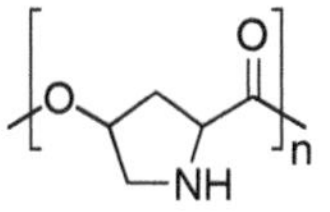

FIGURE 19.10 Poly(4-hydroxy-L-proline ester).

have been used as gene carriers, but their slow degradation rates may limit their applicability in gene therapy.[98] Increasing the hydrophilicity of polyesters by using hydrophilic comonomers is a frequently exploited strategy to accelerate hydrolytic degradation (see the section discussing biodegradable aliphatic polyesters).

Among the most rapidly degrading polyesters are those substituted with carboxylic acid or amine groups. For example, a 90:10 copolymer of lactic acid and α-malic acid degraded within 1 wk at pH 7.2 and 37°C.[99] The influence of amine substitution was shown by Langer et al., who compared the degradation of poly(lactic acid) and poly(lactic acid-co-lysine). The latter polyester appeared to degrade to half its molecular weight after 5 wk (pH 7.1 and 37°C), whereas poly(lactic acid) took 15 weeks under the same conditions to degrade to the same extent.[100] Thus, water-soluble polyamine polyesters may be potentially useful for the delivery of genes because they can form polyion complexes with DNA and may degrade rapidly.

Poly(4-hydroxy-L-proline ester) (PHP; Figure 19.10) was the first water-soluble polycationic biodegradable polymer to be used as a gene carrier, as reported independently by Park et al.[101] and Langer et al.[102]

The degradation of the polymer in aqueous solution was monitored at pH 7 and 37°C using matrix-assisted laser desorption/ionization time-of-flight (MALDI-TOF) mass spectrometry. The polymer showed rapid initial degradation to less than half the molecular weight of intact polymer in less than 2 h. However, due to the formation of acid degradation products, hydrolysis slowed down after the initial degradation phase by decreasing pH of the solution; complete degradation to monomeric units took about 3 mo. PHP was able to bind DNA and protect it against degradation by nucleases for at least 4 h.[101] This indicates that PHP in the complex is not degraded as quickly as when the polymer is not bound to DNA. Poly(α-(4-aminobutyl)-L-glycolic acid) (PAGA; Figure 19.11) is an amine-substituted polyester synthesized by Kim et al.[103,104]

PAGA showed similar degradation behavior as compared to PHP, displaying a rapid initial degradation within 100 min to one third of its starting molecular weight, followed by gradual hydrolysis to the monomers in 6 mo at 37°C.[104] The rapid

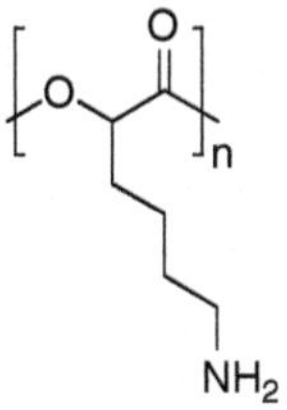

FIGURE 19.11 Poly(α-(4-aminobutyl)-L-glycolic acid) (PAGA).

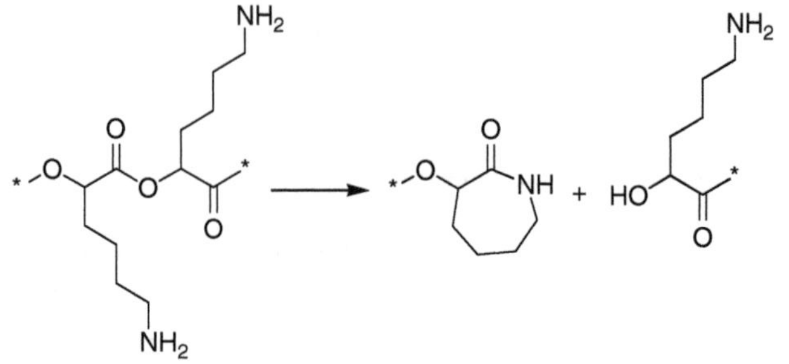

FIGURE 19.12 Intramolecular degradation of PAGA.

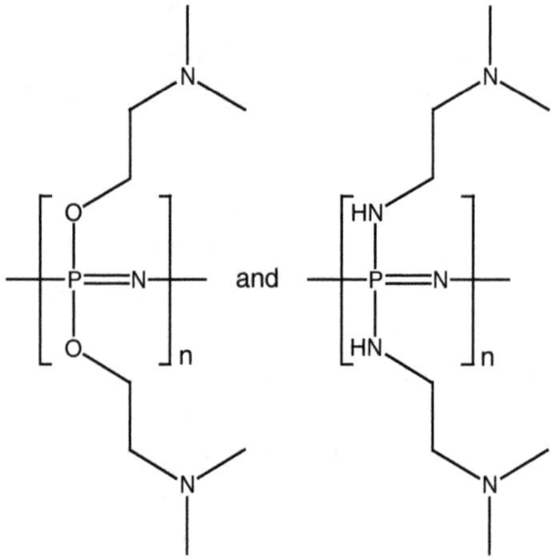

FIGURE 19.13 Cationic water-soluble polyphosphazenes. (From Luten, J. et al., *J. Control. Rel.*, 89, 483, 2003. With permission.)

hydrolysis of PHP and PAGA is attributed to the secondary amine groups in each monomeric unit that act as nucleophiles, probably by the mechanism as shown in Figure 19.12.

In line with the results from PHP, Kim et al. also observed slower degradation of the PAGA:DNA complex than the polymer alone; the complexes were stable for 8 h and dissociated completely in 1 day — a favorable timeframe for *in vivo* gene delivery. As compared with the polyamide analogue of PAGA (polylysine), the polyester was shown to be a more efficient gene delivery vector by *in vitro* tests and displayed less cytotoxicity.[104] This result illustrates the favorable effect of increased biodegradability of a carrier. Successful *in vivo* animal studies have been carried out recently.[105] In our laboratory, cationic polyphosphazenes (Figure 19.13) were synthesized and evaluated as gene delivery systems.[106]

In vitro studies showed that complexes of these polymers with plasmid DNA were able to transfect cells. The cytotoxicities of these polymers were less than those of other polymeric transfectants. The polymers were degradable at physiological conditions (half-life of 5 to 8 days at pH 7.2 and 37°C). However, to use polymer degradation as a tool to release DNA intracellularly, more rapidly degrading polymers are required. Current investigations are aimed at improving the degradation rates of the polymers and involve the synthesis of polyphosphazenes with different amine-bearing side groups and hydrolysis-sensitive cosubstituents.

CONCLUDING REMARKS

When designing fast degrading polymers and hydrogels, one must consider several parameters including the intrinsic hydrolytic sensitivity of the bonds, the extent of hydration of the polymers, and the presence of functional groups in the neighborhood of the labile bonds that may accelerate their degradation. Several examples of the latter phenomenon have been discussed in this chapter, including polyesters containing carboxylic and amine side groups, dextran hydrogels, and lactic acid oligomers whose degradation is influenced by neighboring hydroxyl groups. Suggested mechanisms of degradation enhancement by these functional groups can range from nucleophilic attack by amine groups to stabilization of the transition state by hydroxyl groups. These insights should, in principle, make it possible to modulate and tailor the biodegradation behaviors of polymeric materials.

REFERENCES

1. Uhrich, K.E., Cannizzaro, S.M., Langer, R.S., and Shakesheff, K.M., Polymeric systems for controlled drug release, *Chem. Rev.*, 99, 3181–3198, 1999.
2. Gombotz, W.R. and Pettit, D.K., Biodegradable polymers for protein and peptide drug delivery, *Bioconjugate Chem.*, 6, 332–351, 1995.
3. Jagur-Grodzinski, J., Biomedical applications of polymers, *e-Polymers*, 12, 1–38, 2003.
4. Gupta, P., Vermani, K., and Garg, S., Hydrogels: from controlled release to pH-responsive drug delivery, *Drug Discovery Today*, 7, 569–579, 2002.
5. Weiler, A., Hoffmann, R.F.G, Stahelin, A.C., Helling, H.J., and Sudkamp, N.P., Biodegradable implants in sports medicine: the biological base, *Arthroscopy*, 16, 305–321, 2000.
6. Bostman, O. and Pihlajamaki H., Clinical biocompatibility of biodegradable orthopaedic implants for internal fixation: a review, *Biomaterials*, 21, 2615–2621, 2000.
7. Agrawal, C.M. and Ray, R.B., Biodegradable polymeric scaffolds for musculoskeletal tissue engineering, *J. Biomed. Mater. Res.*, 55, 141–150, 2001.
8. Woodfield, T.B.F., Bezemer, J.M., Pieper, J.S., Van Blitterswijk, C.A., and Riesle, J., Scaffolds for tissue engineering of cartilage, *Crit. Rev. Eukaryot. Gene Expr.*, 12, 209–236, 2002.
9. Ueda, H. and Tabata, Y., Polyhydroxyalkonate derivatives in current clinical applications and trials, *Adv. Drug Del. Rev.*, 55, 501–518, 2003.
10. Van der Walle, G.A., De Koning, G.J., Weusthuis, R.A. and Eggink, G., Properties, modifications and applications of biopolyesters, *Adv. Biochem. Eng. Biotechnol.*, 71, 263–291, 2001.
11. Weber, C.J., Haugaard, V., Festersen, R. and Bertelsen, G., Production and applications of biobased packaging materials for the food industry, *Food Addit. Contam.*, 19, 172–177, 2002.

12. Pagga, U., Compostable packaging materials: test methods and limit values for biodegradation, *Appl. Microbiol. Biotechnol.*, 51, 125–133, 1999.
13. Anderson, J.M., Perspectives on the *in vivo* responses of biodegradable polymers, in *Biomedical Applications of Synthetic Biodegradable Polymers*, Hollinger, J.O., Ed., CRC Press, Boca Raton, FL, 1995, chap. 10.
14. Li, S.M., Garreau, H., and Vert, M., Structure–property relationships in the case of the degradation of massive poly(alpha-hydroxacids) in aqueous media. 3. Influence of the morphology of poly(L-lactic acid), *J. Mater. Sci. Mater. Med.*, 1, 198–206, 1990.
15. Vert, M., Li, S., and Garreau, H., More about the degradation of La/GA-derived matrices in aqueous media, *J. Control. Rel.*, 16, 15–26, 1991.
16. Vert, M., Mauduit, J., and Li, S., Biodegradation of PLA/GA polymers: increasing complexity, *Biomaterials*, 15, 1209–1213, 1994.
17. Vert, M., Schwach, G., Engel, R., and Coudane, J., Something new in the field of PLA/GA bioresorbable polymers? *J. Control. Rel.*, 53, 85–92, 1998.
18. Siepmann, J. and Gopferich, A., Mathematical modeling of bioerodible, polymeric drug delivery systems, *Adv. Drug Del. Rev.*, 48, 229–247, 2001.
19. Gopferich, A. and Tessmar, J., Polyanhydride degradation and erosion, *Adv. Drug Del. Rev.*, 54, 911–931, 2002.
20. Wang, P.P., Frazier, J., and Brem, H., Local drug delivery to the brain, *Adv. Drug Del. Rev.*, 54, 987–1013, 2002.
21. Leong, K.W., Brott, B.C., and Langer, R., Bioerodible polyanhydrides as drug-carrier matrices. I. Characterization, degradation, and release characteristics, *J. Biomed. Mater. Res.*, 19, 941–955, 1985.
22. Heller, J., Barr, J., Ng, S.Y., Shen, H.R., Schwach-Abdelaoui, K.S., Rothen-Weinhold, A., and Gurny, R., Poly(orthoesters): their development and some recent applications, *Eur. J. Pharm. Biopharm.*, 50, 121–128, 2000.
23. Heller, J., Barr, J., Ng, S.Y., Abdelauoi, K.S., and Gurny, R., Poly(orthoesters): synthesis, characterization, properties and uses, *Adv. Drug Del. Rev.*, 54, 1015–1039, 2002.
24. Ng, S.Y., Shen, H.R., Lopez, E., Zherebin, Y., Barr, J., Schacht, E., and Heller, J., Development of a poly(orthoester) prototype with a latent acid in the polymer backbone for 5-fluorouracil delivery, *J. Control. Rel.*, 65, 367–374, 2000.
25. Pitt, C.G., Gratzl, M.M., Kimmel, G.L., Surles, J., and Schindler, A., Aliphatic polyesters. II. The degradation of poly(D,L)-lactide), poly(epsilon-caprolactone), and their copolymers *in vivo*, *Biomaterials*, 2, 215–220, 1981.
26. Therin, M., Christel, P., Li, S., Garreau, H., and Vert, M., *In vivo* degradation of massive poly(α-hydroxy acids): validation of *in vitro* findings, *Biomaterials*, 13, 594–600, 1992.
27. Von Burkersroda, F., Schedl, L., and Gopferich, A., Why degradable polymers undergo surface erosion or bulk erosion, *Biomaterials*, 23, 4221–4231, 2002.
28. Okada, M., Chemical syntheses of biodegradable polymers, *Prog. Polym. Sci.*, 27, 87–133, 2002.
29. Sodergard, A. and Stolt, M., Properties of lactic acid based polymers and their correlation with composition, *Progr. Polym. Sci.*, 27, 1123–1163, 2002.
30. Edlund, U. and Albertsson, A.C., Polyesters based on diacid monomers, *Adv. Drug Del. Rev.*, 55, 585–609, 2003.
31. Kim, Y.B. and Lenz, R.W., Polyesters from microorganisms, *Adv. Biochem. Eng. Biotechnol.*, 71, 51–79, 2001.

32. Lee, S.Y. and Choi, J.L., Production of microbial polyester by fermentation of recombinant microorganisms, *Adv. Biochem. Eng. Biotechnol.*, 71, 183–207, 2001.

33. Shive, M.S. and Anderson, J.M., Biodegradation and biocompatibility of PLA and PL(G)A microspheres, *Adv. Drug Del. Rev.*, 28, 5–24, 1997.

34. Athanasiou, K.A., Niederauer, G.G., and Agrawal, C.M., Sterilization, toxicity, biocompatibility and clinical applications of polylactic acid/polyglycolic acid copolymers, *Biomaterials*, 17, 93–102, 1996.

35. Cadée, J.A., Brouwer, L.A., Den Otter, W., Hennink, W.E., and Van Luyn, M.J.A., A comparative biocompatibility study of microspheres based on crosslinked dextran or poly(lactic-co-glycolic)acid after subcutaneous injection in rats, *J. Biomed. Mater. Res.*, 56, 600–609, 2001.

36. Hyon, S.H., Jamshidi, K., and Ikada, Y., Synthesis of polylactides with different molecular weights, *Biomaterials*, 18, 1503–1508, 1997.

37. Leenslag, J.W. and Pennings, A.J., Synthesis of high-molecular-weight poly(L-lactide) initiated with tin 2-ethylhexanoate. *Makromol. Chem.*, 188, 1809–1814, 1987.

38. Zhong, Z., Dijkstra, P.J., Brig, C., Westerhausen, M., and Feijen, J., A novel and versatile calcium-based initiator system for the ring-opening polymerization of cyclic esters, *Macromolecules*, 34, 3863–3868, 2001.

39. Lewis, D.H., Controlled release of bioactive agents from lactide/glycolide polymers, in *Biodegradable Polymers as Drug Delivery Systems*, Chasin, M. and Langer, R., Eds., Marcel Dekker, New York, 1990.

40. De Jong, S.J., Arias, E.R., Rijkers, D.T.S., Van Nostrum, C.F., Kettenes-van den Bosch, J.J., and Hennink, W.E., New insights into the hydrolytic degradation of (poly(lactic acid): participation of the alcohol terminus, *Polymer*, 42, 2795–2802, 2001.

41. Van de Weert, M., Hennink, W.E., and Jiskoot, W., Protein instability in poly(lactic-co-glycolic acid) microparticles, *Pharm. Res.*, 17, 1159–1167, 2000.

42. Schwendeman, S.P., Recent advances in the stabilization of proteins encapsulated in injectable PL(G)A delivery systems, *Crit. Rev. Ther. Drug Carr. Syst.*, 19, 73–98, 2002.

43. Johansen, P., Men, Y., Merkle, H.P., and Gander, B., Revisiting PLA/PL(G)A microspheres: an analysis of their potential in parenteral vaccination, *Eur. J. Pharm. Biopharm.*, 50, 129–146, 2000.

44. Zhang, Y., Zale, S., Sawyer, L., and Bernstein, H.J., Effects of metal salts on poly(DL-lactide-co-glycolide) polymer hydrolysis, *J. Biomed. Mater. Res.*, 34, 531–538, 1997.

45. Nakamura, T., Hitomi, S., Watanabe, S., Shimizu, Y., Jamshidi, K., Hyon, S.-H., and Ikada, Y., Bioabsorption of polylactides with different molecular properties, *J. Biomed. Mater. Res.* 23, 1115–1130, 1989.

46. Li, S., Girod-Holland, S., and Vert, M., Hydrolytic degradation of poly(DL-lactic acid) in the presence of caffeine base, *J. Control. Rel.*, 40, 40–53, 1996.

47. Juni, K., Ogata, J., Matsui, N., Kubota, M., and Nakano, M., Modification of the release rate of aclarubicin from poly(lactic acid) microspheres by using additives, *Chem. Pharm. Bull.*, 33, 1734–1738, 1985.

48. Lee, K.H., Won, C.Y., Chu, C.C., and Gitsov, I., Hydrolysis of biodegradable polymers by superoxide ions, *J. Polym. Sci. A Polym. Chem.*, 37, 3558–3567, 1999.

49. Swach, G., Coudance, J., Engel, R., and Vert, M., More about the polymerisation of lactides in the presence of stannous octoate, *J. Polym. Sci. A Polym. Chem.*, 35, 3431–3440, 1997.

50. Lou, X.D, Detrembleur, C., and Jerome, R., Novel aliphatic polyesters based on functional cyclic (di)ester, *Macromol. Rapid Commun.*, 24, 161–172, 2003.

51. He, B., Bei, J.Z., and Wang, S.G., Synthesis and characterization of a functionalized biodegradable copolymer: poly(L-lactide-co-RS-β-malic acid), *Polymer*, 44, 989–994, 2003.

52. Ray, W.C. and Grinstaff, M.W., Polycarbonate and poly(carbonate-ester)s synthesized from biocompatible building blocks of glycerol and lactic acid, *Macromolecules*, 36, 3557–3562, 2003.

53. Liu, Y., Yuan, M.L., and Deng, X.M., Study on biodegradable polymers: synthesis and characterization of poly(DL-lactic acid-co-L-lysine) random copolymer, *Eur. Polym. J.*, 39, 977–983, 2003.

54. Zhang, S.P., Yang, J., Liu, X.Y., Chang, J.H., and Cao, A.M., Synthesis and characterization of poly(butylene succinate-co-butylene malate): a new biodegradable copolyester bearing hydroxyl pendant groups, *Biomacromolecules*, 4, 437–445, 2003.

55. Stigers, D.J. and Tew, G.N., Poly(3-hydroxyalkanoates)s functionalized with carboxylic acid groups in the side chain, *Biomacromolecules*, 4, 193–195, 2003.

56. Kopecek, J., Kopeckova, P., Minko, T., Lu, Z.R., and Peterson, C.M., Water soluble polymers in tumor targeted delivery, *J. Control. Rel.*, 74, 147–158, 2001.

57. Nijenhuis, A.J., Colstee, E., Grijpma, D.W., and Pennings, A.J., High molecular weight poly(L-lactide) and poly(ethylene oxide) blends: thermal characterization and physical properties, *Polymer*, 37, 5849–5857, 1996.

58. Zhang, G.B., Zhang, J.M., Zhou, X.S., and Shen, D.Y., Miscibility and phase structure of binary blends of polylactide and poly(vinylpyrrolidone), *J. Appl. Polym. Sci.*, 88, 973–979, 2003.

59. Park, K., Shalaby, W.S.W., and Park, H., *Biodegradable Hydrogels for Drug Delivery*, Technomic Publishing, Basel, 1993.

60. Hennink, W.E. and Van Nostrum, C.F., Novel crosslinking methods to design hydrogels, *Adv. Drug Del. Rev.*, 54, 13–36, 2002.

61. Hennink, W.E., Franssen, O., Van Dijk-Wolthuis, W.N.E., and Talsma, H., Dextran hydrogels for the controlled release of proteins, *J. Control. Rel.*, 48, 107–114, 1997.

62. Simonsen, L., Hovgaard, L., Mortensen, P.B., and Bronsted, H., Dextran hydrogels for colon-specific drug delivery. V. Degradation in human intestinal incubation models, *Eur. J. Pharm. Sci.*, 3, 329–337, 1995.

63. Franssen, O., Vos, O.P., and Hennink, W.E., Delayed release of a model protein from enzymatically degrading dextran hydrogels, *J. Contr. Rel.*, 44, 237–245, 1997.

64. Franssen, O., Van Rooijen, R.D., De Boer, D., Maes, R.A.A., and Hennink, W.E., Enzymatic degradation of crosslinked dextrans, *Macromolecules*, 32, 2896–2902, 1999.

65. Van Dijk-Wolthuis, W.N.E., Franssen, O., Talsma, H., Van Steenbergen, M.J., Kettenes-van den Bosch, J.J., and Hennink, W.E., Synthesis, characterization and polymerization of glycidyl methacrylate derivatized dextran, *Macromolecules*, 28, 6317–6322, 1995.

66. Van Dijk-Wolthuis, W.N.E., Kettenes-van den Bosch, J.J., Van der Kerk-van Hoof, A., and Hennink, W.E., Reaction of dextran with glycidyl methacrylate: an unexpected transesterification, *Macromolecules*, 30, 3411–3413, 1997.

67. Van Dijk-Wolthuis, W.N.E., Hoogeboom, J.A.M., Van Steenbergen, M.J., Tsang, S.K.Y., and Hennink, W.E., Degradation and release behaviour of dextran-based hydrogels, *Macromolecules*, 30, 4639–4645, 1997.

68. De Jong, S.J., De Smedt, S.C., Wahls, M.W.C., Demeester, J., Kettenes-van den Bosch, J.J., and Hennink, W.E., Novel self-assembled hydrogels by stereocomplex formation in aqueous solution of enantiomeric lactic acid oligomers grafted to dextran, *Macromolecules*, 33, 3680–3686, 2000.

69. De Jong, S.J., Van Eerdenbrugh, B., Van Nostrum, C.F., Kettenes-van den Bosch, J.J., and Hennink, W.E., Physically crosslinked dextran hydrogels by stereocomplex formation of lactic acid oligomers: degradation and protein release behavior, *J. Control. Rel.*, 71, 261–275, 2001.

70. Li, Y.X. and Kissel, T., Synthesis and properties of biodegradable ABA triblock copolymers consisting of poly(L-lactic acid) or poly(L-lactic-co-glycolic acid) A-blocks attached to central poly(oxyethylene) B-blocks, *J. Control. Rel.*, 27, 247–257, 1993.

71. Li, Y.X., Volland, C., and Kissel, T., *In vitro* degradation and bovine serum albumin release of the ABA triblock copolymers consisting of poly(L(+) lactic acid) or poly(L(+) lactic acid-co-glycolic acid) A-blocks attached to central polyoxyethylene B-blocks, *J. Control. Rel.*, 32, 121–128, 1994.

72. Kissel, T., Li, Y.X., and Unger, F., ABA-triblock copolymers from biodegradable polyester A-blocks and hydrophilic poly(ethylene oxide) B-blocks as a candidate for *in situ* forming hydrogel delivery systems for proteins, *Adv. Drug Del. Rev.*, 54, 99–134, 2002.

73. Pistel, K.F., Breitenbach, A., Zhange-Volland, R., and Kissel, T., Brush-like branched biodegradable polyesters. III. Protein release from microspheres of poly(vinyl alcohol)-graft-poly(D,L-lactic-co–glycolic acid), *J. Control. Rel.*, 73, 7–20, 2001.

74. Martini, L., Attwood, D., Collett, J.H., Nicholas, C.V., Tanodekaew, S., Deng, N.J., Heatly, F., and Booth, C., Micellization and gelation of triblock copolymer of ethylene oxide and epsilon-caprolactone, $Cl_nE_mCl_n$, in aqueous solution, *J. Chem. Soc. Faraday Trans.*, 90, 1961–1966, 1994.

75. Li, X., Li, J., and Leong, L.W., Preparation and characterization of inclusion complexes of biodegradable amphiphilic poly(ethylene oxide) triblock copolymers with cyclodextrins, *Macromolecules*, 36, 1209–1214, 2003.

76. Rashkov, I., Manolova, N., Li, S.M., Espartero, J.L., and Vert, M., Synthesis, characterization and hydrolytic degradation of PLA/PEO/PLA triblock copolymers with short poly(L-lactic acid) chains, *Macromolecules*, 29, 50–56, 1996.

77. Kissel, T., Li, Y.X., Volland, C., Gorich, S., and Koneberg, R., Parenteral protein delivery systems using biodegradable polyesters of ABA block structure, containing hydrophobic poly(lacticide-coglycolide) A blocks and hydrophilic poly(ethylene oxide) B blocks, *J. Control. Rel.*, 39, 315–326, 1996.

78. Jain, R.A., The manufacturing techniques of various drug-loaded biodegradable poly(lactide-co-glycolide) (PL(G)A) devices, *Biomaterials*, 21, 2475–2490, 2000.

79. Zhou, S., Liao, X., Li, X., Deng, X., and Li, H., Poly-D,L-lactide-co-poly(ethylene glycol) microspheres as potential vaccine delivery systems, *J. Control. Rel.*, 86, 195–205, 2003.

80. Sawhney, A.S., Pathak, C.P., and Hubbell, J.A., Bioerodible hydrogels based on photopolymerized poly(ethyleneglycol)-co-poly(alpha-hydroxy acid) diacrylate macromers, *Macromolecules*, 26, 581–587, 1993.

81. Martens, P., Metters, A.T., Anseth, K.S., and Bowman, C.N., A generalized bulk-degradation model for hydrogel networks formed from multivinyl cross-linking molecules, *J. Phys. Chem. B*, 105, 5131–5138, 2001.

82. Metters, A.T., Anseth, K.S., and Bowman, C.N., A statistical kinetic model for the bulk degradation of PLA-b-PEG-b-PLA hydrogel networks: incorporating network non-idealities, *J. Phys. Chem. B*, 105, 8069–8076, 2001.

83. Jeong, B., Bae, Y.H., Lee, D.S., and Kim, S.W., Biodegradable block copolymers as injectable drug-delivery systems, *Nature*, 388, 860–862, 1997.

84. Jeong, B., Bae, Y.H., and Kim, S.W., Drug release from biodegradable injectable thermosensitive hydrogel of PEG-PL(G)A-PEG triblock copolymers, *J. Control. Rel.*, 63, 155–163, 2000.

85. Kwon, K.W., Park, M.J., Bae, Y.H., Kim, H.D., and Char, K., Gelation behavior of PEO-PL(G)A-PEO triblock copolymers in water, *Polymer*, 43, 3353–3358, 2002.

86. Jeong, B., Bae, Y.H., and Kim, S.W., *In situ* gelation of PEG-PL(G)A-PEG triblock copolymer aqueous solutions and degradation thereof, *J. Biomed. Mater. Res.*, 50, 171–177, 2000.

87. Rypacek, F., Pytela, J., Kotva, R., Skarda, V., and Cifkova, I., Biodegradation of poly(amino acid)s: evaluation methods and structure–function-relationships, *Macromol. Symp.*, 123, 9–24, 1997.

88. Chiu, H.C., Kopeckova, P., Deshmane, S.S., and Kopecek, J., Lysosomal degradability of poly(α-amino acids), *J. Biomed. Mater. Res.*, 34, 381–392, 1997.

89. Mehvar, R. and Shepard, T., Molecular weight-dependent pharmacokinetics of fluorescein-labeled dextrans in rats, *J. Pharm. Sci.*, 81, 908–912, 1992.

90. Duncan, R., Polymer conjugates for tumour targeting and intracytoplasmatic delivery: the EPR effect as a common gateway? *Pharm. Sci. Technol. Today*, 2, 441–449, 1999.

91. Kopecek, J., Kopeckova, P., Minko, T., and Lu, Z.R., HPMA copolymer–anticancer drug conjugates: design, activity and mechanism of action, *Eur. J. Pharm. Biopharm.*, 50, 61–81, 2000.

92. Rihova, B., Etrych, T., Pechar, M., Jelinkova, M., Stastny, M., Hovorka, O., Kovar, M., and Ulbrich, K., Doxorubicin bound to HPMA copolymer carrier through hydrazone bond is effective also in a cancer cell line with a limited content of lysosomes, *J. Control. Rel.*, 74, 225–232, 2001.

93. Blaese, R.M., Gene therapy for cancer, *Sci. Am.*, 6, 91–95, 1997.

94. Prud'homme, G.J., Gene therapy of autoimmune diseases with vectors encoding regulatory cytokines or inflammatory cytokine inhibitors, *J. Gene Med.*, 2, 222–232, 2000.

95. De Smedt, S.C., Demeester, J., and Hennink, W.E., Cationic polymer-based gene delivery systems, *Pharm. Res.*, 17, 113–126, 2000.

96. Boussif, O., Lezoulac'h, F., Zanta, M., Mergny, M., Scherman, D., Demeneix, B., and Behr, J.P., A versatile vector for gene and oligonucleotide transfer into cells in culture and *in vivo*: polyethylenimine, *Proc. Natl. Acad. Sci. USA*, 92, 7297–7301, 1995.

97. Van de Wetering, P., Cherng, J.Y., Talsma, H., and Hennink, W.E., Relation between transfection efficiency and cytotoxicity of poly(2-dimethylaminoethyl methacrylate)/plasmid complexes, *J. Control. Rel.*, 49, 59–69, 1997.

98. Walter, E., Dreher, D., Kok, M., Thiele, L., Kiama, S.G., Gehr, P., and Merkle, H.P., Hydrophilic poly(DL-lactide-co-glycolide) microspheres for the delivery of DNA to human-derived macrophages and dendritic cells, *J. Control. Rel.*, 76, 149–168, 2001.

99. Kimura, Y., Shirotani, K., Yamane, H., and Kitao, T., Copolymerization of 3-(S)-[(benzyloxycarbonyl)methyl]-1,4-dioxane-2,5-dione and L-lactide: a facile synthetic method for functionalized bioabsorbable polymer, *Polymer*, 34, 1741–1748, 1993.

100. Barrera, D.A., Zylstra, E., Lansbury, P.T., and Langer, R., Synthesis and RGD peptide modification of a new biodegradable copolymer: poly(lactic acid-co-lysine), *J. Am. Chem. Soc.*, 115, 11010–11011, 1993.

101. Lim, Y.B., Choi, Y.H., and Park, J.S., A self-destroying polycationic polymer: biodegradable poly(4-hydroxy-L-proline ester), *J. Am. Chem. Soc.*, 121, 5633–5639, 1999.

102. Putman, D. and Langer, R., Poly(4-hydroxy-L-proline ester): low temperature condensation with plasmid DNA complexation, *Macromolecules*, 32, 3658–3662, 1999.

103. Lim, Y.B., Kim, C.H., Kim, K., Kim, S.W., and Park, J.S., Development of a safe gene delivery system using biodegradable polymer, poly([α-(4-aminobutyl)-L-glycolic acid], *J. Am. Chem. Soc.*, 122, 6524–6525, 2000.

104. Lim, Y.B., Han, S.O., Kong, H.U., Lee, Y., Park, J.S., Jeong, B., and Kim, S.W., Biodegradable polyester, poly([α-(4-aminobutyl)-L-glycolic acid], as a non-toxic gene carrier, *Pharm. Res.*, 17, 811–816, 2000.

105. Lee, M., Koh, J.J., Han, S.O., Ko, K.S., and Kim, S.W., Prevention of autoimmune insulitis by delivery of interleukin-4 plasmid using a soluble and biodegradable polymeric carrier, *Pharm. Res*, 19, 246–249, 2003.

106. Luten, J., Van Steenis, J.H., Van Someren, R., Kemmink, J., Schuurmans-Nieuwenbroek, N.M.E., Koning, G.A., Crommelin, D.J.A., Van Nostrum, C.F., and Hennink, W.E., Water-soluble cationic polyphosphazenes for gene delivery, *J. Control. Rel.*, 89, 483–497, 2003.

Section IV

A Perspective on Reflexive Systems

20 A Perspective on Current and Future Synthetic Reflexive Systems

Kinam Park, Nobuhiko Yui, and Randall J. Mrsny

CONTENTS

NEEDS FOR REFLEXIVE (RAPIDLY RESPONSIVE AND REPETITIVE) MATERIALS

Smart polymers and hydrogels respond to environmental changes (see Peppas, Chapter 7, this volume) such as changes in pH, temperature, pressure, salt, organic solvent, and specific molecules.[1,2] Responses by smart water-soluble polymers include precipitation or dissolution, while responses of smart hydrogels take the form of shrinking, swelling, or bending. Advances in the preparation of such environment-responsive materials have been instrumental in the development of various self-regulated drug delivery systems such as modulated insulin delivery systems and biomedical devices such as biosensors.

One of the key properties of environment-responsive materials is that the responses or changes occur by reason of very small changes in environmental factors, as shown in Figure 20.1. For example, for temperature-sensitive hydrogels, shrinking or swelling occurs from a change in temperature of a degree or two. The same is true for pH-sensitive hydrogels. A minute change in pH can result in a substantial change in polymer behavior. Although these types of environment-responsive properties have been well documented, the kinetics of such responses have not been explored in depth.

0-8493-1487-9/04/$0.00+$1.50

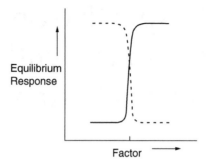

FIGURE 20.1 Responses of smart hydrogel to an environmental factor. The solid and dotted lines indicate positive and negative responses, respectively.

The large changes in responses associated with small changes in environmental factors occur at equilibrium. The time it takes to reach the equilibrium response can be very long. In many applications, a fast response triggered by environmental change is critical and the existing systems have poor ability to perform the same function repetitively. Even if they were able to do so, the recovery time would be too long. Many gaps in the development of smart materials for systems with rapidly responsive and repetitive properties still exist. As shown by the material in this book, many natural systems have the required reflexive properties. Further study of those natural systems and better understanding of the theoretical factors that limit reflexive behavior are expected to improve current synthetic systems with fast responsive properties.

UNDERSTANDING REFLEXIVE SYSTEMS

One of the best approaches to designing new systems such as reflexive materials is to learn from the host of examples provided by Mother Nature. As shown in Chapter 1, the general principles guiding the rapid, repetitive responses of biological systems appear to be simple, at least on the surface. For example, the beta cells of the pancreatic islets respond to rising glucose levels by the increased release of insulin. In fact, synthetic systems based on smart hydrogels can perform the same task. Hydrogels that contain glucose sensors can respond to rising glucose levels by releasing more insulin.[3]

This type of synthetic system, however, is far simpler than its biological counterpart. The increased insulin release by beta cells is a result of an extensive network of intracellular signaling events that are difficult to reproduce in synthetic systems. The lack of an intricate network of intracellular signaling is one of the reasons why existing synthetic systems cannot respond fast and repetitively. As shown in Chapters 2 through 6, all biological systems with rapid, reversible responses involve motor proteins that can be stimulated by electric signals. On the other hand, as discussed in Chapters 7 through 11, synthetic systems present certain limitations in signal transfer ability. The differences between biological and synthetic systems can be best represented by comparing the fast responsive properties of *Mimosa pudica*

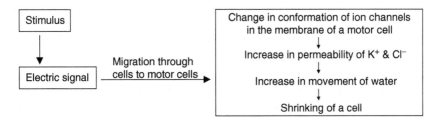

FIGURE 20.2 Sequence of events resulting in rapid response of *Mimosa pudica* to stimulation.

described in Chapter 2 and the fast responses obtainable with a synthetic system (Chapter 11).

RESPONSES TO STIMULI IN BIOLOGICAL AND SYNTHETIC SYSTEMS

When mechanical, thermal, electrical, and chemical stimuli are applied to *Mimosa pudica*, the leaflets close or fold and the petioles bend quickly. Mechanical stimuli in the form of gentle touching and shaking produce immediate folding of leaves and bending of petioles. These rapid movements are caused by rapid changes in the motor organ known as the pulvinus and located at the base of each leaf or leaflet. Upon stimulation, an electrical signal is generated and spread to the motor cells in the pulvinus. The electrical signal is then converted into a chemical signal that makes the motor cells in the lower side of the pulvinus shrink.

The shrinking of the motor cells occurs because of increased permeability of the cell membranes to K^+ and Cl^- ions, leading to loss of water. (The movement of ions accompanies the movement of water.) Changes in ion permeability through the cell membranes are known to result from changes in conformation of ion channels affecting the rates of ion migration through the membranes. The process of response by *Mimosa pudica* in a simplified form is shown in Figure 20.2. The electric signal generated by a stimulus will migrate through cells to the motor cells of the pulvinus. This process and subsequent conformational changes in the ion channels in the motor cell membranes occur very quickly. Thus, the rate-limiting step is the movement of water (following the movement of ions). Even the rate-limiting step occurs quickly, as we know from the rapid response of *Mimosa pudica* to touching.

A synthetic system designed to simulate the process illustrated in Figure 20.2 should have the ability to transform environmental signals into electrical signals that can migrate to an actuator where the intended action occurs. When considering the use of smart hydrogels, one must deal with the fast movement of water to elicit fast responses. The analysis described in Chapter 11 of this book shows that diffusion-limited networks of macroscopic size swell or shrink rather slowly.

The diffusion coefficient of a polymer network in water is on the order of 10^{-7} cm^2/s and is relatively insensitive to the type of polymer network. This means that the swelling would take hours for a gel membrane as thin as 1 mm. Making the sample size smaller has circumvented this problem. It is difficult, however, to reduce the sample size to the level of motor cells and align them to function as a unit. For this reason, most efforts have been directed toward making porous smart hydrogel systems in which the dominant mass transfer mechanism is convection. Following convection through the pores, water molecules can diffuse quickly through the thin walls of the hydrogels. Chapter 13 deals with such an approach for making fast swelling hydrogels. By combining additional features such as fast shrinking properties, it may be possible to engineer smart hydrogels that can mimic natural systems. The realization of this possibility should not be far away as we gain better understanding of biological systems and utilize nanotechnology to build molecular devices and machines.[4]

KEY PROPERTIES OF REFLEXIVE SYSTEMS

The first part of this book deals with the mechanisms of fast responsive systems from nature. It provides a basis for understanding the progress of biological systems that have highly organized hierarchies designed to respond to any changes in surrounding environment for the purpose of survival and proliferation. Randall J. Mrsny described the overall theme of this book and summarized the common mechanisms of several stimuli-responsive systems in nature. The responsiveness of nerve cells is established by the large potential energy across the plasma membranes. Ca^{2+} levels regulate the rapid actions of muscles and the coordination of myofibrils is used to generate mechanical forces. Endocrine tissues are also regulated by Ca^{2+} flux across cell membranes.

Nobuyuki Kanzawa and Takahide Tsuchiya described the details of seismonastic movements of plants. The well-known seismonastic bending movements of *Mimosa pudica* are controllable by Ca^{2+} levels that initiate water flux across the cell membranes. Madoka Suzuki and Shin'ichi Ishiwata described mechanochemical energy transduction in myofibrils as found in the contractile systems of muscles. Spatiotemporal synchronization in protein assemblies of actin–myosin couples is emphasized in creating mechanical forces. Michio Homma and Toshiharu Yokushi described a bacterial flagellar motor — another example of a mechanical system. A flagellar filament with a spiral structure rotates like a screw to create a propulsive force. Bacterial cells undergo these actions via the electrochemical potential of protons and sodium ions for energy conversion.

Teruo Shimmen and Etsuo Yokota described cytoplasmic streaming of plant cells, an alternative action of plants. The motive force for streaming is generated by the sliding functions of actin filaments in internodal cells surrounded by cell walls. The most distinguishable point in a comparison with muscle contraction is that actin–myosin sliding continues to generate the motive force of the streaming in the resting states of plant cells.

Namjin Baek and Kinam Park described natural polymeric gel systems in nature. The common mechanism of such natural systems is that transient Ca^{2+} release regulates Ca^{2+}-dependent protein kinase. Ca^{2+} plays a common role in almost all natural systems that respond to external signals. It is inspiring to learn that natural systems are regulated mainly by ionic exchanges through cell membranes. Many natural systems utilize Ca^{2+} and related ions as electrochemical potentials and also as triggers for activating protein kinase to reorganize skeletal components in cells. Another important point to learn from nature is the existence of highly organized hierarchical structures in all natural systems. They cannot change or switch their functions so quickly and repetitively in response to external stimuli if they do not have organized structures such as myofibrils in muscles.

The second part of this book focuses on the theoretical analysis of fast and repetitive responses of smart polymers and hydrogels. It contributes to our understanding of the fundamentals involved in designing rapidly responsive polymeric systems for their possible applications in biomedical and pharmaceutical fields. Nicholas A. Peppas described the fundamentals of the dynamic behavior of polymeric hydrogel systems; it is possible to predict the exact swelling behaviors of both neutral and ionic hydrogels under different conditions. Hiroshi Frusawa and Kohzo Ito described theoretical aspects of polyelectrolyte solutions and hydrogels. In particular, the effects of counterion fluctuations and polyion conformations on solution properties were emphasized to explain the natures of these systems.

Ryo Yoshida described kinetics of cyclic hydrogel systems that exhibit autonomous oscillating swelling behaviors. A representative hydrogel system using the Belousov–Zhabotinsky reaction enables one to generate periodic mechanical energy. Further studies on synchronizing such systems with biological clock systems may create a new field of stimuli-responsive polymeric systems.

Rupali Gangopadhyay, Jian Ping Gong, and Yoshihito Osada described theoretical and experimental aspects of cooperative binding in surfactant–polymer associations for chemomechanical hydrogel systems. Their approach provided a new idea for the design of artificial muscle systems based on soft gels for robots and other machines. Norihiro Kato and Stevin H. Gehrke described kinetic limitations of fast responsive polymeric systems. In particular, they proposed the potential of microporous hydrogels as fast responsive systems. It was calculated that the responses of microporous hydrogels are more than a thousand times faster than those of nonporous systems. This section provides information on the kinetic limitations of fast responses by synthetic systems based on conventional polymers and/or hydrogel systems.

The third section of the book surveys synthetic polymeric systems that exhibit some reflexive properties. It discusses variations of fast responsive mechanisms, such as shrinking, swelling, slide motion, light-induced orientation, liquid crystals, dissociation, and degradation. Mitsuhiro Ebara, Akihiko Kikuchi, Kiyotaka Sakai, and Teruo Okano described fast shrinkable hydrogel systems and emphasized the concept of introducing freely mobile temperature-responsive graft chains into hydrogel networks to accelerate the shrinking process. The rate of shrinking was markedly improved. Richard A. Gemeinhart and Chunqiang Guo discussed fast swelling hydrogel systems. They presented a rapidly swelling system based on superporous hydrogels. Their work relates to Chapter 11 by Norihiro Kato and Stevin H. Gehrke in Section II. Swelling of porous hydrogel systems is not limited by diffusion of water through the hydrogel matrix, and thus porous hydrogels can quickly respond to environmental changes.

Nobuhiko Yui and Tooru Ooya explained fast sliding motions of supramolecular assemblies. To mimic sliding motions of actin–myosin myofibrils seen in muscle contraction, cyclic compounds were threaded onto linear polymeric chains of a polyrotaxane structure. Sliding motions of the cyclic compounds differed from the simple polymer relaxation or aggregation phenomena observed in three-dimensional polymer networks or solutions, and thus, they may be used for designing new stimuli-responsive polymers and hydrogels.

Kunihiro Ichimura described light-induced molecular orientation systems and introduced a variety of photo-induced generations of light anisotropy using photo-alignment phenomena of azobenzene groups linked to polymeric surfaces. It deserves special attention that such optical anisotropy is markedly amplified by the self-assembling nature of liquid crystals at the polymer surfaces. Seiji Kurihara introduced fast responsive liquid crystalline polymer systems and described the details of thermotropic liquid crystalline side-chain polymers with photochromic low molecular weight compounds such as azobenzene. Such an optical switching system makes real-time holographic data processing possible.

Eduardo Jule and Kazunori Kataoka examined copolymer micelles as drug targeting systems. They introduced the fundamental properties of polymeric micelles, in particular the effect of their stability on pharmaceutical applications. The relationship between micelle stability and micelle association can be used to design rapidly dissociating micelle systems.

Jong-Duk Kim, Seung Rim Yang, Yong Woo Cho, and Kinam Park reviewed fast responsive proteinoid systems. External stimuli-responsive properties of self-assembled amphiphilic poly(amino acid)s and nanoparticulate proteinoids were described. Wim E. Hennink, Jan Hein van Steenis, and Cornelus F. van Nostrum explored rapidly biodegradable polymeric systems. The focus was on how labile bonds in polymeric systems can accelerate degradation. These insights make it possible to modulate and tailor the biodegradation of polymers and hydrogels.

Reflexive Systems with Advanced Functions

All the chapters in the third section showed that relatively simple synthetic polymeric systems can possess fast responsive properties. The synthetic systems described may appear primitive when compared with systems found in the nature. However, comparison of two different types of systems related to their fast responsive properties shows that one of the key parameters for fast responsiveness is using molecular assemblies constructed by intermolecular forces.

Combining molecular forces with the design of specific molecular architectures can lead to anisotropic assemblies or alignments of macromolecules that may determine how quickly and accurately a system can function. For most useful applications of reflexive systems, we should consider the accuracy and the speed of the response. For improved accuracy, it may be necessary to provide multisensing properties by designing, for example, synchronized stimuli-responsive systems. This idea was applied to the designs of dual-stimuli-responsive degradation systems by using interpenetrating polymer networks consisting of polysaccharide and protein chains.[5-7] Two different molecular forces between host polymers and guest molecules were used.[8,9]

A combination of β-cyclodextrin-conjugated poly(ε-lysine) and a guest molecule with hydrophobic head and anionic tail showed gelation only at physiological pH and limited temperature range within milliseconds. Since this system does not show the gelation behavior when pH or temperature is deviated from the tight range, it may provide more accurate responses than the single-stimulus-responsive systems. Clearly, systems can be designed to respond to more than two stimuli, and such multistimuli systems based on multiple intermolecular forces and architectures can be used to develop extremely fast diagnostic devices and drug delivery systems.

In sensing biological stimuli, multivalent interaction can be used to amplify an initiation signal. In biological systems, at least in principle, each receptor is designed to transmit a signal through the activation of cytoplasmic (sometimes enzymatic) pathways via ligand binding. In order to accelerate and amplify the signal, however, multiple copies of the same ligand attached to a polymeric backbone have been used.[10] While this approach increases the binding constant to some extent, excess increase in the number of ligands causes the spatial mismatching with receptors, resulting in a decrease in the binding ability per ligand unit. In order to overcome this, a supramolecular approach has been proposed.[11-13]

Multiple copies of ligands are introduced to cyclodextrins that are threaded onto a linear polymeric chain with both terminals capped with bulky end groups (poly-rotaxanes). The ligands are freely mobile along the polymeric chain, and thus they can bind to receptors several thousand times stronger than a single ligand does. The binding ability of ligands in the polyrotaxanes is linearly related to the degree of ligand mobility estimated by a pulsed NMR technique. The rate of cyclodextrin threading onto a linear polymeric chain in these polyrotaxanes seems to be much higher than the rate of diffusion of polymeric chains in water.

The dynamic responses of polymers and hydrogels follow their relaxation and diffusion phenomena in water. For example, the swelling and shrinking kinetics of hydrogels are governed by diffusion-limited polymeric network transport in water, and thus, the rate of swelling or shrinking is inversely proportional to the square root of the hydrogel dimension. One way of overcoming this rate-limiting step and shortening the response time is to use dynamic motion of molecular assembling systems through controlling noncovalent interactions.

APPLICATIONS OF REFLEXIVE SYSTEMS

Controlled drug delivery systems with fast responsive, repetitive properties are critical in developing clinically useful systems. One of the holy grails of controlled drug delivery is development of modulated (or self-regulated) insulin delivery systems. The fast responsive property is critical for such systems based on glucose-sensitive hydogels. The increase in glucose level in blood must be counteracted by the release of insulin in a matter of a few minutes. Unfortunately, the responses of most of the existing modulated insulin delivery systems based on smart materials are too slow.

The release of insulin 20 to 30 min after a rise of the blood glucose level may be too late. For any system to be clinically useful, it should respond within 5 min of the rise in glucose. Furthermore, the repetitive property is not always reliable in existing systems. As discussed in Chapter 1, biological systems utilize a complex array of sensors and actuators, and for any synthetic systems to reproduce biological systems, the bottom-up nanotechnology may have to be utilized, instead of smart hydrogels based on one property such as pH-sensitivity.

Another holy grail of drug delivery is the development of reliable gene delivery systems. While viral gene delivery is known to be effective, using live viruses is also dangerous. For this reason, active research utilizing nonviral gene delivery systems is continuing. Most of the nonviral gene delivery systems are known to end up in endosomes where genes are broken down by enzymes.[14] Due to the slightly lower pH levels of endosomes, a number of approaches have been developed to exploit the pH differences between endosomes and cytosols. In this type of application, fast responses of breaking the endosomeal membranes are critical for successful gene delivery.

pH-sensitive, fast responsive systems can also be used in the development of tumor-targeted delivery systems. The extracellular pH of solid tumors is known to be on average 0.2 pH units lower than the pH of surrounding tissues.[15] pH-sensitive polymeric micelles based on pH-sensitive poly(L-histidine) that respond to pH shifts from 7.4 to 6.6 through 7.2 can be used effectively in tumor-targeting drug delivery systems.[16] For any of these systems to be useful, the response to changes in environmental factors must be fast. Combining the fast responsive property with repetitive function would make the best combination for developing clinically effective controlled drug delivery systems.

Several recent articles describe biomimetic materials and systems.[17–19] The focus of biomimetic materials is biocompatibility so that they can interact with biological molecules and/or to elicit desired biological responses. For some biomimetic materials, fast responses may be prerequisites for their functions. Molecular imprinting has been used widely to prepare molecular assemblies of desired structures and properties, usually for interacting with target molecules.[20] One application of molecular imprints is biosensor development in which fast responsiveness is critical. This is even more so if the sensing is tied to subsequent actions such as delivery of insulin after sensing glucose levels. Use of novel polymeric systems such as the polyrotaxane systems described above would make it possible to overcome the limitations set by the diffusion process.

FUTURE OF REFLEXIVE SYSTEMS

As is often the case, functional aspects of a system observed in nature provide what has been determined through experimental studies as the optimal method of achieving a goal. In essence, what we learn over and over is that nature has used time and selective pressure to develop methods to establish the minimum requirements of components and energy to achieve an outcome that is no more and no less than required. In some cases such as phage display screening,[21] humans have learned from nature and used its approaches to find an optimal solution to an interfacial binding problem using selective pressure. One day we might also utilize methods to identify optimal ways to recapitulate what nature has already achieved when defining synthetic reflexive systems. Ultimately, we may find the solution to be near identical to what nature has already defined, except for a few important differences.

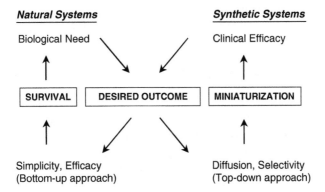

FIGURE 20.3 Drivers for natural and synthetic reflexive systems differ in several respects. The overwhelming concern in a natural system is survival; a synthetic system is concerned with functional parameters. For synthetic systems to achieve the efficiency and simplicity that drives survival in a natural system, they must focus on complexities such as diffusion and selectivity. In both cases, an iterative process is used to derive the desired outcome.

Identification of an optimal outcome to any problem is based on the parameters defined as critical to the problem. In our efforts to solve problems associated with synthetic reflexive systems, we can appreciate neither the priority nor the required complexity of system components that nature has determined using the ultimate criterion: survival. We can only study outcomes of reflexive systems observed in nature and try to emulate what we perceive as the critical components required for successful functioning. It is important to appreciate that in the establishment of natural systems and in the development of synthetic systems, the iterative process preceding a successful outcome has unique drivers — drivers motivated by the essential features of systems in these two cases (Figure 20.3). So what are these essential features? Observations made in the first section of this book (Chapters 1 through 6) reiterate several themes. In general, reflexive systems seem to have (1) triggers, (2) thresholds for responses to the triggers, (3) amplification steps, (4) dissemination (or dispersion) components, and (5) resolution events that activate or facilitate recovery. All these components are required for a system to be rapid, repetitive, and responsive or *reflexive*.

Do these natural systems break down these steps into stages as has been done here? Not really. The summation of these events occurring in a cumulative fashion determines the success of a reflexive system in nature. However, in our efforts to understand reflexive systems sufficiently to recreate them synthetically, we must first deconstruct them. As this dismantling occurs, it is obvious that natural systems have all components listed above and also identified methods to accelerate rate-limiting events associated with the systems. This may mean the rapid resynthesis of a critical material or the recocking of a trigger mechanism. In any case, nature has made sure that the ability to keep these systems running is not compromised.

Any hope we might have to create a truly reflexive system comparable to those observed in nature would require us to identify and overcome rate-limiting steps in the action and/or recovery phases of the material being designed. Nature has already determined these for the systems present in plants and animals. Since any synthetic system can never be as complex as a natural system, it is likely that synthetic systems designed to emulate natural ones may have distinct rate-limiting steps. This means that our ability to learn from natural systems will only go to the point where the limiting steps diverge and novel approaches to maximize the potential of the synthetic system must be determined.

Why is this likely to be the case? The motivation for this point comes from the difficulty we will encounter in miniaturizing these systems the way nature has. Both natural and synthetic reflexive systems are designed and constructed at the molecular level. However, nature also has the luxury of using molecular-sized workers to fabricate systems while man must use much less efficient and less refined methods of production. Nature can also assess quality control at the molecular level and organize components of a reflexive system at the same level. Nature can compress highly complex individual units of a reflexive system into minute areas and in doing so dramatically increase sensitivity, efficiency, and speed through close approximation of critical components.

Nanofabrication[22] of synthetic reflexive systems may provide a solution to achieving the propinquity required to approach the capabilities of natural systems. Manufacturing such systems should be possible, but we still do not know every component needed to fabricate an optimal synthetic reflexive system. Thus, it is difficult to say fabrication will be feasible with any degree of certainty. What is certain is that the success of any effort to create synthetic reflexive systems will require improvements in the quality, quantity, and scale of manufacturing processes currently in use.

REFERENCES

1. Qiu, Y. and Park, K., Environment-sensitive hydrogels for drug delivery, *Adv. Drug Del. Rev.*, 53, 321–339, 2001.
2. Qiu, Y. and Park, K., Modulated drug delivery, in *Supramolecular Design for Biological Applications,* N. Yui, Ed., CRC Press, Boca Raton, 2002, pp. 227–243.
3. Obaidat, A.A. and Park, K., Characterization of protein release through glucose-sensitive hydrogel membranes, *Biomaterials*, 18, 801–806, 1997.
4. Balzani, V., Venturi, M., and Credi, A., *Molecular Devices and Machines: A Journey into the Nanoworld*, Wiley-VCH, Weinheim, Germany, 2002.
5. Kurisawa, M., Terano, M., and Yui, N., Double stimuli-responsive degradable hydrogels for drug delivery: interpenetrating polymer networks composed of oligopeptide-terminated poly(ethylene glycol) and dextran, *Macromol. Rapid Commun.*, 16, 663–666, 1995.
6. Kurisawa, M. and Yui, N., Gelatin/dextran hydrogels with an interpenetrating polymer network for intelligent drug delivery: dual-stimuli-responsive degradation in relation to miscibility between two different polymers, *Macromol. Chem. Phys.*, 199, 1547–1554, 1998.
7. Kurisawa, M. and Yui, N., Dual-stimuli-responsive drug release from IPN-structured hydrogels consisting of gelatin and dextran, *J. Control. Rel.*, 54, 191–200, 1998.

8. Choi, H.S., Huh, K.M., Ooya, T., and Yui, N., pH- and thermo-sensitive supramolecular assembling system: rapidly responsive properties of β-cyclodextrin-conjugated poly(ε-lysin), *J. Am. Chem. Soc.*, 125, 6350–6351, 2003.

9. Choi, H.S., Ooya, T., Sasaki, S., and Yui, N., Control of rapid phase transition induced by supramolecular complexation of β-cyclodextrin-conjugated poly(ε-lysin) with specific guest, *Macromolecules*, 36, 5342–5347, 2003.

10. Mammen, M., Choi, S.-K., and Whiteside, G.M., Polyvalent interactions in biological systems: implications for design and use of multivalent ligands and inhibitors, *Angew. Chem. Int. Ed.*, 37, 2754–2794, 1998.

11. Yui, N., Ooya, T., Kawashima, T., Saito, Y., Tamai, I., Sai, Y., and Tsuji, A., Inhibitory effect of supramolecular polyrotaxane-dipeptide conjugates on digested peptide uptake via human peptide transporter, *Bioconj. Chem.*, 13, 582–587, 2002.

12. Yui, N. and Ooya, T., Polyrotaxanes: challenge to multivalent binding with biological receptors on cell surfaces, *Mater. Sci. Forum*, 426–432, 3242–3248, 2003.

13. Ooya, T., Eguchi, M., and Yui, N., Supramolecular design for multivalent interaction: maltose mobility along polyrotaxane enhanced binding with concanavalin A, *J. Am. Chem. Soc.*, 125, 13016–13017, 2003.

14. Cho, Y.W., Kim, J.D., and Park, K., Polycation gene delivery systems: escape from endosomes to cytosol, *J. Pharm. Pharmacol.*, 55, 721–734, 2003.

15. Stubbs, M., McSheehy, P.M.J., and Griffiths, J.R., Causes and consequences of acidic pH in tumors: a magnetic resonance study, *Adv. Enzyme Reg.*, 39, 13–30, 1999.

16. Lee, E.S., Na, K., and Bae, Y.H., Polymeric micelle for tumor pH- and folate-mediated targeting, *J. Control. Rel.*, 91, 103–113, 2003.

17. Dillow, A.K. and Lowman, A.M., *Biomimetic Materials and Design: Biointerfacial Strategies, Tissue Engineering, and Targeted Drug Delivery*, Marcel Dekker, New York, 2002.

18. Aizenbert, J., McKittrick, J.M., and Orme, C.A., *Biological and Biomimetic Materials: Properties to Function*, Symposium Proceedings, Vol. 724, Material Research Society, Warrendale, PA, 2002.

19. Simon, U., Schmid, G., Hong, S., Stranick, S.J., and Arrivo, S.M., *Bioinspired Nanoscale Hybrid Systems*, Symposium Proceedings, Vol. 735, Material Research Society, Warrendale, PA, 2003.

20. Komiyama, M., Takeuchi, T., Mukawa, T., and Asanuma, H., *Molecular Imprinting: From Fundamentals to Applications*, Wiley-VCH, Weinheim, Germany, 2002.

21. Sarikaya, M., Tamerler, C.J., Schulten, K., and Baneyx, F., Molecular biomimetics: nanotechnology through biology, *Nature Mater.*, 2, 577–585, 2003.

22. Quake, S.R. and Scherer, A., From micro- to nanofabrication with soft materials, *Science*, 290, 1536–1540, 2000.

Index

A

A-band, 36–37
A-band motility assay system, 40–42
Actin
    description of, 24–25
    in *Mimosa pudica*, 24–26
    phosphorylation of, 26–27
Actin filaments
    bundling of, 71
    in *Characeae*, 71
    description of, 24
    flexibility of, 38
    fluorescence microscopy imaging of, 38
    gelsolin effects on, 87
    imaging of, 38
    myosin S1 movement along, 42
    organization of, 78
    phalloidin binding to, 75
    in plants, 70–71
    in pollen tubes, 78
    sliding movement of, in A-band motility assay
        system, 41
    tension development, 43
Actin inhibitors, 24
Actin-activated ATPase, 75
Actin–fragmin kinase, 27
Actinogelin, 87
Action potentials
    description of, 6–7
    in plants, 21
Active targeting by drug delivery systems
    carbohydrates, 361–362
    description of, 359
    kinetic constants, 363
    ligand densities, 363
    moieties of, 359–364
    multivalency, 362–364
    peptides, 359–361
    receptor-mediated endocytosis, 359
Adenosine diphosphate, 9
Adenosine diphosphate-spontaneous oscillatory
        contraction, 39
Adenosine triphosphate
    description of, 7
    hydrolysis of, 8–9
Adenosine triphosphate synthase, 260

B

Basal body proteins, 57
Belousov–Zhabotinsky reaction, 151–153
Beta cells, 428
Bifurcation, 157
Biodegradable aliphatic polyesters, 405–409
Biodegradable hydrogels
    advantages of, 409
    amphiphilic copolymers, 412–413
    bulk hydrolysis of, 409–410
    description of, 409
    dextran
        chemically crosslinked, 410–411
        physically crosslinked, 411–412
    surface erosion of, 409–410

Agitation, 67
Aliphatic polyesters, 405–409
Alkyltrimethyl ammonium bromide, 168
α-Amino acid-N-carboxyanhydrides, 375–376
Amphiphilic lyotropic liquid crystals, 313
Amphiphilic polymers, 174
Annealed polyions, 124
Arginine-rich peptides, 392
Aspartic acid, 376
Atomic force microscope, 33
Autocrine factors, 10
Azobenzene
    chemical structure of, 288
    chromophores, 307
    description of, 287, 324
    geometrical isomers of, 316
    in-plane photoorientation of
        background, 287–288
        excitation wavelength, 288–292
        photodichroism, 287
        sample temperatures, 293–295
        thermal enhancement, 295–297
    liquid crystal photoalignment by, 301–302
    liquid-crystalline polymers, 291
    photochemistry, 316
    photoisomerization of, 324, 339
    photoresponsive behaviors of, 330–334
    structures of, 334–338

T

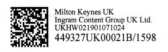